MEDICINES FOR
CHILDREN

MEDICINES FOR
CHILDREN

The Comprehensive Guide

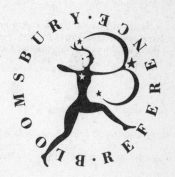

BLOOMSBURY

CONSULTANTS AND CONTRIBUTORS

Dr Ian K. M. Morton BSc, PhD, *King's College London*
(Series Consultant)
Dr William Barry MB, BCh, DCh, MRCP (Consultant Editor)
Dr Judith M. Hall BSc, PhD, *King's College London*
(Technical Editor)
Alyson Fox BSc, *King's College London*

While the creators of this work have made every effort to be as
accurate and up-to-date as possible, medical and pharmaceutical
knowledge is constantly changing and the application of it to
particular circumstances depends on many factors. Therefore readers
are urged always to consult a qualified medical specialist for
individual advice. The contributors, editors, consultants and
publishers of this book can not be held liable for any errors and
omissions, or actions that may be taken as a consequence of using it.

First published 1990

Copyright © 1990 by Clark Robinson Limited

Bloomsbury Publishing Limited, 2 Soho Square, London W1V 5DE

The CIP record for this book is available from the British Library.

10 9 8 7 6 5 4 3 2 1

ISBN 0 7475 0624 8

Designed by Malcolm Smythe
Typeset by Action Typesetting Limited, Gloucester
Printed in Great Britain by
Richard Clay Ltd, Bungay, Suffolk

PREFACE

This dictionary is a comprehensive guide to the range of medicines that may be used in the treatment of children in the United Kingdom today. It is not intended to be a guide to the prescription or administration of drugs; a qualified practitioner should always be consulted before any medicine is taken.

How to use this book
The book begins with an introduction to the ways in which the treatment of children with drugs is special, and to the considerations that are involved in prescribing drugs to children. The introduction also discusses the management of some common childhood ailments. This is followed by the A to Z. The articles in the A to Z describe the drugs listed under their generic and proprietary names. There are also articles describing the major drug types (indicated by *).

The A to Z is cross-referenced so that further information may be found quickly. Cross-references are indicated by SMALL CAPITALS. Many of the articles list warnings (indicated by ✚) about the use of a particular drug, and a description the possible side-effects (indicated by ▲).

INTRODUCTION

This dictionary describes a wide and varied selection of medicines for children that might either be prescribed by a doctor or which can be bought over the counter at a chemist.

The medicines in the book are listed alphabetically under both their generic names and their proprietary (or trade) names. The generic name of a drug is its approved chemical name, while the proprietary name is that given by a manufacturer to a preparation of a drug or a mixture of drugs. For example, paracetamol is the generic name of a well-known and commonly used pain killer (analgesic). There are many manufacturers of paracetamol and therefore a great number of proprietary preparations that contain it, such as Calpol, Disprol, Paldesic, Panadol, Panaleve and Salzone. Readers of this book may well be familiar with some of these names, but are unlikely to have come across them all.

Clearly such a system of names is a recipe for confusion. The dictionary, however, makes things easier to understand by using a system of cross-references that allows quick identification of the main active components and actions of a medicine when looked up under either its generic or its trade names. There is also cross-referencing that relates medicines to the major classes of drug to which they belong. This allows the reader to get a deeper understanding of both the drug itself and of other drugs with similar actions.

In addition to drugs, the dictionary includes vitamins and dietary supplements. Such dietary supplements range from high-calorie foods to special milks for babies who, for instance, cannot tolerate cows' milk. Under certain circumstances these "borderline substances" (so called because they are not exactly medicines but are given for medical reasons) can often be prescribed for children under the National Health Service, and therefore are included in this book.

This introduction will mainly discuss how children, especially newborn babies, differ from adults in their response to drugs, how medicines can be administered to children and babies, some side-effects of drugs used in childhood and the management of some common problems encountered in children.

Children and adults differ greatly in how they react to medication. Such differences are even greater in the very young, and particularly in premature babies. Drugs may be absorbed and broken down by a child's body in quite a different way than by an adult's. This is particularly so in the first month of life, because the functioning of the liver and kidneys tends to be immature. Such factors must be taken into consideration when deciding which medicines should be given to children and what dosage of a drug they should be given.

The administration of medicines to children

Medicine can be given in many ways: by mouth in the form of liquids, capsules or tablets; as suppositories; by injection; by inhalation or by application to the surface of the body (known as topical application). Most medicines are administered to children by mouth. For babies and toddlers the medicine is usually in the form of a liquid. Many such liquids are syrups, which means that they contain sugar. Often the sugar is present to mask an unpleasant taste or to encourage the child to take the medication. Where a medicine is to be given for only a few days, the sugar content is of little importance; but if treatment is to be given for a long time, the sugar may cause dental decay.

Drug companies are becoming increasingly aware of this problem and try to produce preparations of medicines that contain less sugar or have alternative flavourings and sweeteners. If they are to be taken over a long period, sugar-free tablets (particularly if they are sucked or chewed) or liquids should be used when possible. It may be a good idea to discuss this with your pharmacist or doctor.

Liquid medicines

Often only a very small quantity of a medicine is required, in which case the preparation will often be supplied to you in diluted form to make it easier to give to a child. The dilution will usually be enough to increase the volume per dose to five millilitres, which is approximately a teaspoonful. Usually a plastic spoon is provided with the bottle of medicine. It is important to use this because household teaspoons vary in size.

Most babies and children will take medicine from a spoon, but if giving a liquid in this way proves difficult, or where it is not possible to dilute the medicine, a disposable plastic syringe can be useful. The liquid medicine is drawn up into the syringe and then gently placed into the child's mouth. This technique provides great accuracy and is particularly useful for premature babies. Other useful devices are available for administering small volumes, and a chemist can be consulted about this. Liquid medicines should not be added to a baby's bottle.

Tablets and capsules

The age at which children become able to swallow tablets or capsules varies greatly. Capsules usually must be swallowed whole. An exception to this rule is the use of Slophyllin capsules (a preparation of theophylline used in the treatment of asthma). These capsules can be broken open to release many tiny granules which can be mixed with soft food, such as yoghurt. Some tablets can be crushed, dissolved in water or broken in two. Your pharmacist's advice about this can be very helpful. One form of tablet that must be swallowed whole is the "sustained release" variety. These tablets are designed so that, once swallowed, they release medication at a gradual rate throughout the

day or night. If they are chewed or crushed, they may lose this
important property.

Suppositories

Suppositories are special tablets or capsules that are inserted into the
rectum (back passage), where the drug is absorbed into the body. In the
United Kingdom, suppositories are not as commonly used for children
as they are in some other countries. Suppositories can be used to treat
constipation, but it is usually more pleasant for the child to take
laxatives by mouth. Administering drugs by the rectum can, however,
be very useful when treating convulsions in children. Clearly, a child
who is convulsing can not swallow medication, but drugs such as
diazepam are very rapidly absorbed into the bloodstream when given
by way of the rectum. Diazepam (in the form of Stesolid) can easily be
administered as a suppository, and parents whose children suffer from
frequent convulsions may be provided with Stesolid rectal tubes so that
they can administer such treatment at home in an emergency.

Injections

Injections can be given into the skin (intradermally), under the skin
(subcutaneously), into a muscle (intramuscularly) or into the
bloodstream by way of a vein (intravenously). Intradermal injections
may be used to administer the BCG vaccine (which provides protection
against tuberculosis), but are rarely used for other purposes. Insulin is
usually given to diabetic children subcutaneously. Medication is
absorbed slowly from the site and this helps to reduce the number of
injections a child needs. Most injections, however, are given either
intramuscularly or intravenously. In hospital, a needle with a tube
attached known as a drip is sometimes inserted into a vein, and once
this is in place further doses can be given through the drip without
causing distress to the child.

Injections are distressing to children, but there are often good reasons
why they cannot be avoided. Some medications (such as insulin) are not
absorbed if given by mouth, or the child may be vomiting and so
unable to take medicine by mouth. Injections also have the advantage
that larger doses can often be given. For example, if a child has a
serious bacterial infection, it is possible to give more of an antibiotic by
injection than would be tolerated by mouth.

It is now possible to reduce some of the distress of inserting
intravenous drips by first applying a local anaesthetic to the skin. Such
a preparation is Emla cream but this needs to be applied about half an
hour before the injection is administered.

Topical applications

All the methods of giving medication discussed so far apply to
medicines that are taken into the body. This is often referred to as
giving the medicine "systemically". Topical treatment does not usually
involve significant absorption into the body and is often by means of
ointments and creams applied to the skin. Examples include topical
antibiotics and steroids. Steroids are usually used to treat conditions
such as atopic eczema. Provided the steroid cream is sufficiently dilute,
no significant systemic absorption should take place. It is rarely, if

ever, necessary to use very potent steroid creams or ointments on a child's skin. Many forms of therapy are given topically, and children can often be given a drug topically which cannot be given to them systemically. For example, sticky eyes are a common problem in the newborn. Infection is usually the cause, and the problem can be treated by the use of topical antibiotic drops or eye ointments. Drops are a little easier to place in the infant's eyes than ointment and tend to be more popular. Topical treatment can also be used for external ear infections.

Saline nose drops (a preparation made from the correct amount of salt dissolved in water) applied to the inside of the nose are useful, particularly for a baby with a blocked nose. (Babies tend to breathe through their noses more than older children so a blocked nose can interfere with their ability to suck and feed.) These drops can be obtained from a chemist.

Probably the most frequent use of topical therapy is in the treatment of thrush. In children thrush occurs most commonly in the mouth and on the nappy area (often exacerbating nappy rash). The therapy may be given in the form of drops to the mouth and by the application of ointment or cream to the nappy area.

Inhalers and nebulizers

Asthma is the commonest reason for administering drugs by inhalation. Inhalation is the best way of giving the drug because the medication gets to the required site (the airways) more quickly and a smaller amount of the drug is required. Furthermore, little of the medicine is absorbed into the body.

A very efficient method of treating asthma is the use of a nebulizer. This is a machine that generates a fine aerosol mist of medication. Nebulizers are usually used in hospitals, but are also used at home, in particular for toddlers who are too young to use inhalers. Unfortunately, doctors are not able to prescribe nebulizers on the National Health Service. Occasionally, hospitals can lend nebulizers, but usually parents have to purchase the nebulizer themselves.

For older children, a wide variety of inhalers is available. Many children have difficulties in using the standard meter-dosed inhaler, which tends to be favoured by adults. A child with asthma needs to be able to use an inhaler even when short of breath. Dry powder inhalers, such as the Rotahaler, Diskhaler and Turbohaler, are extremely useful for children and can be used reliably from the age of five, even during an asthmatic attack.

Spacer devices are used in young children, sometimes as young as two years old. They help children who cannot manage to co-ordinate breathing in with releasing a dose from an aerosol inhaler. Examples of spacer devices include the Nebuhaler and Volumatic.

The correct choice of inhaler is very important for children with asthma. Some time spent practising and perfecting your child's inhaler technique is well spent. It is a good idea to get your doctor to check that your child is using his or her inhaler properly, because if it is being used badly, treatment will be less effective or even useless.

Children should be told that their inhaler (or any other medicine) is special, and only for them. It is by no means unknown for children to "share" their inhalers with friends at school.

Drug dosage

One of the biggest differences between giving drug therapy to adults and giving it to children is that children, being smaller, require less of a particular medicine. Dosages are generally based on a child's age or weight. Inclusion of age on a prescription is a legal requirement in the case of prescription-only medicines for children under 12 years of age. When great accuracy is required (for example, in giving potentially toxic medication such as anticancer drugs), dosage may be calculated according to a child's surface area. The surface area can be estimated using the child's height and weight. Drug dosage is specified in terms of the weight of the drug to be administered. The weight is expressed in metric measurements.

Drug dosage can be critical in managing certain conditions such as epilepsy, because the effect of the medicine is usually directly related to the amount that there is in the bloodstream. This amount can vary from one child to another, even though they have both received the same weight-related dose. It is possible to measure the amount of certain drugs (including anti-epileptic drugs) in the bloodstream, and the dose can then be adjusted to the individual child's needs. Measurement of the level of drugs in the blood can also be useful for ensuring that a child does not receive too much of a drug that might be toxic if given in excess. Gentamicin, for example, is a powerful antibiotic used to treat serious infections. If a patient is given too large a dose it can affect the hearing and kidneys. By measuring the blood level of gentamicin, it is possible to ensure that a safe dosage is being administered, and also that sufficient is being given to eradicate the infection.

It is important to realise that a course of antibiotic therapy should always be finished. If it is not, there is a risk of the infection re-establishing itself.

Ensuring that a child who goes to school receives a consistent and regular dose of a medicine requires a common sense approach. Sending a child to school with a preparation is often not very satisfactory because few schools are able to provide suitable medical supervision. Thus, for example, if the prescription calls for dosing three times a day, it may be best to give the medicine to the child on rising, on return from school and at bedtime. It is a good idea to discuss this with your doctor or pharmacist.

Choice of medication

Most childhood infections are caused by viruses and are self-limiting — that is, the child gets better without any treatment. It is sometimes said that a cold will last for a week with treatment and seven days if left alone. Also, there are many infections for which there are no specific remedies. It is sometimes difficult for doctors to decide whether a specific infection needs treatment. The commonest reason for a child to visit a doctor is a cold or some other respiratory infection. Most chest infections are caused by viruses for which there are no specific treatments, but a few are caused by bacteria, in which case the infection should respond well to antibiotics.

The problem is that there is no easy method of telling which chest infections are bacterial. Many doctors prescribe an antibiotic in such a situation rather than risk a potentially serious deterioration in the child's condition. Although such antibiotic treatment is often unnecessary, one can see why it is given. The decision is not always easy, and may explain why doctors' prescribing habits differ.

Side-effects and interactions

All drugs may have some form of potential side-effect. No drug should be used unless there is good reason and the benefits of using it are thought to outweigh any disadvantages. While adults may worry about the possibility of side-effects for themselves, they are often more concerned for their children. Doctors dealing with children tend to be conservative in their prescribing habits and generally stick to a few well-tried medications with which they are familiar.

Adults who are chronically ill sometimes take a number of medications at the same time, and this leads to the possibility of adverse affects caused by interactions between drugs. A child may visit the doctor and be given no medication at all, and will rarely be given much more than one medicine at a time. The problem of drug interaction is therefore less common in children.

The side-effects of certain medicines cause particular concern to parents. One such group of drugs is the corticosteroids, which are more commonly referred to simply as steroids. They can have unwanted effects if taken systemically in sufficient dosage and for a long period. In particular, parents are worried that these drugs may have a harmful effect on a child's growth. Steroids are used for their powerful anti-inflammatory effect, and are often used to treat acute asthmatic attacks. In such cases, however, they are usually used only for a few days, and such a short course will have no effect on growth.

There are many other conditions for which steroids are used in childhood, most of which are potentially serious. One such is nephrotic syndrome − a condition in which the child's kidneys leak protein and he or she becomes very puffy. This condition may require oral steroid treatment for some weeks. It is usual to give a relatively large dose of steroids to begin with and then tail off the course over perhaps six weeks. While such a course of treatment may make the child gain weight and become temporarily rather "moon-faced", it should not have a permanent effect on growth. Problems might occur if the child requires such courses of treatment frequently, which can happen because some children with nephrotic syndrome have a tendency to relapse when the steroid therapy is stopped. Under these circumstances, it is usual to tail the dose down to the minimum required to control the symptoms, and administration on an alternate day basis is thought to be helpful in reducing the potential for side-effects. Prolonged courses of steroid therapy may have some effect on growth, but in some unfortunate children they are essential to maintain well-being. It is worth remembering that any chronic illness, if untreated, can in itself have an adverse effect on growth. A doctor will not recommend a prolonged course of oral steroid therapy unless there is a good reason.

Inhaled corticosteroids, such as beclomethasone or budesonide, are used to prevent asthmatic symptoms in moderately to severely affected children. The effective dosage is usually so low that the steroid merely acts on the lining of the airways and there is no significant absorption. Such treatment can have a dramatic effect on a child's lifestyle and state of well-being. Sometimes, with control of chronic asthma by means of inhaled steroids, growth may actually improve. However, if a child has very severe asthma and requires very large doses of inhaled steroid, some absorption may take place. Nevertheless, this is much preferable to the probable alternative of having to take steroids by mouth on a long-term basis.

Topical steroids are most commonly applied to the skin in such conditions as atopic eczema. As long as the more potent preparations are avoided, no significant absorption into the body takes place.

Medicines restricted for use in children

Certain medicines that are in common use with adults are not recommended or are restricted for use with children. For instance, it has been known for a long time that tetracycline antibiotics, if taken into the body, are deposited in growing bone and teeth, which can result in permanent staining of the teeth if given to a young child. Consequently, tetracycline preparations should normally not be given to children under the age of twelve, and in particular to children under eight. On the other hand, tetracycline ointments and eye drops can safely be used in children because there is no significant systemic absorption. One of the more common uses for tetracycline antibiotics is in the treatment of acne. Fortunately, acne tends to come on after puberty, and tetracyclines can safely be used for older children.

Recently the Committee on Safety of Medicines has advised against the use of aspirin for minor illnesses in children under the age of twelve because a possible link has been found between the use of aspirin in feverish children and a rare condition called Reye's Syndrome. This condition is characterized by swelling of the brain and fatty change in the liver, and can be fatal. Because paracetamol is an effective alternative treatment for fever in children, there seems little point in risking such a serious, if very rare, complication. However, aspirin and aspirin-like drugs can still be prescribed for such conditions as juvenile rheumatoid arthritis.

Newborn babies differ considerably in their responses to medicines from older children and adults. As already mentioned, the liver and kidneys are quite immature and this can affect the way they handle certain drugs. The liver has an important role in breaking down medicines and the kidneys are important in their excretion.

Furthermore, many newborn babies are jaundiced. Jaundice is caused by an excess of a yellow pigment called bilirubin. Most of this pigment is attached to protein in the bloodstream and in this form does no harm. Certain medicines – such as sulphonamide-containing antibiotics – detach bilirubin from protein and can therefore cause problems by increasing the amount of free bilirubin in the bloodstream. Such free bilirubin can get into the brain and, if it does so in sufficient quantity, can result in deafness or brain damage. Therefore antibiotics containing sulphonamides are not used in newborn children.

Because of the immaturity of the liver, powerful antibiotics such as chloramphenicol can accumulate and result in toxic effects. Similarly, antibiotics such as gentamicin, which are normally excreted by the kidney, may accumulate because of immaturity of the kidneys in the newborn. Such effects can be anticipated by reducing the dosage and by monitoring the amount of these drugs in the bloodstream.

Another group of drugs that can cause problems in newborn and young children is the opiate group. Some cough mixtures used in adults contain mild opiates such as codeine. Generally these are best avoided in babies and young children because they can sometimes depress breathing. Alternative cough mixtures that do not contain any opiate-like drug should be used. Similarly, some proprietary antidiarrhoeal medications contain opiates, and again they should not be used in young children.

The more powerful opiates are good analgesics. Again, there is a problem with the newborn. Opiate analgesics (such as morphine) are frequently given to older children and adults who have had operations and are in pain. Such medication can also relieve pain in the newborn under similar circumstances. However, drugs such as morphine can give unpredictable results in the newborn, because there is a risk of depressing the breathing; in some cases breathing may actually stop and the baby has to be to be placed on a ventilator. Thus powerful opiate analgesics are only prescribed to a newborn baby with considerable caution.

Other medications can depress breathing in the newborn, including drugs used to stop convulsions, such as phenobarbitone and diazepam. These effects are exaggerated when two such medicines need to be used in combination. Stopping convulsions in a newborn baby can sometimes require large doses of anticonvulsants, but fortunately the advent of neonatal intensive care has made the placing of a baby on a ventilator, to counteract breathing difficulties, a well practised technique.

Anti-emetic medication helps to stop vomiting. Commonly used drugs include metoclopramide and the phenothiazine group. These are usually well tolerated in adults, but some children and teenagers can develop bizarre neurological effects when given these drugs. Although these side-effects are self-limiting, the use of such medication should be restricted to severe intractable vomiting with a known cause, such as vomiting associated with radiotherapy and anticancer drug therapy, and a few other specific indicators.

THE MANAGEMENT OF SOME COMMON CHILDHOOD PROBLEMS

Diarrhoea and vomiting

The management of diarrhoea and vomiting (caused by gastroenteritis) has greatly improved in recent years with the widespread use of rehydration solutions, which help to replace water and important salts. Rehydration solutions consist of glucose and electrolytes (such as sodium and potassium) dissolved in water. Babies are particularly prone to dehydration if they develop gastroenteritis. Absorption of sodium and water from the intestine is enhanced by glucose, and therefore rehydration solutions provide all the fluid and salts the baby needs. You can consult yur pharmacist about the non-prescription preparations available. It is now becoming quite rare for babies to be admitted to hospital in the United Kingdom with severe dehydration caused by gastroenteritis. Worldwide, the proper use of oral rehydration solutions is probably saving as many lives as all the rest of the medicines in this book put together. Furthermore, such treatment is extremely cheap.

Gastroenteritis is more common in babies who are bottle-fed than those who are breast fed. If the bottle-fed infant develops diarrhoea, then milk feeds and solid food (if the baby is eating it) should be stopped. When oral rehydration therapy is started, it is important that the baby is given a sufficient quantity. Giving the therapy in frequent small quantities may actually help to prevent vomiting. Once the diarrhoea has settled, perhaps after a day, the baby is gradually weaned back on to milk. Some doctors recommend that the infant is given quarter-strength milk, then half-strength, then three-quarters, followed by full-strength milk. The quarter-strength milk should be made up using the rehydration solution, but the other strengths are made up with water in the usual way. Other doctors feel that in most cases this slow re-grading is over-complicated and recommend that a baby should go to half-strength milk when the diarrhoea settles and then, if all remains well, proceed to full-strength milk. In all cases, solids are reintroduced later. Breast-fed babies can also develop diarrhoea. The usual advice here is different. Mothers should continue to breast feed, but offer the oral rehydration solution after a feed. The solution can be given either from a bottle or by spoon.

There is really no place for drug therapy in diarrhoea in babies and young children. Most drugs that are available either simply produce a more solid looking stool or slow the time it takes for faeces to pass through the bowel. They do not help the main problem, which is fluid loss from the bowel.

The child with a fever

Infections are often associated with a high temperature. The response of young children to a fever can be quite different to that of adults. About four per cent of children will suffer a convulsion associated with fever (known as febrile convulsions) between the ages of six months and five years. The fever is often caused by a relatively trivial illness, such as a cold. Measures to lower the temperature can sometimes help to prevent a fit. Clothes should be removed and the administration of paracetamol is very helpful. Other useful measures include sponging the child's body with tepid water. The water will then evaporate, which causes cooling of the body. Cold water should not be used as this can reduce the blood flow to the skin and actually result in raising the temperature of the centre of the body. Gentle fanning may also help.

When children have convulsions, they should be placed on their sides. Most convulsions soon stop, but there are few things that frighten parents more than the sight of their child having a convulsion for the first time. Medical assistance should be sought, and if the convulsion does not stop quickly, it may be better to call an ambulance. Most children who have had their first convulsion are admitted to hospital for a period of observation because very rarely there may be a serious underlying infection. Fortunately, febrile convulsions cause no long-term problems in otherwise healthy children, and do not mean that the child has epilepsy. Unfortunately, there is often a tendency for convulsions to recur if the child has another fever, at least until the age of about five years.

Children with fevers tend to look unwell. A doctor may give a child with a temperature some paracetamol to lower the fever and then re-examine the child later. If the child looks much better when the temperature comes down, a serious infection is much less likely.

Respiratory infections

Colds and coughs caused by viruses have no specific treatment. However, the symptoms can be alleviated. If there is a fever, paracetamol may help to lower the patient's temperature, and there is a wide variety of non-prescription cough mixtures available from your pharmacist, but care should be taken to use only paediatric preparations. It is doubtful whether any of these actually produce much benefit, although soothing substances such as syrup or glycerol may relieve a dry, irritating cough. It should be borne in mind that none of the preparations will actually hasten a child's recovery from a cough. As we have already seen, the use of cough suppressants containing codeine or similar opiate analgesics is not generally recommended for children and should be avoided altogether for those under one year old.

Other useful preparations are decongestants for a blocked-up nose. These can either be topically applied inside the nose, or given by mouth. Most preparations contain one of the sympathomimetic group of drugs. If these are used topically, they can cause rebound swelling of the lining of the nose once treatment is stopped, if used for too long a period. However, saline nose drops are usually as effective as those containing sympathomimetic drugs and are preferred. Oral decongestants are of marginal benefit, but will not produce any nasal swelling. Many preparations also contain antihistamines which may lead to some drowsiness.

Nappy rash

Nappy rash is a very common problem. Usually it clears up with the use of a barrier cream and by exposing the nappy area to the air as much as is possible. Nappies should be changed frequently and the use of tightly fitting rubber and plastic pants is best avoided. The most common reason for nappy rash failing to recover when these simple measures are applied is that there is also a thrush infection. This fungal infection usually responds well to the use of an ointment or cream containing an antifungal agent, such as nystatin. Commonly, the ointment or cream also contains a weak corticosteroid because this reduces the inflammation and redness.

Sometimes there may be thrush present in the mouth and this also requires treatment. Such a thrush infection is not found as often in breast-fed babies as in those fed by bottle. Thrush can be a side-effect of antibiotic treatment. Antibiotics disrupt the population of harmless bacteria that normally live in the gut, and this allows other organisms, such as yeasts, to proliferate.

Accidental poisoning

It must be emphasized that drugs can be very dangerous if taken in overdose. All medicines in the home should be kept under lock and key. It is not sufficient just to place them on a high shelf because young children soon learn to climb up on chairs. Medicines are now dispensed in "child-proof" containers. These are no guarantee that a child cannot get at the contents. Some children, frustrated at not being able to open the bottle, have been known to smash the container open using a hammer or another similar object. When children are away from home it is important that any medicines they need are entrusted to a responsible adult, so that neither the child concerned nor any other child can misuse them.

If your child has taken an overdose, you should always seek medical advice. Under such circumstances children are often admitted to hospital for a period of observation and treatment. It is important to bring the medicine that has been taken (and its container) with you to the hospital so that the doctors will know exactly what the substance is.

The most common form of therapy given for an overdose is the administration of syrup of ipecacuanha; this induces vomiting. Only a few medications have specific antidotes or treatments. Fortunately, although overdoses in children cause considerable distress, fatalities are rare. Prevention is clearly important, not only in one's own home, but also when one is visiting people who may not be aware of the dangers.

Dr William Barry
Consultant Paediatrician
Queen Mary's Hospital, Sidcup, Kent
and King's College Hospital, London

Abidec (*Parke-Davis*) is a proprietary non-prescription MULTIVITAMIN compound that is not available from the National Health Service. Produced in the form of capsules and drops, Abidec contains RETINOL (vitamin A), several forms of vitamin B (thiamine, riboflavine, PYRIDOXINE and nicotinamide), ASCORBIC ACID (vitamin C) and ERGOCALCIFEROL (vitamin D).

acetazolamide is a mild diuretic drug used to treat pressure in the eyeball (glaucoma) by reducing the formation of the aqueous humour in adults. Secondary uses include the treatment of grand mal and focal epilepsy, particularly in cases resistant to more commonly used medications. Administration is usually oral in the form of tablets or capsules.
▲ side-effects: there may be drowsiness, numbness and tingling of the hands and feet, flushes and headache, thirst and frequency of urination.
✚ warning: acetazolamide should not be administered to patients with sodium or potassium deficiency, or with malfunction of the adrenal glands.
Related article: DIAMOX.

Acetoxyl (*Stiefel*) is a proprietary, non-prescription, topical preparation for the treatment of acne. Produced in the form of a gel (in two strengths − 2.5% and 5%), its active constituent is benzoyl peroxide, which has both KERATOLYTIC and ANTIMICROBIAL properties.
▲/✚ side-effects/warning: *see* BENZOYL PEROXIDE.

acetylcysteine is a mucolytic drug. In theory it might be helpful in reducing the viscosity of sputum and so facilitate expectoration (the coughing up of sputum) in children with cystic fibrosis. Experience has proven it to be disappointing. It is also used to treat abdominal complications associated with cystic fibrosis; or as an antidote to overdosage of PARACETAMOL. Administration is oral in the form of a solution of dissolved granules, by injection or infusion, or by nebulisation through a face-mask or mouthpiece.
▲ side-effects: there may be nausea and vomiting, and stomatitis (inflammation of the mouth).
✚ warning: acetylcysteine should be administered with caution to patients with severe respiratory insufficiency.
Related article: PARVOLEX.

Achromycin (*Lederle*) is a proprietary form of the broad- spectrum ANTIBIOTIC tetracycline hydrochloride, available only on prescription. It is used to treat many types of microbial infection and is applied systemically, on the skin and in the ears and eyes (not recommended for children under 12). Achromycin is produced in many forms: as tablets (in two types), as a syrup, as an ointment (in two strengths), as an ophthalmic oil suspension (for use as drops), and powdered in vials for reconstitution and injection.
▲/✚ side-effects/warning: *see* TETRACYCLINE.

Achromycin V (*Lederle*) is a form of the proprietary tetracycline ANTIBIOTIC Achromycin that also contains a buffer − a substance that does not change its acid-alkali balance (pH) if it is diluted. It is produced in the form of capsules and as a syrup.

▲/✚ side-effects/warning: *see* TETRACYCLINE.

Acnegel (*Kirby-Warrick*) is a proprietary non-prescription topical preparation for the treatment of acne. Produced in the form of a gel (in two strengths − 5% and 10% − the latter under the trade name Acnegel Forte), its active constituent is benzoyl peroxide, which has both KERATOLYTIC and ANTIMICROBIAL properties.

▲/✚ side-effects/warning: *see* BENZOYL PEROXIDE.

Acnidazil (*Janssen*) is a proprietary, non-prescription, topical preparation for the treatment of acne. Produced in the form of a cream, its active constituents are benzoyl peroxide, which has both KERATOLYTIC and ANTIBACTERIAL properties, and the ANTIFUNGAL agent miconazole nitrate.

▲/✚ side-effects/warning: *see* BENZOYL PEROXIDE; MICONAZOLE

Acthar Gel (*Armour*) is a proprietary preparation of adrenocorticotrophic HORMONE (ACTH, or corticotrophin), available only on prescription. The hormone controls the secretions of corticosteroids by the adrenal glands. In the form of injections of the hormone in a hydrolysed gelatin base, Acthar Gel is used to treat infantile spasms (a rare but serious form of fit in infancy).

Actidil (*Wellcome*) is a proprietary non-prescription ANTIHISTAMINE drug used to treat various allergic conditions, particularly conditions of the nose (allergic rhinitis) and skin (urticaria). It may also be used to assist sedation or as a premedication before surgery. Produced in the form of tablets and as a syrup for dilution (the syrup once dilute retains potency for 14 days), Actidil is a preparation of triprolidine hydrochloride.

▲/✚ side-effects/warning: *see* TRIPROLIDINE.

Actifed (*Wellcome*) is a proprietary, non-prescription, compound nasal and respiratory DECONGESTANT that is not available from the National Health Service. Produced in the form of tablets and as a syrup for dilution (the syrup once dilute retains potency for 14 days), Actifed contains the SYMPATHOMIMETIC VASOCONSTRICTOR ephedrine and the ANTIHISTAMINE triprolidine.

▲/✚ side-effects/warning: *see* EPHEDRINE HYDROCHLORIDE; TRIPROLIDINE.

Actifed Compound Linctus (*Wellcome*) is a proprietary, non-prescription, compound cough preparation that is not available from the National Health Service. Produced in the form of an elixir for dilution (the elixir once dilute retains potency for 14 days), the Compound Linctus contains the SYMPATHOMIMETIC VASOCONSTRICTOR ephedrine, the ANTIHISTAMINE triprolidine, and the narcotic ANTITUSSIVE dextromethorphan. It is not recommended for children under the age of two years.

▲/✚ side-effects/warning: *see* DEXTROMETHORPHAN; EPHEDRINE HYDROCHLORIDE; TRIPROLIDINE

Actifed Expectorant (*Wellcome*) is a proprietary, non-prescription, compound EXPECTORANT that is not available from the National Health Service. Produced in the form of an elixir for dilution (the elixir once dilute retains potency for 14 days), the preparation contains the VASOCONSTRICTOR ephedrine, the ANTIHISTAMINE triprolidine, and the expectorant guaiphenesin. It is not recommended for children under the age of two years.
▲/✚ side-effects/warning: *see* EPHEDRINE HYDROCHLORIDE; TRIPROLIDINE.

Actinac (*Roussel*) is a proprietary lotion, to be made up from powder and a diluent solvent, used as a topical treatment for acne. Available only on prescription, Actinac's active constituents include the broad-spectrum ANTIBIOTIC chloramphenicol and the STEROID hydrocortisone.
▲/✚ side-effects/warning: *see* CHLORAMPHENICOL; HYDROCORTISONE.

actinomycin D is an ANTIBIOTIC drug that is also CYTOTOXIC, and therefore used to treat cancer. Dosage is critical to each patient. Administration is by injection of a bolus of the drug into a vein.
▲ side-effects: hair loss is common, even to total baldness; there may be inflammation of the mucous lining of the mouth (stomatitis), nausea and vomiting. There may also be increased sensitivity to radiotherapy.
✚ warning: suppression of the bone-marrow's function of producing red blood cells is inevitable, and regular blood counts are essential. *Related article:* COSMEGEN LYOVAC.

Actraphane (*Novo*) is a proprietary intermediate-duration combination of mixed INSULINS (isophane insulin 70%, neutral insulin 30%) used to treat patients with diabetes mellitus.

Actrapid (*Novo*) is a proprietary quick-acting preparation of neutral INSULIN, used to treat patients with diabetes mellitus.

Acupan (*Carnegie*) is a proprietary non-narcotic ANALGESIC, available only on prescription, used to treat severe pain (such as that following surgery, or in cancer or toothache). Produced in the form of tablets and in ampoules for injection, Acupan is a preparation of nefopam hydrochloride. It is not usually recommended for children under the age of 12 years.
▲/✚ side-effects/warning: *see* NEFOPAM.

AC Vax (*SK&F*) is a VACCINE designed to give protection against the organism meningococcus, which can cause serious infection including meningitis. It may be indicated for travellers intending to go areas where the risk of meningococcal infection is much higher than in the United Kingdom, such as parts of Africa. It may be given to adults and children over two months.

acyclovir is an ANTIVIRAL agent used to treat chicken-pox in children considered to be at high risk of becoming seriously ill from the disease, for example some new-born infants and children with problems related to their immune systems. It is also used to treat infection caused by the

Herpes simplex virus, such as encephalitis (infection of the brain), stomatitis (infection of the mouth), eye infections and in children with underlying eczema or immune disorders. It works by inhibiting the action of one of the enzymes in cells used by the virus to replicate itself. To be effective, however, treatment of an infection must begin early. Administration is oral, topical or by infusion.

▲ side-effects: applied topically, there may be a temporary burning or stinging sensation; some patients experience a localized drying of the skin. Taken orally, acyclovir may give rise to gastrointestinal disturbance and various blood deficiencies; there may also be fatigue and a rash.

✚ warning: acyclovir should be administered with caution to patients who are pregnant or who have impaired kidney function. Adequate fluid intake must be maintained.

Related article: ZOVIRAX

Adcortyl (*Squibb*) is a proprietary form of the ANTI-INFLAMMATORY glucocorticoid (CORTICOSTEROID) drug triamcinolone acetonide, available only on prescription. Produced in the form of an ointment or cream, Adcortyl is used to treat skin infections (such as dermatitis), psoriasis, insect bites and sunburn; a version is available that includes the ANTIBIOTIC neomycin and the antimicrobial agent gramicidin, and which is known as Adcortyl with Graneodin. In ORABASE paste, Adcortyl is used to treat oral and dental inflammations. Produced as injections, Adcortyl is used in two different ways in order to achieve either of two distinct purposes: intradermal injection relieves some scaly skin diseases (such as lichen planus); injection direction into a joint relieves pain, swelling and stiffness (such as with rheumatoid arthritis, bursitis and tenosynovitis). Adcortyl is a very potent corticosteroid and is rarely used in children.

▲/✚ side-effects/warning: *see* TRIAMCINOLONE ACETONIDE.

Addamel (*Kabi Vitrum*) contains additional electrolytes and trace elements for use in association with VAMIN infusion fluids, for the intravenous nutrition of a patient in whom feeding via the alimentary tract is not possible.

Addiphos (*Kabi Vitrum*) contains additional phosphate for use in association with VAMIN infusion fluids, for the intravenous nutrition of a patient in whom feeding via the alimentary tract is not possible.

adrenaline is a hormone (a catecholamine) produced and secreted by the central core (medulla) of the adrenal glands. It is involved in the response to stress and is a powerful stimulant. Adrenaline may be injected to restart the heart in an emergency. It is given directly into the heart, into a vein or down an endotracheal tube (a tube passed into the windpipe). It can also be given subcutaneously (under the skin) in asthmatic attacks and in severe allergic reactions. However, it is regarded as rather an obsolete form of treatment in asthma. Adrenaline can also produce temporary benefit when given by nebulization (an aerosol) to children with croup. In addition, adrenaline administered simultaneously with a local anaesthetic

A

considerably lengthens the effective duration of the local anaesthetic.

▲ side-effects: there is an increase in heart rate; there may also be headache, anxiety, and coldness in the fingertips and toes. High dosage may lead to tremor and the accumulation of fluid in the lungs. Adrenaline in eye-drops may cause redness of the eye.

✚ warning: adrenaline should be administered with caution to patients who suffer from insufficient blood supply to the heart, from high blood pressure (hypertension), from diabetes, from overactivity of the thyroid gland (hyperthyroidism), or who are already taking drugs that affect the heart or mood.
Related articles: MARCAIN; MIN-I-JET ADRENALINE; XYLOCAINE; XYLOTOX.

adsorbed diphtheria and tetanus vaccine is diphtheria and tetanus VACCINE adsorbed on to a mineral carrier.
see DIPHTHERIA AND TETANUS VACCINE.

adsorbed diphtheria, tetanus and pertussis vaccine is diphtheria, pertussis and tetanus (DPT) VACCINE adsorbed on to a mineral carrier.
see DIPHTHERIA, PERTUSSIS AND TETANUS (DPT) VACCINE.

adsorbed tetanus vaccine is tetanus VACCINE adsorbed on to a mineral carrier.
see TETANUS VACCINE.

Aerolin Autohaler (*Riker*) is a metered dose inhaler for use in asthma. It differs from an ordinary aerosol inhaler in that it is breath-activated, which means that whenever a patient sucks on the inhaler a metered inhalation is automatically delivered. It may help overcome some problems encountered by children in co-ordinating their breathing with an inhaler, but a sudden delivery of a dose of aerosol can make the unwary gag. The inhaler delivers the BETA-RECEPTOR STIMULANT salbutamol, which is a BRONCHODILATOR.
▲/✚ side-effects/warning: *see* SALBUTAMOL.

Aerosporin (*Calmic*) is a proprietary form of the ANTIBIOTIC drug polymyxin B sulphate, available only on prescription, which is used to treat many infective organisms (particularly in the urinary tract), but which is also fairly toxic. It is produced in the form of powder for reconstitution as a medium for injection.
▲/✚ side-effects/warning: *see* POLYMYXIN B SULPHATE.

Afrazine (*Kirby-Warrick*) is a proprietary non-prescription preparation of the nasal DECONGESTANT oxymetazoline hydrochloride, a SYMPATHOMIMETIC, that is not available from the National Health Service. It is produced in the form of nose-drops (in two strengths) and as a nasal spray.
▲/✚ side-effects/warning: *see* OXYMETAZOLINE HYDROCHLORIDE.

Agarol (*Warner-Lambert*) is a proprietary, non-prescription, compound LAXATIVE that is not available from the National Health Service.

Produced in the form of a liquid for dilution (the mixture once dilute retains potency for 28 days), Agarol contains the seaweed extract gel, agar, together with phenolphthalein and liquid paraffin.
▲ side-effects: laxative effects may continue for several days; there may be dysfunction of the kidneys, leading possibly to discoloration of the urine. A mild skin rash may appear.

Agiolax (*Radiol*) is a proprietary non-prescription form of the stimulant LAXATIVE senna together with the bulking-agent laxative ispaghula; it is not available from the National Health Service. Produced in the form of granules for solution in water, Agiolax is not recommended for children aged under five years.
▲/✚ side-effects/warning: *see* ISPAGHULA HUSK; SENNA

Aglutella Azeta (*G F Dietary Supplies*) is a proprietary non-prescription brand of gluten-free cream-filled wafers which are also low in protein, sodium and potassium. They are intended for consumption by patients with gluten sensitivity (as with coeliac disease), amino-acid abnormalities (such as phenylketonuria), or kidney or liver failure.

Aglutella Gentili (*G F Dietary Supplies*) is a proprietary non-prescription brand of gluten-, sucrose- and lactose-free pasta — spaghetti, spaghetti rings, macaroni, macaroni spirals, and tagliatelle — intended for consumption by patients with gluten sensitivity (as with coeliac disease), amino-acid abnormalities (such as phenylketonuria), or kidney or liver failure.

Albucid (*Nicholas*) is a proprietary ANTIBIOTIC of the SULPHONAMIDE family, available only on prescription, used to treat eye infections. Produced in the form of eye-drops and (under the trade name Albucid Ointment) as an ointment (in either a water-miscible base or an oily base), Albucid's active constituent is the sulphonamide sulphacetamide sodium.
▲/✚ side-effects/warning: *see* SULPHACETAMIDE.

Albumaid (*Scientific Hospital Supplies*) is the brand name of a series of proprietary foods for special diets, as required mostly in hospitals and clinics. They are produced as powders for reconstitution. Albumaid Complete contains protein, amino acids, vitamins, minerals, trace, elements and has no carbohydrate or fat. Albumaid XP contains protein, carbohydrate, vitamins, minerals and amino acids, but less than 0.01% phenylalanine and no fat. Albumaid XP Concentrate contains protein, vitamins, minerals, trace elements, amino acids, but less than 0.025% phenylalanine and no carbohydrate or fat. Other Albumaid preparations generally follow the pattern of Albumaid XP, but instead of a minimum content of phenylalanine contain minimum quantities of the amino acids cystine, histidine, methionine or tyrosine.

alclometasone dipropionate is a mild CORTICOSTEROID drug used for topical application to treat inflammatory skin disorders in which the cause of inflammation is deemed not to be infection — in particular to treat eczema. Administration is as a cream or an ointment. Dosage should be the minimum effective dose.

▲ side-effects: side-effects are rare, but may include skin sensitivity and hair growth.

✚ warning: as with all corticosteroids, alclometasone diproprionate treats the symptoms and does not treat any underlying disorder. An undetected infection may thus become worse although its symptoms may be suppressed by the drug.

Related article: MODRASONE.

Alcobon (*Roche*) is a proprietary ANTIFUNGAL drug, available only on prescription, used to treat systemic infections by yeasts (such as candidiasis, or thrush). Produced for hospital use only, in the form of tablets and in infusion flasks, Alcobon is a preparation of flucytosine.

▲/✚ side-effects/warning: *see* FLUCYTOSINE.

Alcoderm (*Alcon*) is a proprietary non-prescription skin emollient (softener and soother), used to treat dry or itchy skin. Produced in the form of a cream and a lotion, Alcoderm's major constituents are liquid paraffin and a moisturizer.

alcohol is the name of a class of compounds derived from hydrocarbons. The alcohol in alcoholic drinks is ethyl alcohol (or ethanol) and is produced by the fermentation of sugar by yeast. Alcohol is ultimately a depressant, at high doses producing sleep (HYPNOTIC), general anaesthesia (ANAESTHETIC), and eventually coma and death. At low doses (consumption) it reduces social inhibitions, so can be effectively a stimulant. It has marked diuretic actions, and produces vasodilatation, particularly in the skin. As a food, alcohol has calorific values between carbohydrates and fats. It is particularly dangerous in children because it lowers blood sugar levels.

For medical purposes, a strong solution of ethyl alcohol can be used as an ANTISEPTIC (particularly to prepare skin before injection, where it has the advantage that it evaporates) or as a preservative. However, it should not be used on broken skin as it will sting. Another form of alcohol, methyl alcohol (or methanol) is perhaps better known as wood alcohol. In the body it is oxidized more slowly than ethyl alcohol, forming poisonous products that may cause blindness and/or death. Methylated spirits is a mixture of ethanol with a little methanol and other petroleum hydrocarbons; one form is alternatively called surgical spirit or rubbing alcohol.

Alcopar (*Wellcome*) is a proprietary non-prescription ANTHELMINTIC drug, used to treat infections by roundworms, specifically by hookworms. Produced in the form of granules in sachets for solution in water, Alcopar is a preparation of bephenium hydroxynaphthoate.

▲ side-effects: *see* BEPHENIUM.

alcuronium chloride is a SKELETAL MUSCLE RELAXANT, of the type known as competitive or non-depolarizing. It is used during surgical operations to achieve long-duration paralysis. Administration is by injection, but only after the patient has been rendered unconscious. *Related article:* ALLOFERIN.

Aldactone (*Searle*) is a proprietary potassium-sparing DIURETIC drug, available only on prescription, used to treat congestive heart failure, cirrhosis of the liver, and the accumulation of fluids within the tissues (oedema). Produced in the form of tablets, Aldactone is a preparation of the comparatively weak diuretic spironolactone. Spironolactone is commonly used in combination with potassium-losing diuretics such as FRUSEMIDE.
▲/✚ side-effects/warning: *see* SPIRONOLACTONE.

alfacalcidol is a powerful synthesized form of CALCIFEROL (vitamin D), used to make up body deficiencies, particularly in the treatment of types of hypoparathyroidism and rickets. It tends to be used in chronic renal failure or rickets which do not respond to ordinary vitamin D. Calcium levels in the body should be regularly monitored during treatment. Administration is oral in the form of capsules or drops.
✚warning: overdosage may cause kidney damage.
Related article: ONE-ALPHA.

Allbee with C (*Robins*) is a proprietary, non-prescription MULTIVITAMIN preparation that is not available from the National Health Service. Used to treat vitamin deficiencies and produced in the form of capsules, Allbee with C − as its name indicates − consists of several forms of vitamin B (thiamine, riboflavine, PYRIDOXINE, nicotinamide and pantothenic acid) together with ASCORBIC ACID (vitamin C).

Aller-eze is a proprietary non-prescription ANTIHISTAMINE, in which the active constituent is clemastine. It is used to give relief from allergies such as hay fever.
▲/✚ side-effects/warning: *see* CLEMASTINE.

Alloferin (*Roche*) is a proprietary SKELETAL MUSCLE RELAXANT, available only on prescription, of the type known as competitive or non-depolarizing. It is used during surgical operations, but only after the patient has been rendered unconscious. Produced in ampoules for injection, Alloferin is a preparation of alcuronium chloride.
▲/✚ side-effects/warning: *see* ALCURONIUM CHLORIDE.

allopurinol is a xanthine-oxidase inhibitor, a drug used to combat an excess of uric acid in the blood, and thus to try to prevent gout. Gout is very rare in children, but allopurinol is used to counteract high levels of uric acid produced during cancer or leukaemia chemotherapy.
▲side-effects: there may be gastrointestinal disturbances. Rarely, there may be headache, dizziness, high blood pressure (hypertension), hair loss, and/or problems with the sense of taste.
✚warning: allopurinol should be administered with caution to patients who suffer from liver or kidney disease.
Related articles: ALORAL; ALULINE; COSURIC; ZYLORIC.

A

Almevax (*Wellcome*) is a proprietary VACCINE against German measles (rubella) in the form of a solution containing live but attenuated viruses of the Wistar RA27/3 strain. Available only on prescription, and administered as injections, it is intended specifically for the immunization of non-pregnant women.

Almodan (*Berk*) is a proprietary ANTIBIOTIC available only on prescription, used to treat systemic bacterial infections of the upper respiratory tract, the ear, the sinuses and the urinary tract; it is sometimes used to treat typhoid fever. Produced in the form of capsules, as a syrup for dilution and as a powder for reconstitution as a medium for injection, Almodan is a preparation of the broad-spectrum penicillin, amoxycillin.
▲/✚ side-effects/warning: *see* AMOXYCILLIN.

Aloral (*Lagap*) is a proprietary form of the xanthine-oxidase inhibitor, allopurinol, used to treat high levels of uric acid in the bloodstream. Available only on prescription, Aloral is produced in the form of tablets (in two strengths).
▲/✚ side-effects/warning: *see* ALLOPURINOL.

Alphaderm (*Norwich Eaton*) is a proprietary cream preparation containing urea (10%) with the CORTICOSTEROID hydrocortisone (1%) dispersed in a slightly oily base. Available only on prescription, the cream is used as a topical application for the treatment of ichthyosis (dry and horny epidermis) and other mild inflammations of the skin.
▲/✚ side-effects/warning: *see* HYDROCORTISONE.

Alpha Keri (*Bristol-Myers*) is a proprietary non-prescription skin emollient (softener and soother) for use in the bath. Containing mineral and lanolin oils, it can also be massaged into the skin to treat dry or itchy areas.

alpha tocopheryl acetate is a form of VITAMIN E (tocopherol), used to treat body deficiency and generally as a vitamin supplement. Administration is oral in the form of tablets for chewing, capsules and in suspension, or as a paraffin-based ointment. Alpha tocopheryl acetate may be given to very premature infants suffering anaemia due to vitamin E deficiency. It may also be given to children to prevent neuromuscular problems (such as cystic fibrosis) associated with low vitamin E levels due to long-standing problems with fat absorption.
Related articles: EPHYNAL; VITA-E.

Alphosyl (*Stafford-Miller*) is a proprietary non-prescription preparation used to treat eczema and psoriasis. Produced in the form of a water-based cream and as a lotion, Alphosyl's major active constituent is COAL TAR extract.

Alphosyl HC (*Stafford-Miller*) is a proprietary COAL TAR and CORTICOSTEROID preparation, available only on prescription, used to treat psoriasis. Produced in the form of a water-based cream, Alphosyl HC's steroid constituent is hydrocortisone.
▲/✚ side-effects/warning: *see* HYDROCORTISONE.

alprostadil is a hormonal drug (a prostaglandin) used to maintain life in babies born with various congenital heart defects (it keeps the ductus arteriosus open), while emergency preparations are made for corrective surgery and intensive care. Administration is by infusion in dilute solution.

▲ side-effects: in addition to the symptoms of the congenital defect, administration of the drug may cause breathing difficulties, low blood pressure (hypotension) and slow or fast heart rate, high temperature and flushing. Prolonged use may cause bone deformity and damage to the pulmonary artery.

✚ warning: monitoring of arterial pressure is essential; a close watch must also be kept for haemorrhage.
Related article: PROSTIN VR.

Altacite (*Roussel*) is a proprietary non-prescription ANTACID that is not available from the National Health Service. Produced in the form of tablets for chewing and as a sugar-free suspension, Altacite's active constituent is HYDROTALCITE, a compound that also has deflatulent properties.

Altacite Plus (*Roussel*) is a proprietary non-prescription ANTACID preparation used to soothe acid stomach, indigestion, flatulence and peptic ulcer. Produced in the form of a suspension, Altacite Plus contains the antacid-deflatulent HYDROTALCITE together with the antifoaming agent DIMETHICONE, and is not recommended for children aged under eight years. A version of Altacite Plus is produced in the form of tablets, but is not available from the National Health Service.

Aludrox (*Wyeth*) is a proprietary non-prescription ANTACID preparation used to soothe acid stomach, indigestion and peptic ulcer. It is produced in the form of a gel containing aluminium hydroxide, and is not recommended for children aged under two years. Versions of Aludrox available only on prescription are produced in the form of tablets under the trade name Aludrox Tablets; and as a gel or a suspension (incorporating ambutonium bromide and magnesium salts) under the trade name Aludrox SA. Aludrox SA suspension is not recommended for children.

▲/✚ side-effects/warning: *see* ALUMINIUM HYDROXIDE.

Aluline (*Steinhard*) is a proprietary form of the xanthine-oxidase inhibitor allopurinol, used to treat high levels of uric acid in the bloodstream. Available only on prescription, Aluline is produced in the form of tablets (in two strengths).

▲/✚ side-effects/warning: *see* ALLOPURINOL

alum is used therapeutically as an astringent, particularly to treat mouth-pain and in mouth-washes.

▲/✚ side-effects/warning: treatment with alum may in fact cause tissue damage and actually delay healing.

aluminium hydroxide is an ANTACID which, because it is relatively insoluble in water, is long-acting when retained in the stomach. It is

used to treat digestive problems from acid stomach to peptic ulcers and oesophageal reflux. Administration is oral in the form of tablets for chewing or sucking, as a gel, or in a compound liquid mixture. Aluminium hydroxide is also used in kidney failure to bind phosphate in order to keep the body's phosphate level low. Some proprietary preparations are not recommended for children.
Related articles: ALUDROX; ASILONE; DIOVOL; GAVISCON; MUCAINE.

Alunex (*Steinhard*) is a proprietary non-prescription ANTIHISTAMINE, used to treat allergic conditions such as hay fever and urticaria. Produced in the form of tablets, Alunex is a preparation of chlorpheniramine maleate.
▲/✚ side-effects/warning: *see* CHLORPHENIRAMINE.

Alupent (*Boehringer Ingelheim*) is a proprietary compound BRONCHODILATOR, available only on prescription, which works as a selective SMOOTH MUSCLE RELAXANT. Administered orally in the form of tablets, as an aerosol spray (under the trade name Alupent Aerosol) or as a sugar-free syrup (under the trade name Alupent Syrup), it is used to treat bronchospasm, and thus relieves the effects of asthma. It contains the BETA-RECEPTOR STIMULANT, orciprenaline, which is not usually used to treat asthma in children because it tends to stimulate other systems (for example, the heart), more than the highly selective beta-receptor stimulants such as salbutamol or terbutaline.
▲/✚ side-effects/warning: *see* ORCIPRENALINE.

Alupram (*Steinhard*) is a proprietary ANXIOLYTIC and SKELETAL MUSCLE RELAXANT, available only on prescription. Produced for both purposes in the form of tablets (in three strengths), Alupram is a preparation of the BENZODIAZEPINE diazepam.
▲/✚ side-effects/warning: *see* DIAZEPAM.

Aluzine (*Steinhard*) is a proprietary DIURETIC drug, available only on prescription, used to treat the accumulation of fluids in the tissues (oedema), particularly when caused by kidney failure. Produced in the form of tablets (in three strengths), Aluzine is a preparation of frusemide.
▲/✚ side-effects/warning: *see* FRUSEMIDE.

Ambaxin (*Upjohn*) is a proprietary ANTIBIOTIC, available only on prescription, used to treat systemic bacterial infections and infections of the upper respiratory tract, the ear, nose and throat, and the urinary tract. Produced in the form of tablets, Ambaxin is a preparation of the broad-spectrum penicillin, bacampicillin.
▲/✚ side-effects/warning: *see* BACAMPICILLIN HYDROCHLORIDE.

amethocaine hydrochloride is a local ANAESTHETIC used in creams and in solution for topical application or instillation into the bladder, and in eye-drops for ophthalmic treatment. It is absorbed rapidly from mucous membrane surfaces.
▲ side-effects: rarely, there are hypersensitive reactions.
✚ warning: topical administration may cause initial stinging. It should be given with caution to patients with epilepsy, impaired

cardiac conduction or respiratory damage, or with liver damage.
Related articles: MINIMS AMETHOCAINE HYDROCHLORIDE.

Amfipen (*Brocades*) is a proprietary ANTIBIOTIC, available only on
prescription, used to treat systemic bacterial infections and infections
of the upper respiratory tract, the ear, nose and throat, and the
urinary tracts. Produced in the form of capsules (in two strengths), as
a powder for reconstitution, as a syrup (in two strengths, under the
trade name Amfipen Syrup), and in vials for injection (in two
strengths, under the name Amfipen Injection), Amfipen is a
preparation of the broad-spectrum penicillin, ampicillin.
▲/✚ side-effects/warning: *see* AMPICILLIN.

amikacin is an ANTIBIOTIC drug (of the aminoglycoside family), used to
treat several serious bacterial infections, particularly those due to
gram-negative organisms that prove to be resistant to the more
generally used aminoglycosides GENTAMICIN, TOBRAMYCIN and NETILMICIN.
Administration is by intramuscular or intravenous injection.
▲ side-effects: extended and/or high dosage may cause irreversible
deafness; temporary kidney malfunction may occur.
✚ warning: amikacin should be administered with caution to patients
with impaired function of the kidney. Careful monitoring for
toxicity is advisable during treatment.
Related article: AMIKIN.

Amikin (*Bristol-Myers*) is a proprietary preparation of the
aminoglycoside ANTIBIOTIC amikacin, available only on prescription,
used to treat several serious bacterial infections, particularly those
that prove to be resistant to the more generally used aminoglycoside
GENTAMICIN. Amikin is produced in vials for injection or infusion (as
amikacin sulphate) in two strengths.
▲/✚ side-effects/warning: *see* AMIKACIN.

Aminex (*Cow & Gate*) is a brand of non-prescription lactose- and
sucrose-free biscuits intended for consumption by patients suffering
from lactose or sucrose intolerance, amino-acid abnormalities (such as
phenylketonuria), kidney failure, or cirrhosis of the liver. Mostly
carbohydrate, the biscuits contain a small proportion of fat, and less
than 1% protein.

Aminofusin L Forte (*Merck*) is a proprietary form of nutrition for
intravenous infusion into patients who are unable to take in food via
the alimentary canal. Available only on prescription it contains
amino acids, vitamins and electrolytes.

Aminogran (*Allen & Hanburys*) is a proprietary non-prescription form
of nutritional supplement for patients with amino-acid abnormalities
(such as phenylketonuria). It comprises a food supplement containing
all essential amino acids except for phenylalanine. There is in
addition a mineral mixture − intended to be combined with the food
supplement, or for use with independent synthetic diets − containing
all necessary minerals.

aminophylline is a BRONCHODILATOR used by slow intravenous injection or infusion to treat severe asthmatic attacks. It is a mixture of THEOPHYLLINE and ethylenediamine (which makes it more water soluble). Aminophylline is also used in sustained release form by mouth to treat and prevent the symptoms of chronic asthma. Tablets are usually taken twice daily, and determination of blood levels of theophylline can be performed to optimize an individual's dosage. It can also be given as a suppository, but this practice has fallen out of favour because of uncertain absorption and a general disinclination from giving treatment this way unless it is considered essential. It is also used to treat neonatal apnoea (a tendency to stop breathing).
▲ side-effects: there may be nausea and gastrointestinal disturbances, an increase or irregularity in the heartbeat, and/or insomnia. Treatment in the form of suppositories may cause proctitis.
✚ warning: treatment should initially be gradually progressive in quantity administered. Aminophylline should be administered with caution to patients who suffer from heart or liver disease.
Related articles: PHYLLOCONTIN CONTINUS; THEOPHYLLINE

Aminoplasmal (*Braun*) is a proprietary form of nutrition for intravenous infusion into patients who are unable to take in food via the alimentary canal. Available only on prescription, it contains amino acids and electrolytes. Various strengths are produced, differentiated by suffixes to the trade name: Ped, L3, L5 and L10.

Aminoplex 12 (*Geistlich*) is a proprietary form of nutrition for intravenous infusion into patients who are unable to take in food via the alimentary canal. Available only on prescription, it contains amino acids, malic acid and electrolytes. Another version, Aminoplex 5, additionally contains the sugar-substitute sorbitol and ethanol (ethyl alcohol); a third version, Aminoplex 14, additionally contains vitamins.

Aminoven 12 (*MCP Pharmaceuticals*) is a proprietary form of nutrition for intravenous infusion into patients who are unable to take in food via the alimentary canal. Available only on prescription, it contains synthesized amino acids and electrolytes.

amiodarone is a potentially toxic drug used to treat severe irregularity of the heartbeat, especially in cases where for one reason or another alternative drugs cannot be used. Administration is oral in the form of tablets, or by injection.
▲ side-effects: deposits on the cornea of the eyes and associated sensitivity to light are inevitable, but reversible on withdrawal of treatment. There may be other neurological effects.
✚ warning: amiodarone should not be administered to patients who suffer from very slow heartbeat, thyroid dysfunction, or shock. Dosage in each individual case should be the minimum to achieve the desired results. Patients should shield their skin from bright light because of the possibility of phototoxic reactions.

amitriptyline is an ANTIDEPRESSANT drug that also has sedative properties. As well as the treatment of depressive illness, however, the drug may be used to prevent bedwetting at night in children. While the treatment is often effective for bedwetting, children frequently relapse on stopping the medicine. It may be particularly useful for when a child is staying away from home, to avoid embarrassment. Administration is oral in the form of tablets, capsules or a dilute mixture. It is not recommended for young children.

▲/✚ side-effects/warning: there may be drowsiness and dry mouth, although there are few or no side-effects in the dosages for bedwetting.

Related articles: ELAVIL; TRYPTIZOL.

amoebicidal drugs prevent or treat infection by the microscopic protozoan organisms known as amoebae. Best known and most used are CHLOROQUINE and METRONIDAZOLE — metronidazole particularly to counter intestinal forms of infection (amoebic dysentery) and chloroquine to treat infection of the liver. Both subject their patients to some potentially unpleasant side-effects. Chloroquine is not prescribed for this purpose in children.

▲/✚ side-effects/warning: *see* METRONIDAZOLE.

Related articles: AVLOCLOR; FLAGYL; METROLYL; NIDAZOL; ZADSTAT.

Amoxil *(Bencard)* is a proprietary ANTIBIOTIC, available only on prescription, used to treat systemic bacterial infections and infections of the upper respiratory tract, of the ear, nose and throat, and of the urinary tracts. It is produced in the form of capsules (in two strengths), as sugar-free soluble (dispersible) tablets, as a syrup for dilution (in two strengths; the potency of the syrup once diluted is retained for 14 days), as a suspension for children, in the form of powder in sachets, as a sugar-free powder in sachets, and as a powder in vials for reconstitution as a medium for injection. Amoxil is a preparation of the broad-spectrum PENICILLIN amoxycillin.

▲/✚ side-effects/warning: *see* AMOXYCILLIN

amoxycillin is a broad-spectrum penicillin-type ANTIBIOTIC, closely related to AMPICILLIN. Readily absorbed orally, it is used to treat many infections especially infections of the respiratory tract and the middle ear. It is also sometimes used to prevent infection in dental surgery. Administration is oral in the form of capsules or liquids, or by injection.

▲ side-effects: there may be sensitivity reactions such as rashes, high temperature and joint pain. Allergic patients may suffer very severe reactions. The most common side-effect, however, is diarrhoea.

✚ warning: amoxycillin should not be administered to patients who are known to be allergic to penicillin-type antibiotics; it should be administered with caution to those with impaired kidney function.

Related articles: AMOXIL; AUGMENTIN.

amphotericin is a broad spectrum ANTIMICROBIAL used particularly to treat infection by fungal organisms. It can be given by infusion, and is extremely important in the treatment of systemic fungal infections and is active against almost all fungi and yeasts. However, it is a toxic drug and side-effects are common. Administration is oral in the form of tablets, lozenges or liquids, or by infusion.

▲ side-effects: treatment by infusion may cause nausea, vomiting, severe weight loss, ringing in the ears (tinnitus) and fever; some patients have a marked reduction in blood potassium. Prolonged or high dosage may cause kidney damage.

✚ warning: amphotericin should not be administered to patients who are already undergoing drug treatment that may affect kidney function. During treatment by infusion, tests on kidney function are essential; the site of injection must be changed frequently.
Related articles: FUNGILIN; FUNGIZONE.

ampicillin is a broad-spectrum penicillin-type ANTIBIOTIC. Easily absorbed — although absorption is reduced by the presence of food in the stomach or intestine — it is used to treat many infections and especially infections of the respiratory tract and middle ear. It is also used in high dosage by injection to treat bacterial meningitis, and is the drug of choice in Listeria infections. However, many bacteria have, over the past two decades, become resistant to ampicillin, and other antibiotics have to be used. Administration is oral in the form of capsules or liquids, or by injection.

▲ side-effects: there may be sensitivity reactions such as minor rashes, high temperature and joint pain. Allergic patients may suffer very severe reactions. The most common side-effect, however, is diarrhoea.

✚ warning: ampicillin should not be administered to patients who are known to be allergic to penicillin-type antibiotics in case anaphylactic shock ensues; it should not be given to patients with glandular fever because administration of the drug may result in a widespread rash.
Related articles: AMPICLOX; BRITCIN; FLU-AMP; MAGNAPEN; PENBRITIN; VIDOPEN.

Ampiclox (*Beecham*) is a proprietary ANTIBIOTIC, available only on prescription, used to treat systemic bacterial infections and infections of the upper respiratory tract, ear, nose and throat. Produced in vials for injection, Ampiclox is a compound preparation of the broad-spectrum ANTIBIOTIC ampicillin and cloxacillin. A smaller dose version (under the trade name Ampiclox Neonatal) is produced in the form of a sugar-free suspension and as a powder for reconstitution as a medium for injection, and is used to treat or prevent infections in newborn or premature babies. However, Ampiclox Neonatal is rarely used in the newborn period as most infections at this age are resistant to it.

▲/✚ side-effects/warning: *see* AMPICILLIN; CLOXACILLIN.

Anadin (*Whitehall Laboratories*) is a proprietary, non-prescription compound non-narcotic ANALGESIC produced in the form of tablets and as capsules. Anadin is a preparation of aspirin, caffeine and quinine sulphate.

It is not recommended for children under 12 years old because of the aspirin content.

▲/✚ side-effects/warning: *see* ASPIRIN; CAFFEINE; QUININE.

Anadin Extra (*Whitehall Laboratories*) is a proprietary, non-prescription compound non-narcotic ANALGESIC produced in the form of tablets and as capsules. Anadin Extra is a preparation of aspirin, caffeine and paracetamol. Not recommended for children under 12 years old because of the aspirin content.

▲/✚ side-effects/warning: *see* ASPIRIN; CAFFEINE; PARACETAMOL.

*anaesthetics are drugs that reduce sensation; such drugs affect either a specific local area − a local anaesthetic − or the whole body with loss of consciousness − a general anaesthetic.

The drug used to induce general anesthesia is generally different from the drug or drugs used to continue it. Frequently used drugs for the induction of anaesthesia include THIOPENTONE SODIUM and ETOMIDATE. For the continuance of anaesthesia, common drugs include oxygen-nitrous oxide mixtures and HALOTHANE. Prior to induction, a patient is usually given a premedication, a drug to calm the nerves, an hour or so before an operation is due. Such premedications include OPIATES, BENZODIAZEPINES and also HYOSCINE or ATROPINE. The later two may help to reduce salivary production and secretions from the chest. They also prevent excessive slowing of the heart, which might result from other medications. Other drugs in addition to general anaesthetics are used during surgery; for most internal surgery a SKELETAL MUSCLE RELAXANT, or perhaps a narcotic ANALGESIC, is also required.

Local anaesthetics are injected or absorbed in the area of the body where they are intended to take effect; they work by temporarily impairing the functioning of local nerves. Frequently used local anaesthetics include LIGNOCAINE, which is often used in dental surgery. Recently an effective topical anaesthetic (Emla cream) has become available. This can greatly reduce discomfort associated with blood tests or the siting of an intravenous drip. However, it needs to be applied to the skin under a dressing for at least 30 minutes to be effective.

*analgesics are drugs that relieve pain. Because pain is a subjective experience that can arise from many causes, there are many ways that drugs can be used to relieve it. However, the term analgesic is best restricted to two main classes of drug.

First, narcotic analgesics are drugs such as MORPHINE that have powerful actions on the central nervous system and alter the perception of pain. Because of the numerous possible side-effects, the most important of which is drug dependence (habituation), this class is usually used under medical supervision, and normally the drugs are only available on prescription. Other notable side-effects commonly include depression of respiration, nausea and sometimes hypotension, constipation, inhibition of coughing, and constriction of the pupils. Other members of this class include DIAMORPHINE, PENTAZOCINE, METHADONE, PETHIDINE and CODEINE, in descending order of potency with respect to their ability to deal with severe pain. Narcotic analgesics (such as pethidine) given to a mother in labour may depress the infants breathing at birth.

Second, non-narcotic analgesics, of which the most commonly used is PARACETAMOL. Paracetamol also has the ability to lower body temperature (antipyretic action). ASPIRIN is no longer used as an analgesic in children under 12 years old. Other analgesics occasionally used in childhood include MEFANAMIC ACID. Often drugs in this class are used in combination with each other (such as paracetamol and codeine) or with drugs of other classes (such as CAFFEINE). Some analgesics also have an anti-inflammatory action as well, and are referred to as non-steroidal anti-inflammatory drugs (NSAID), an example being IBUPROFEN.

Apart from this two main classes, there are other drugs that are sometimes referred to as analgesics because of their ability to relieve pain (such as local anaesthetics in the USA). To achieve the degree of pain relief necessary for major surgical operations, general ANAESTHETICS are used, but often in conjunction with narcotic analgesics.

Andrews (*Sterling Health*) is a proprietary, non-prescription ANTACID, produced in the form of a powder. By dissolving various amounts in water, the solution may also be used as a laxative or simply a refreshing drink. Andrews contains sodium bicarbonate and magnesium sulphate.
▲/✚ side-effects/warning: *see* MAGNESIUM SULPHATE; SODIUM BICARBONATE.

Anectine (*Calmic*) is a proprietary MUSCLE RELAXANT, available only on prescription, that has an effect for only five minutes. It is used to relax muscles during surgical anaesthesia and this facilitates some surgical procedures (such as inserting a ventilation tube into the windpipe). Produced in ampoules for injection, Anectine is a preparation of suxamethonium chloride.
▲/✚ side-effects/warning: *see* SUXAMETHONIUM CHLORIDE.

Anethaine (*Evans*) is a proprietary non-prescription local ANAESTHETIC used to treat painful skin conditions and itching. Produced in the form of a water-miscible cream for topical application, Anethaine is a preparation of amethocaine hydrochloride.
▲/✚ side-effects/warning: *see* AMETHOCAINE HYDROCHLORIDE.

Anexate (*Roche*) is a proprietary preparation of the BENZODIAZAPINE antagonist, flumazanil, available only on prescription. It is used to reverse the sedative effects of benzodiazapines used in anaesthetic, intensive care and diagnostic procedures. Anexate is produced in ampoules for injection.
▲/✚ side-effects/warning: *see* FLUMAZANIL.

Angilol (*DDSA Pharmaceuticals*) is a proprietary BETA-BLOCKER, available only on prescription. In adults it is used to lower blood pressure (anti-hypertensive). It may be used in childhood to slow and regularize the heartbeat, to counter the effects of excess thyroid

hormone in the blood stream (thyrotoxicosis) or to help prevent
migraine attacks. The medication can also help block the symptoms of
anxiety. Produced in the form of tablets (in four strengths), Angilol is
a preparation of propranolol hydrochloride.
▲/✚ side-effects/warning: *see* PROPRANOLOL.

*antacids are drugs that effectively neutralize the hydrochloric acid
that the stomach produces as a means of digestion. Much of
indigestion is caused by an excessive quantity of acids in the stomach,
and simple indigestion can be complicated by the effects of stomach
acids on peptic ulcers. Antacids thus reduce acidity, but may
themselves cause flatulence or diarrhoea as side-effects. Antacids may
also impair the absorption of other drugs. Most used and best known
antacids include ALUMINIUM HYDROXIDE, SODIUM BICARBONATE, MAGNESIUM
HYDROXIDE and calcium carbonate.

antazoline is an ANTIHISTAMINE used to treat topical allergic conditions.
It is used in combination with other drugs to treat allergic skin
irritations, stings and bites, and in combination with other
antihistamines to relieve the symptoms of allergic conjunctivitis.
Administration is in the form of a cream or as eye-drops.
Related articles: OTRIVINE-ANTISTIN; R.B.C.; VASOCON A.

Antepar (*Wellcome*) is a proprietary non-prescription ANTHELMINTIC drug
used to treat infestation by threadworms or roundworms. A laxative
administered simultaneously is often expedient. Produced in the form of
tablets and as an elixir for dilution (the potency of the elixir once diluted
is retained for 14 days), Antepar is a preparation of piperazine hydrate.
▲/✚ side-effects/warning: *see* PIPERAZINE.

*anthelmintic drugs are used to treat infections caused by parasitic
organisms of the helminth (worm) family. The threadworm and the
roundworm are most commonly responsible for helminth infections in
the UK. In the warmer, underdeveloped countries illness caused by
helminths, such as hookworms (anaemia and debilitation), schistosomes
(bilharzia) and filaria (elephantiasis and anchocerciasis), is a major
health problem. Most worms infest the intestines; diagnosis often
corresponds to evidence of their presence as shown in the faeces. Drugs
can then be administered, and the worms are killed or anaesthetized and
excreted in the normal way. Complications arise if the worms migrate
within the body, in which case in order to make the body's environment
untenable for the worms, the treatment becomes severely unpleasant for
the patient. In the case of threadworms, medication should be combined
with hygienic measures (such as short clean finger nails), and also the
whole family should be treated. Most used and best known anthelmintics
include MEBENDAZOLE, PIPERAZINE and THIABENDAZOLE.

Anthical (*May & Baker*) is a proprietary non-prescription
ANTIHISTAMINE, used to treat allergic symptoms of itching and rashes.
Produced in the form of a cream, Anthical is a preparation of
mepyramine maleate and ZINC OXIDE.
▲/✚ side-effects/warning: *see* MEPYRAMINE.

Anthranol (*Stiefel*) is a proprietary preparation, available only on prescription, used to treat serious non-infective skin inflammation, in particular psoriasis. Produced in the form of an ointment (in three strengths), Anthranol is a preparation of the powerful drug dithranol with salicylic acid.

▲/✚ side-effects/warning: *see* DITHRANOL; SALICYLIC ACID.

*anti-allergic drugs relieve the symptoms of allergic sensitivity to specific substances. These substances may be endogenous (in the patient's body), or they may be exogenous (present in the environment). Because allergic reactions generally cause the internal release of histamine, the most effective drugs for the purpose are the ANTIHISTAMINES. However, some allergic reactions include inflammatory symptoms, and in such cases the CORTICOSTEROIDS may afford useful relief. How certain of the corticosteroids may relieve asthmatic symptoms is not fully understood, but the effect may be due to the reduction of inflammatory responses in the lining of the airways. There are many other types of drugs that also treat the symptoms of asthma, including the SYMPATHOMIMETICS and the ANTICHOLINERGIC or xanthine BRONCHODILATORS. In allergic emergencies – anaphylactic shock – blood pressure is severely lowered and initial treatment is generally an injection of ADRENALINE (which may have to be repeated), followed by intravenous infusion of an antihistamine (such as CHLORPHENIRAMINE). SODIUM CROMOGLYCATE is an anti-allergic drug that prevents the release of histamine from cells, unlike antihistamines which antagonize histamine.

*antiarrhythmic drugs strengthen and regularize a heartbeat that has become unsteady and is not showing its usual pattern of activity. But because there are many ways in which the heartbeat can falter – atrial tachycardia, ventricular tachycardia, atrial flutter or fibrillation – there is a variety of drugs available, each for a fairly specific use. Best known and most used antiarrhythmic drugs include DIGOXIN (a CARDIAC GLYCOSIDE), VERAPAMIL (a calcium antagonist) and the BETA-BLOCKERS.

*anti-asthmatic drugs relieve the symptoms of bronchial asthma or prevent recurrent attacks. The symptoms of asthma include spasm of the muscles in the bronchial passages and make breathing difficult, so some anti-asthmatic drugs are BRONCHODILATORS and some are also SMOOTH MUSCLE RELAXANTS. The SYMPATHOMIMETICS are drugs in common use, notable examples being SALBUTAMOL and TERBUTALINE. In an emergency situation, CORTICOSTEROIDS may also be required to limit inflammatory responses in the mucous membranes of the air passages, and are being increasingly used by inhalation in the prevention of asthmatic attacks. But there are many other types of drugs used in the treatment of asthma. In the prevention of asthmatic attacks, regular dosage of SODIUM CHROMOGLYCATE is often the preferred initial therapy. If this fails then inhaled steroids are usually effective. AMINOPHYLLINE or THEOPHYLLINE taken by mouth may help to prevent asthmatic symptoms.
see ANTI-ALLERGIC.

*antibacterial drugs have a selectively toxic action on bacteria. They can be used both topically to treat infections of superficial tissues; or systemically, being carried by the blood, following oral absorption or injection, to the site of the infection. As bacteria are the largest and most diverse group of pathogenic micro-organisms, antibacterials form the major constituent group of ANTIBIOTICS.

*antibiotics are, strictly speaking, natural products secreted by micro-organisms into their environment where they inhibit the growth of competing micro-organisms of different species. But in common usage, and in this book, the term is applied to any drug – natural or synthetic – that has a selectively toxic action on bacteria or similar non-nucleated, single-celled micro-organisms (inlcuding chlamydia, rickettsia and mycoplasma); such drugs have no effect on viruses. Most synthetic antibiotics are modelled on natural substances. When administered by an appropriate route, such as orally, by injection or by infusion, antibiotics kill infective bacteria (bactericidal action) or inhibit their growth (bacteriostatic action). The selectively toxic action on invading bacteria exploits differences between bacteria and their human host cells. Major target sites are the bacterial cell wall located outside the cell membrane (human cells have only a cell membrane), and the bacterial ribosome (the protein-synthesizing organelle within its cell), which is different in bacteria and in human cells. Antibiotics of the PENICILLIN and CEPHALOSPORIN families (collectively known as beta-lactam antibiotics) attack the bacterial cell wall, whereas aminoglycoside and TETRACYCLINE antibiotics attack the bacterial ribosomes. Viruses, which lack both cell walls and ribosomes, are therefore resistant to these and other similar antibiotics.

Because there is such a diversity of disease-causing (pathogenic) bacteria, it is not surprising that specific infections are best treated using specific antibiotics, developed to combat them. But unfortunately, with the continuing widespread use of antiobiotics, certain strains of common bacteria have developed resistance to antibiotics that were formerly effective against them. This is now a major problem. Another problem is the occurrence of "superinfections", in which the use of a broad-spectrum antibiotic disturbs the normal, harmless bacterial population in the body as well as the pathogenic ones. In mild cases this may allow, for example, an existing but latent oral or vaginal thrush infection to become worse, or mild diarrhoea to develop. In rare cases the superinfection that develops is more serious than the disorder for which the antibiotic was administered.

*anticancer drugs are mostly CYTOTOXIC: they work by interfering one way or another with cell replication or production, so preventing the growth of new tissue. Inevitably, this means that normal cell production is also affected and thus there may be some severe side-effects. They are generally administered in combination in a series of treatments known collectively as chemotherapy. But there are other forms of anticancer drug therapy, such as the corticosteroids prednisone and prednisolone used as anticancer drugs in the treatment of leukaemia and lymphoma.

A

*anticholinergic drugs inhibit the action, release or production of the substance acetylcholine (a neurotransmitter), which plays an important part in the nervous system. The drugs tend to relax smooth muscle, to reduce the secretion of saliva, digestive juices and sweat, and to dilate the pupil of the eye. Atropine is an example of an anticholinergic drug. It is used as a premedication before a general anaesthetic

*anticoagulants are agents that prevent the clotting of blood and dissolve blood clots that have formed. The blood's own natural anticoagulant is heparin, probably still the most effective anticoagulant known. Heparin is often added in small quantities to solutions being infused through vascular lines to prevent blood from clotting and causing blockage.

*anticonvulsant drugs prevent the onset of epileptic seizures or reduce their severity if they do occur.
SODIUM VALPROATE is used to treat all forms of epilepsy; others include those used solely to treat grand mal forms of epilepsy, such as CARBAMAZEPINE and PHENYTOIN and those used solely to treat petit mal forms, such as ETHOSUXIMIDE. PHENOBARBITONE is commonly used in the newborn, but less so in older children, to treat major convulsions. In every case, dosage must be adjusted to the requirements of each individual patient.

*antidepressants are drugs that relieve the symptoms of depressive illness. There are two main groups of drugs used for the purpose. One is the group nominally called tricyclic antidepressants, which include AMITRYPTILINE, IMIPRAMINE and doxepin, and are effective in alleviating a number of symptoms – although they have ANTICHOLINERGIC side-effects. The other group consists of the monoamine-oxidase inhibitors (MAOIs), which include isocarboxazid, tranylcypromine and phenelzine, and are now used less commonly because they have severe side-effects. A third type of antidepressant consists of the amino acid, tryptophan. Caution must be taken in prescribing antidepressant drugs.

*antidiarrhoeal drugs prevent the onset of diarrhoea or assist in treating it if the symptom is already present. Yet the main medical treatment while diarrhoea lasts is always the replacement of fluids and minerals. Commercial preparations of fluid and minerals are readily available, such as DIORALYTE and REHIDRAT. These should form the basis of the treatment of diarrhoea, and there should really be no need to use drugs. Because there is a perceived need on the part of the general public, however, antidiarrhoeals are generally available, without prescription. Many are adsorbent mixtures that bind faecal material into solid masses; such mixtures include those containing KAOLIN, chalk or METHYLCELLULOSE – preparations which may also be useful in controlling faecal consistency for patients who have undergone colostomy or ileostomy. Other antidiarrhoeals work by reducing the movement of the intestines (peristalsis) and this slows down the movement of faecal material: OPIATES such as CODEINE

PHOSPHATE and MORPHINE are efficient at this. Diarrhoea caused by inflammatory disorders may be relieved by treatment with CORTICOSTEROIDS.

*anti-emetic (or antinauseant) drugs prevent vomiting, and are therefore used primarily to prevent travel sickness, to relieve vertigo experienced by patients with infection of the organs of balance in the ears, or to alleviate nausea in patients undergoing chemotherapy for cancer. No specific type of drug is used for the purpose, although most of the ANTIHISTAMINES are effective. HYOSCINE is also useful, as in many cases are the PHENOTHIAZINE derivatives (such as CHLORPROMAZINE and PROCHLORPERAZINE). In all cases, treatment causes drowsiness and reduces concentration.

*antifungal drugs are used to treat infections caused by fungal micro-organisms; they may be naturally or synthetically produced. Usually fungal infections are not a major problem in healthy, well-nourished patients. However, superficial, localized infections, such as thrush (caused by *Candida albicans*) athlete's foot or ringworm (caused by fungi of the derematophyte group), are common. Severe infections occur most frequently where the host's immunity is low, for example, following immunosuppression for transplant surgery. Under such conditions fungi that are not normally pathogenic can exploit the situation and generate a life-threatening infection. Unfortunately the most potent antifungal drugs also tend to be highly toxic, and therefore severe systemic fungal infections remain a considerable danger. NYSTATIN and IMIDAZOLES such as CLOTRIMAZOLE are used for local treatment, with GRISEOFULVIN as an alternative. AMPHOTERICIN and FLUCYTOSINE are reserved for systemic fungal infections. The most common form of fungal infection in childhood is thrush. It usually occurs in the mouth and in the nappy area of infants. The treatment most often used involves topical nystatin or MICONAZOLE.

*antihistamines are drugs that inhibit the effects in the body of histamine. Histamine release occurs naturally as the result of a patient's coming into contact with a substance to which he or she is allergically sensitive, and the resultant symptoms, if not more serious, may be those of hay fever, urticaria, itching (pruritus) or even asthma. Many antihistamines also have ANTI-EMETIC properties, and are thus used to prevent travel sickness, vertigo, or the effects of chemotherapy in the treatment of cancer. Side-effects following administration commonly include drowsiness (and a small number of antihistamines are used as sedatives), dizziness, blurred vision, gastrointestinal disturbances and a lack of muscular co-ordination.

Conventionally, only the earlier discovered drugs that act on histamine's H_1 receptors are referred to by the general name "antihistamines". Somewhat confusingly, however, the recently discovered drugs used in the treatment of peptic ulcers (such as CIMETIDINE and RANTIDINE) are also antihistamines, but act on another class of receptor (H_2) that is involved in gastric secretion.

see ASTEMIZOLE; AZATADINE MALEATE; BROMPHENIRAMINE MALEATE; CINNARIZINE; CLEMASTINE; CYCLIZINE; CYPROHEPTADINE HYDROCHLORIDE; DIMENHYDRINATE; DIMETHINDENE MALEATE; DIPHENHYDRAMINE HYDROCHLORIDE

HYDROXYZINE HYDROCHLORIDE; MEBHYDROLIN; MEPYRAMINE MALEATE; MEQUITAZINE; OXATOMIDE; PHENIRAMINE MALEATE; PROMETHAZINE HYDROCHLORIDE; TERFENADINE; TRIMEPRAZINE TARTRATE; TRIPROLIDINE HYDROCHLORIDE.

*__antihypertensive__ drugs reduce high blood pressure. Many DIURETICS have an antihypertensive action, as do the BETA-BLOCKERS.

*__anti-inflammatory__ drugs are those used to reduce inflammation (the body's defensive reaction when tissue is injured). The way they work depends on the type of drug (such as CORITCOSTEROID or NSAID), but may involve actions such as the reduction of blood flow to the inflamed area, or an inhibitory effect on the chemicals released in the tissue that cause the inflammation.

*__antimalarial__ drugs are used to treat or prevent malaria. The disease is caused by infection of the red blood cells with a small organism called a protozoon (of the genus *Plasmodium*) which is carried by the *Anopheles* mosquito. Infection occurs as a result of the female mosquito's bite. The class of drug most frequently used to treat or prevent infection by the malaria protozoon are the quinidines, of which CHLOROQUINE is the standard. However, in many parts of the world, some forms of the protozoon that causes malaria are resistant to chloroquine; in such cases, the traditional remedy for malaria, QUININE, is used. Quinine may also be used in patients who cannot tolerate chloroquine. The prevention of malaria by drugs cannot be guaranteed. However, administration of chloroquine, PROGUANIL or PYRIMETHAMINE before, and for a period after, travelling to a tropical place, is thought to provide reasonable protection.

*__antimicrobials__ are drugs used to treat infections caused by microbes. These include the major classes of pathogenic micro-organisms covered in this book − viruses, mycoplasma, rickettsia, chlamydia, protozoa, bacteria and fungi, but not helminths (worms). Antimicrobial is therefore a wide term embracing ANTIBACTERIALS, ANTIBIOTICS, ANTIPROTOZOALS, ANTIVIRALS and ANTIFUNGALS. A drug that combines both the properties of an antibacterial and an antifungal could be more concisely termed an antimicrobial. However, in this text more specific terms will be used where possible.

*__antinauseants__ are usually described as anti-emetics, although theoretically they remedy nausea (the sensation that makes people feel as if they are about to vomit) rather than prevent vomiting. The term is used occasionally to make this distinction. *see* ANTI-EMETIC.

*__antiprotozoal__ drugs are used to treat or prevent infections caused by micro-organisms called protozoa. Of these the most important, in terms of illness and death, are the protozoa of the genus *Plasmodium*, which cause malaria. Other major protozoal diseases found in tropical countries include trypanosomiasis, leishmaniasis and amoebic dysentery. Protozoal infections more familiar in this country include, toxoplasmosis, trichomoniasis and giardiasis. A common form of pneumonia in immunosuppressed patients (including those suffering from AIDS) is caused by the protozoon, *Pnuemocytes cariniu*. *see* ANTIMALARIAL.

***antipsychotic** (or neuroleptic) drugs calm and soothe patients without impairing consciousness. They are used mainly to treat psychologically disturbed patients, particularly those who manifest the complex behavioural patterns of schizophrenia, but in the short term they may also be used to treat severe anxiety. Affecting mood, they may also worsen or help to alleviate depression. Antipsychotics exert their effect by acting in the brain. They exhibit many side-effects, including abnormal face and body movements, and restlessness; these may resemble the symptoms of the condition being treated. The use of other drugs may be required to control these side-effects. Antipsychotic drugs include haloperidol, flupenthixol decanoate and the PHENOTHIAZINE derivatives, especially CHLORPROMAZINE and thioridazine. Those antipsychotics with markedly depressant side-effects are known as major TRANQUILLIZERS.

***antipyretic** drugs reduce high body temperature. Some children between the ages of six months and five years are prone to convulsions associated with fever (febrile convulsions), and the use of PARACETAMOL to lower the temperature helps prevent such fits.

***antirheumatic** drugs are used to relieve the pain and the inflammation of rheumatism and arthritis, and sometimes of other musculo-skeletal disorders. The primary form of treatment is with non-steroidal ANTI-INFLAMMATORY (NSAID) non-narcotic ANALGESICS such as ASPIRIN, SODIUM SALICYLATE, INDOMETHACIN, fenoprofen, IBUPROFEN and PHENYLBUTAZONE. CORTICOSTEROIDS may also be used for their notable anti-inflammatory properties. Suitable steroids include PREDNISOLONE and TRIAMCINOLONE. Corticosteroids are only used in the most severe cases because of the undesirable side-effects (such as stunting of growth). Finally, there are some drugs that seem to halt the progressive advance of rheumatism; some have unpleasant side-effects, others may take up to six months to have any effect. They include gold (in the form of SODIUM AUROTHIOMALATE) and PENICILLAMINE, and some drugs otherwise mostly used as immunosuppressants.

***antiseptics** are agents that destroy micro-organisms, or inhibit their activity to a level such that they are less or no longer harmful to health. Antiseptics may be applied to the skin, burns and wounds and to limit the spread of pathogenic micro-organisms. The term antiseptic is often used synonymously with DISINFECTANT.

***antiserum** is a general term used to describe certain preparations of blood serum. Antiserums are used to provide (passive) immunity to diseases, or to provide some measure of treatment if the disease has already been contracted. The general term used to describe the disease-causing entity is "antigen". If an antigen is injected into an animal, the animal produces antibodies in response to the antigen. An antiserum is a sample of blood serum containing these antibodies.

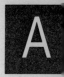

Most antiserums are prepared from the blood of antigen-treated horses, and when the purified antiserums are used to immunize humans they often cause hypersensitivity reactions. For this reason, use of such preparations is now very rare, and they have to a large extent been replaced by preparations of human antibodies.

*antitubercular (or antituberculous) drugs are used in combination to treat tuberculosis. The initial phase of treatment usually employs three drugs (ordinarily ISONIAZID, RIFAMPICIN and PYRAZINAMIDE STREPTOMYCIN or ETHAMBUTOL HYDROCHLORIDE) in order to tackle the disease as efficiently as possible, while reducing the risk of encountering bacterial resistance. If the first line of treatment is successful, after about two months, treatment usually continues with only two of the initial three drugs (one of which is generally isoniazid).
  If the first line of treatment was not successful, for example because the patient suffered intolerable side-effects or because the disease was resistant to drugs, then other drugs (such as CAPREOMYCIN and CYCLOSERINE) are used to treat the patient. The duration of treatment depends on the combination of drugs used.

*antitussives are drugs that assist in the treatment of coughs. Sometimes the term antitussive is used to describe only those drugs that suppress coughing rather than drugs used to treat the cause of coughing. Cough suppressants include OPIATES such as DEXTROMETHORPHAN, noscapine, METHADONE and CODEINE. They tend to cause constipation as a side-effect and so should not be used for prolonged periods. Other antitussive preparations are EXPECTORANTS and demulcents. Expectorants are drugs used to decrease the viscosity of mucus or to increase the secretion of liquid mucus in dry, unproductive coughs, the idea being that air passages will become lubricated, thereby making the cough more productive. Expectorants include ammonium chloride and IPECACUANHA. These expectorants are included in many proprietary compound cough medicines. Demulcents also help to reduce the viscosity of mucus and relieve dry, unproductive coughs. All of these drugs are used to soothe coughs rather than treat the underlying cause of the cough, such as an infection. The use of cough suppressants containing opiates in the very young may be dangerous and is best avoided.

*antivenin is an antidote to the poison in a snake-bite, a scorpion's sting, or a bite from any other poisonous creature (such as a spider). Normally, it is an ANTISERUM, and is injected into the bloodstream for immediate relief. Identification of the poisonous creature is important so that the right antidote can be selected.

*antiviral drugs are relatively few in number and their effectiveness is often restricted to preventative or disease limitation treatment. This is perhaps not surprising as viruses reproduce by taking over the biochemical machinery of the host cells and perverting it to their own needs. Therefore, it is extremely difficult to design a drug that can differentiate between attacking a vital viral mechanism and the host cell itslf. However, some antiviral drugs can be life-saving, especially in immunocompromised patients. Infections due to the herpes viruses (such as cold sores, genital herpes and chicken pox) may be prevented or contained by early treatment with ACYCLOVIR. Serious cytomegaloviral infections may also be contained by treatment with ganciclovir. Severe respiratory infections in children, caused by the respiratory syncytial virus, are treated with RIBAVIRIN. As more of the molecular biology of the virus-host interactions becomes known, more selective antivirals will be possible.

Antraderm (*Brocades*) is a proprietary form of the powerful drug dithranol, used to treat serious non-infective skin inflammations, particularly psoriasis. It is produced in the form of a wax stick for topical application. In three strengths, the strongest under the trade name Antraderm Forte, the weakest under the name Antraderm Mild, it is available only on prescription, except for Antraderm Mild.
▲/✚ side-effects/warning: *see* DITHRANOL.

*anxiolytic drugs relieve medically diagnosed anxiety states and should be prescribed only for patients whose anxiety in the face of stress is actually hindering the prospect of its resolution. Treatment should be at the lowest dosage effective, and must not be prolonged: psychological dependence (if not physical addiction) readily occurs and may make withdrawal difficult. Best known and most used anxiolytic drugs are the BENZODIAZEPINES, such as DIAZEPAM, chlordiazepoxide, LORAZEPAM and CLOBAZAM; others include meprobamate and some of the ANTIPSYCHOTIC drugs used in low dosage. Drugs of this class may also be referred to as minor TRANQUILLIZERS.

Apresoline (*Ciba*) is a proprietary vasodilator, available only on prescription, used to treat moderate to severe high blood pressure (hypertension) in adults. It can also be used to treat heart failure. It is a useful adjunct to diuretic therapy. Produced in the form of tablets (in two strengths) and as a powder for reconstitution as a medium for injection, Apresoline is a preparation of hydralazine hydrochloride.
▲/✚ side-effects/warning: *see* HYDRALAZINE.

Aprinox (*Boots*) is a proprietary DIURETIC, available only on prescription, used to treat high blood pressure (*see* ANTIHYPERTENSIVE) and the accumulation of fluid within the tissues (oedema). Produced in the form of tablets (in two strengths), Aprinox is a preparation of the THIAZIDE bendrofluazide.
▲/✚ side-effects/warning: *see* BENDROFLUAZIDE.

Aproten (*Ultrapharm*) is a proprietary non-prescription brand of gluten-free, low protein food preparations, for the use of patients with phenylketonuria and similar amino acid abnormalities, kidney or liver failure, cirrhosis of the liver, coeliac disease, or gluten sensitivity. It is produced in the form of various types of pasta, as biscuits, as crispbread and as flour.

Apsifen (*Approved Prescription Services*) is a proprietary non-narcotic ANALGESIC, available only on prescription, used to relieve pain, particularly the pain of rheumatic disease and other musculo-skeletal disorders. It is produced in the form of tablets, which can be film- or sugar-coated; the film-coated are available in 3 strengths and the sugar-coated in two strengths. Apsifen is a preparation of the ANTI-INFLAMMATORY drug ibuprofen.

▲/✚ side-effects/warning: *see* IBUPROFEN.

Apsin V.K. (*Approved Prescription Services*) is a proprietary ANTIBIOTIC, available only on prescription, used to treat bacterial infections of the ear, nose and throat. Produced in the form of tablets and as a syrup (in two strengths) for dilution (the potency of the syrup once dilute is retained for 7 days if stored at a temperature below 15 degrees centigrade), Apsin V.K. is a preparation of the PENICILLIN phenoxymethylpenicillin.

▲/✚ side-effects/warning: *see* PHENOXYMETHYLPENICILLIN.

aqueous cream is an emollient used to soothe and hydrate the skin. It is used in conditions where the skin is dry; most commonly atopic eczema where, like other emollients, it should be applied generously.

aqueous iodine solution is a non-proprietary solution of iodine and potassium iodide in water (and is known also as Lugol's solution). It is used as an iodine supplement for patients suffering from an excess of thyroid HORMONES in the bloodstream (thyrotoxicosis), especially prior to thyroid surgery.

▲/✚ side-effects/warning: *see* IODINE

arachis oil is peanut oil, used primarily as an emollient in treating crusts on skin surfaces in such conditions as psoriasis, cradle cap, dandruff and eczema (often in combination with CALAMINE). It is also a constituent in many anal suppositories, and is used as a vehicle for the rectal administration of the anticonvulsant PARALDEHYDE to young children with uncontrollable fits.

Arilvax (*Wellcome*) is a proprietary form of VACCINE against yellow fever. It consists of a suspension containing live but attenuated viruses, which are cultured in chick embryos. Available only on prescription, it is produced in vials with a diluent. It is not recommended for children under the age of nine months.

Arobon (*Nestlé*) is a proprietary non-prescription preparation used to treat diarrhoea. Produced in the form of a sugar-free powder (to be taken orally in liquid), Arobon is a preparation of the adsorbent substance ceratonia in a mixture of starch and cocoa.

Arpimycin (*RP Drugs*) is a proprietary ANTIBIOTIC, available only on prescription, used to treat many forms of infection (particularly pneumonia and Legionnaires' disease) and to prevent others (particularly whooping cough); it is also used as an alternative to penicillin-type antibiotics in patients who are allergic or whose infections are resistant to penicillins. Produced in the form of a mixture (in three strengths) for dilution (the potency of the syrup once

diluted is retained for seven days), Arpimycin is a preparation of the macrolide antibiotic erythromycin.
▲/✚ side-effects/warning: *see* ERYTHROMYCIN.

Arret (*Janssen*) is a proprietary ANTIDIARRHOEAL drug, which works by reducing the rate at which material travels along the intestines. Produced in the form of capsules and as a syrup (for adults), Arret is a preparation of the OPIATE loperamide hydrochloride. It is not recommended for children aged under four years.
▲/✚ side-effects/warning: *see* LOPERAMIDE HYDROCHLORIDE

Ascabiol (*May & Baker*) is a proprietary non-prescription preparation of benzyl benzoate in suspension, used to treat infestation of the skin of the trunk and limbs by itch-mites (scabies) or sometimes to treat infestation by lice. A skin irritant, it is not suitable for use on the head, face and neck; for children it should be in diluted form (or another preparation should be used).
▲/✚ side-effects/warning: *see* BENZYL BENZOATE.

Ascalix (*Wallace*) is a proprietary non-prescription ANTHELMINTIC drug used to treat infestation by threadworms or roundworms. Produced in the form of syrup (in bottles and in sachets), Ascalix is a preparation of piperazine hydrate.
▲/✚ side-effects/warning: *see* PIPERAZINE.

ascorbic acid is the chemical name of the water-soluble VITAMIN C. Essential in the diet, the vitamin is instrumental in the development and maintenance of cells and tissues. Deficiency leads to scurvy and to certain other disorders associated particularly with the elderly. Good food sources are green vegetables and citrus fruits. Vitamin C supplements are rarely necessary; when they are, it is only in small quantities. Administration is in the form of tablets, or by injection.
✚ warning: ascorbic acid in food is lost by over-cooking or through the action of ultraviolet light.

Aserbine (*Bencard*) is a proprietary non-prescription cream containing three acids (malic, benzoic and salicylic) and other additives, used to cleanse and remove hard, dry, dead skin from ulcers, burns and bedsores so that natural healing can take place. The same preparation is also available in the form of a solution.
✚ warning: contact with the eyes should be avoided, and Aserbine should only be applied externally.

Asilone (*Berk*) is a proprietary non-prescription ANTACID compound that is not available from the National Health Service. It is used to treat acid stomach, flatulence, heartburn and gastritis, and to soothe peptic ulcers. It is produced in the form of tablets, as a gel for dilution, and as a suspension for children (under the trade name Asilone Infant Suspension) for dilution. The potency of Asilone once dilute is retained for 14 days. Asilone is a combination of the ANTACIDS aluminium hydroxide and magnesium oxide ("magnesia") together with the antifoaming agent DIMETHICONE.

Asmaven (*Approved Prescription Services*) is a proprietary form of the
BETA-RECEPTOR STIMULANT BRONCHODILATOR salbutamol, available only on
prescription. It is able to relax the muscles of the airways and is thus
used in the treatment of asthma. It is produced in the form of tablets
(in two strengths) and as an inhalant. As with all drugs, patients
should not exceed the prescribed dose and should be careful to follow
the manufacturer's directions.
▲/✚ side-effects/warning: *see* SALBUTAMOL.

aspirin (or acetylsalicylic acid) is a well known and widely used non-
narcotic ANALGESIC that also has ANTI-INFLAMMATORY properties and is
useful in reducing high body temperature (ANTIPYRETIC). As an analgesic
it relieves mild to moderate pain, particularly headache, toothache,
menstrual pain and the aches of rheumatic disease. Its temperature-
reducing capacity helps in the treatment of the common cold, fevers or
influenza. Aspirin is also used as an ANTICOAGULANT. In tablet form,
aspirin may irritate the stomach lining and many forms of soluble
aspirin, in trying to avoid this drawback, include chalk. Other
proprietary forms combine aspirin with such drugs as codeine or
paracetamol. Administration is oral. Recently a link has been suggested
between aspirin and a rare but serious disorder called Reye's syndrome
(that causes inflammation of the brain and liver). Therefore it is advised
that aspirin should not be administered to children aged under 12 years
old. It may still be prescribed in special situations, such as juvenile
rheumatoid arthritis. Some people are allergic to aspirin.
▲ side-effects: gastric irritation with or without haemorrhage is
   common, although such effects may be neutralized to some extent
   by taking the drug after food. Aspirin may enhance the effect of
   some hypoglycaemic and anticoagulant drugs.
✚ warning: irritation of the stomach lining may, in susceptible patients,
   cause nausea, vomiting, pain and bleeding (which may lead to anaemia
   if prolonged). Overdosage may cause ringing in the ears (tinnitus), dizziness, nausea, vomiting, headache, hyperventilation, and sometimes a
   state of confusion or delirium followed by coma. Aspirin may also
   dispose a patient to bronchospasm, which in asthmatic patients may
   prove problematic. Repeated overdosage may result in kidney damage.
   Related article: MIGRAVESS.

astemizole is an ANTIHISTAMINE drug used primarily to treat allergic
symptoms such as hay fever, conjunctivitis and skin rashes.
Administration is oral in the form of tablets, or as a suspension.
▲ side-effects: sedation is minimal for an antihistamine, although
   there may be headaches and/or weight gain.
✚ warning: astemizole should be administered with caution to those
   with epilepsy or liver disease.

A.T.10 (*Sterling Research*) is a proprietary non-prescription
preparation of CALCIFEROL (vitamin D) in the form of its analogue
dihydrotachysterol. Used to increase the absorption and improve the
use of calcium in the body, A.T.10 is produced as a solution in a
dropper bottle; administration is oral only.
✚ warning: see DIHYDROTACHYSTEROL.

Atarax (*Pfizer*) is a proprietary ANTIHISTAMINE, available only on
prescription. It is used to treat emotional disturbances and anxiety
(*see* ANXIOLYTIC) which may manifest as physical symptoms. It is also
used to treat physical conditions caused by allergy (such as itching
and mild rashes). Atarax may also be used as a sedative (for example,
before or after surgery), and as an ANTI-EMETIC. Produced in the form
of tablets (in two strengths) and as a syrup (under the trade name
Atarax Syrup), Atarax is a preparation of hydroxyzine hydrochloride.

Ativan (*Wyeth*) is a proprietary ANXIOLYTIC, available only on
prescription, used to treat anxiety and phobias, as a HYPNOTIC in
insomnia, as a sedative or premedication before surgery, and — as an
emergency treatment — to control status epilepticus (in which
epileptic fits succeed each other so closely that the patient does not
recover consciousness and is gradually deprived of oxygen). Produced
in the form of tablets (in two strengths) and in ampoules for injection,
Ativan is a preparation of the BENZODIAZEPINE lorazepam.
▲/✚ side-effects/warning: *see* LORAZEPAM.

Atkinson and Barkers (*Strenol*) is a proprietary, non-prescription
preparation of infant's gripe mixture. It contains the ANTACIDS sodium
bicarbonate and magnesium carbonate.
▲/✚ side-effects/warning: *see* SODIUM BICARBONATE; MAGNESIUM
  CARBONATE.

atropine is a powerful ANTICHOLINERGIC drug obtained from plants
including belladonna (deadly nightshade). It is able to depress certain
functions of the autonomic nervous system, and is a useful
antispasmodic. In combination with morphine it may be used as a
premedication to relax the muscles prior to surgery. It is also used to
dilate the pupil of the eye for ophthalmic surgery (although this
requires care in order not to trigger off latent glaucoma).
▲ side-effects: there is commonly dry mouth and thirst; there may also
  be visual disturbances, and constipation.

atropine methonitrate is a less toxic salt of the ANTICHOLINERGIC,
ATROPINE, which used to be used in the
treatment of pyloric stenosis (a muscular obstruction at the exit of the
stomach). Surgery is now the preferred method for treating this
condition.
▲ side-effects: there is commonly dry mouth and thirst; there may
  also be visual disturbances (including sensitivity to light), flushing,
  irregular heartbeat, dry skin, rashes, difficulty in urinating and
  constipation. Rarely, there may be high temperature accompanied
  by delirium.
  Related article: EUMYDRIN.

Atrovent (*Boehringer Ingelheim*) is a proprietary preparation of the
ANTICHOLINERGIC BRONCHODILATOR ipratropium bromide, available only
on prescription, used to treat asthma. It is produced in the form of an
aerosol spray (in two strengths, the stronger under the name
Atrovent Forte) and as a solution for use in a nebulizer. Using either

method, patients should not exceed the prescribed dose and should be careful to follow the manufacturer's directions; treatment should be initiated under hospital supervision. It may also be particularly useful in children under 18 months with wheezing.

▲/✚ side-effects/warning: *see* IPRATROPIUM.

Attenuvax (*Morson*) is a proprietary VACCINE against measles (rubeola), available only on prescription. It is a powdered preparation of live but attenuated measles viruses for administration by injection. Attenuvax is not usually recommended for children aged under 12 months.

▲ side-effects: there may be inflammation at the site of injection. Occasionally a mild measles-like illness may develop about a week after the vaccination.

✚ warning: attenuvax should not be administered to patients who suffer from any infection, particularly tuberculosis; who have known immune-system abnormalities; who are pregnant; or who are already taking corticosteroid drugs (except for replacement therapy), cytotoxic drugs or undergoing radiation treatment.

Audax (*Napp*) is a proprietary non-prescription non-narcotic ANALGESIC in the form of ear-drops, used to soothe pain associated with infection of the outer or middle ear. Its active constituent is choline salicylate.

Audicort (*Lederle*) is a proprietary ANTI-INFLAMMATORY ANTI-BACTERIAL and ANTIFUNGAL, available only on prescription, used in the treatment of bacterial and/or fungal infections of the outer ear. It contains the CORTICOSTEROID triamcinolone acetonide, the local ANAESTHETIC benzocaine, the ANTIBIOTIC neomycin, and the antifungal drug undecenoic acid.

▲/✚ side-effects/warning: *see* BENZOCAINE; NEOMYCIN; TRIAMCINOLONE ACETONIDE.

Augmentin (*Beecham*) is a proprietary preparation of the penicillin-like ANTIBIOTIC amoxycillin together with an "extending agent", clavulanic acid, which extends amoxycillin's action and power. It is used primarily to treat infections of the skin, ear, nose and throat, and urinary tract, and is produced in a number of forms: as tablets, as a solution (under the name Augmentin Dispersible), in milder versions as a powder for solution (under the names Augmentin Paediatric and Augmentin Junior), and in vials for injection or infusion (under the trade name Augmentin Intravenous).

▲/✚ side-effects/warning: *see* AMOXYCILLIN.

Auralgicin (*Fisons*) is a proprietary non-prescription ear-drop used to soothe pain and treat bacterial infections of the middle ear. In a glycerol base, its active constituents include the local ANAESTHETIC benzocaine, the VASOCONSTRICTOR ephedrine hydrochloride, the ANTIBACTERIAL chlorbutol, and the ANALGESIC phenazone.

▲/✚ side-effects/warning: *see* BENZOCAINE; EPHEDRINE HYDROCHLORIDE.

Auraltone (*Radiol*) is a proprietary non-prescription ear-drop used to soothe the pain of an inflamed eardrum or of an infection of the

middle ear. In a glycerol base, it contains the ANALGESIC phenazone
and local ANAESTHETIC benzocaine.

▲/✚ side-effects/warning: *see* BENZOCAINE.

Aureocort (*Lederle*) is a proprietary ANTIBIOTIC preparation for topical
application, available only on prescription, used to treat
inflammations of the skin where infection is also present. Produced as
a water-miscible cream, an anhydrous ointment, and an aerosol spray,
Aureocort contains the CORTICOSTEROID triamcinolone acetonide and
the ANTIBIOTIC chlortetracycline hydrochloride.

▲/✚ side-effects/warning: *see* CHLORTETRACYCLINE; TRIAMCINOLONE
ACETONIDE.

Aureomycin (*Lederle*) is a proprietary broad-spectrum ANTIBIOTIC,
available only on prescription, used to treat a wide range of bacterial
infections. It is produced in the form of capsules (in which form it is
not recommended for children under 12 years) as a cream and as an
ointment. In every form it is a preparation of the antibiotic
TETRACYCLINE chlortetracycline hydrochloride.

▲/✚ side-effects/warning: *see* CHLORTETRACYCLINE.

Avloclor (*ICI*) is a proprietary ANTIMALARIAL drug, available only on
prescription, used primarily to prevent or treat certain forms of malaria,
but also used as an AMOEBICIDAL drug to treat amoebic hepatitis, and to
treat rheumatoid arthritis. Produced in the form of tablets, Avloclor is a
preparation of chloroquine phosphate. In children under 12 years old,
Avloclor is used only to prevent or to suppress malaria.

▲/✚ side-effects/warning: *see* CHLOROQUINE.

Avomine (*May & Baker*) is a proprietary non-prescription
ANTINAUSEANT drug used to treat symptoms of nausea, vomiting and/or
vertigo caused by certain diseases, motion sickness, or some forms of
drug therapy. Produced in the form of tablets, Avomine is a
preparation of promethazine theoclate.

▲/✚ side-effects/warning: *see* PROMETHAZINE THEOCLATE

Azactam (*Squibb*) is a proprietary ANTIBIOTIC, available only on
prescription, used to treat severe bacterial infections. Produced in the
form of powder for reconstitution as a medium for injection or
infusion, Azactam is a preparation of aztreonam.

▲/✚ side-effects/warning: *see* AZTREONAM.

Azamune (*Penn*) is a proprietary IMMUNOSUPPRESSANT drug, available
only on prescription, used to reduce the possibility of tissue rejection
in patients who undergo organ transplants. It may also be used to
treat other conditions where the more usual forms of corticosteroid
therapies have failed. Produced in the form of tablets, Azamune is a
preparation of the CYTOTOXIC drug azathioprine.

▲/✚ side-effects/warning: *see* AZATHIOPRINE.

azatadine maleate is an ANTIHISTAMINE drug, used primarily to treat
allergic symptoms such as hay fever and urticaria, and those arising

A

from insect bites and stings. Administration is oral in the form of
tablets, or as a syrup. Its proprietary form is not recommended for
children aged under 12 months.
▲ side-effects: sedation may affect the patient's capacity for speed of
thought and movement; there may be nausea, headaches and/or
weight gain, dry mouth, gastrointestinal disturbances and visual
problems.
Related article: OPTIMINE.

azathioprine is a powerful IMMUNOSUPPRESSANT drug used mostly to
reduce the possibility of tissue rejection in patients who undergo
organ transplants. It may also be used to treat autoimmune diseases,
some collagen disorders, and other conditions where the more usual
steroid therapies have failed. Administration is oral in the form of
tablets, or by injection.
▲ side-effects: there may be suppression of the bone-marrow's
function, rashes and liver damage.
✚ warning: as with all CYTOTOXIC drugs, patients receiving
azathioprine are prone to infections. Constant checking of blood
counts is essential to monitor and adjust dosage to cope with any
bone-marrow toxicity.
Related articles: AZAMUNE; IMURAN.

azlocillin is a penicillin-type ANTIBIOTIC used primarily to treat
infections by a type of bacteria called *Pseudomonas*, and particularly
in serious infections of the urinary tract and respiratory tract, and for
septicaemia. Administration is by injection or infusion.
▲ side-effects: there may be some allergic reactions – such as a rash
– and high temperature; some patients experience pain in the
joints. Diarrhoea may occur.
✚ warning: azlocillin should not be administered to patients who are
known to be allergic to penicillins; it should be administered with
caution to those who have impaired kidney function, or who are
pregnant.
Related article: SECUROPEN.

aztreonam is an ANTIBIOTIC used to treat severe bacterial infections.
Administration is by injection or infusion. A relatively recent
addition to the pharmacopoeia, aztreonam is thought to arouse fewer
sensitivity reactions than are caused by many other antibiotics of the
beta lactam type.
▲ side-effects: there may be diarrhoea and vomiting; skin rashes may
occur, with pain or inflammation at the site of injection or infusion.
Rarely, there may be reduction in the number of white cells in the
blood causing bleeding and lowered resistance to infection.
✚ warning: aztreonam should be administered with caution to those
who are known to be sensitive to penicillin or cephalosporin, who
have impaired kidney or liver function, or who are lactating.
Related article: AZACTAM.

B

bacampicillin hydrochloride is a broad-spectrum penicillin-type ANTIBIOTIC, a derivative of AMPICILLIN that is converted to ampicillin in the bloodstream. Used to treat many infections, especially those of the respiratory tract and middle ear, it is administered orally in the form of tablets.

▲ side-effects: there may be sensitivity reactions, ranging from a minor rash to urticaria, high temperature and joint pain, or even to anaphylactic shock. The most common side-effect, however, is simply diarrhoea.

✚ warning: bacampicillin hydrochloride should not be administered to patients who are known to be allergic to penicillin-type antibiotics; it should be administered with caution to those with impaired kidney function.

Related article: AMBAXIN.

baclofen is a drug used as a SKELETAL MUSCLE RELAXANT that relaxes muscles which are in spasm, especially muscles in the limbs, and particularly when caused by injury or disease in the central nervous system. In childhood its most common use is in sufferers from severe spasticity associated with cerebral palsy. Although it is chemically unrelated to any other antispasmodic drug, it has similar clinical uses to certain of the BENZODIAZEPINE group of drugs. Administration is oral in the form of tablets or a dilute sugar-free liquid.

▲ side-effects: there may be drowsiness and fatigue, weakness and low blood pressure (hypotension). Nausea and vomiting may occur.

✚ warning: baclofen should be administered with caution to patients with any form of cerebrovascular disease, epilepsy, or psychiatric conditions. Initial dosage should be gradually increased (to avoid sedation); withdrawal of treatment should be equally gradual.

Related article: LIORESAL.

Bacticlens (*Smith & Nephew*) is a proprietary non-prescription DISINFECTANT, used to treat minor wounds and burns on the skin. Produced in the form of a solution in sachets, Bacticlens is a preparation of chlorhexidine gluconate.

▲/✚ side-effects/warning: *see* CHLORHEXIDINE.

Bactigras (*Smith & Nephew*) is a proprietary non-prescription dressing in the form of gauze impregnated with chlorhexidine acetate. It is used to treat wounds and ulcers.

▲/✚ side-effects/warning: *see* CHLORHEXIDINE.

Bactrian (*Loveridge*) is a proprietary non-prescription ANTISEPTIC cream used in the treatment of minor burns and abrasions. It contains the antiseptic CETRIMIDE in very dilute solution.

Bactrim (*Roche*) is a proprietary ANTIBACTERIAL available only on prescription, used to treat bacterial infections, especially infections of the urinary tract, sinusitis and bronchitis, and infections of bones and joints. Produced in the form of tablets (in three strengths), as soluble (dispersible) tablets, as a suspension for dilution (the potency of the suspension once dilute is retained for 14 days), as a sugar-free syrup for dilution (the potency of the syrup once dilute is retained for 14 days), in ampoules for injection, and in ampoules for intravenous infusion (following dilution), Bactrim is a preparation of the SULPHONAMIDE compound co-trimoxazole.

▲/✚ side-effects/warning: *see* CO-TRIMOXAZOLE.

Bactroban (*Beecham*) is a proprietary ANTIBIOTIC, available only on prescription, used in topical application to treat bacterial infections of the skin. Produced in the form of a water-miscible ointment, Bactroban is a preparation of MUPIROCIN in dilute solution. It is also effective against a highly resistant organism, methicillin resistant *Staphylococus aureus* (MRSA).

✚warning: the ointment may sting on application.

Bactroban nasal (*Beecham*) is a proprietary ANTIBIOTIC ointment, available only prescription. It is most commonly used to eliminate organisms such as *Staphylococci*, which may be carried by the nose. Bactroban nasal is a preparation of the antibiotic drug mupirocin.

▲/✚ side-effects/warning: *see* MUPIROCIN.

Balanced Salt Solution (*Alcon; Cooper Vision Optics*) is a proprietary non-prescription sterile solution, used as an eye-wash. It is a preparation of SODIUM CHLORIDE, sodium citrate, sodium acetate, MAGNESIUM CHLORIDE and POTASSIUM CHLORIDE.

Balneum (*Merck*) is a proprietary non-prescription skin emollient (softener and soother) for use in the bath; it is a preparation of soya oil in a fragrant solution.

Balneum with tar (*Merck*) is a proprietary non-prescription preparation, used to treat non-infective skin inflammations including psoriasis and eczema. It is produced in the form of a bath oil and is a preparation of natural oils, including COAL TAR and soya oil.

Baltar (*Merck*) is a proprietary non-prescription preparation used to treat psoriasis and other scaly disorders of the scalp, produced in the form of a soap-free shampoo. Baltar's active constituent is COAL TAR DISTILLATE.

barbiturates are a group of drugs derived from barbituric acid, with a wide range of essentially depressant actions. They are used mostly as ANTICONVULSANTS and ANAESTHETICS. They work by direct action on the brain, depressing specific centres, and may be slow- or fast-acting; all are extremely effective. Best known and most used barbiturates include the sedative and anticonvulsasnt phenobarbitone, and the anaesthetic thiopentone. Administration is oral in the form of tablets, or by injection.

▲ side-effects: there is drowsiness and dizziness within a hangover effect; there may be shallow breathing and headache. Some patients experience sensitivity reactions, which may be serious. When used as an anticonvulsant, phenobarbitone can cause hyperactivity.

see PHENOBARBITONE; THIOPENTONE SODIUM.

B

Barquinol HC (*Fisons*) is a proprietary non-prescription CORTICOSTEROID cream used to treat mild inflammations of the skin. Apart from its ANTI-INFLAMMATORY properties it also has some ANTIBACTERIAL and ANTIFUNGAL activity because, in addition to the steroid hydrocortisone acetate, it contains the iodine-based ANTISEPTIC clioquinol.
▲/✚ side-effects/warning: *see* CLIOQUINOL; HYDROCORTISONE.

Baxan (*Bristol-Myers*) is a proprietary ANTIBIOTIC, available only on prescription, used to treat many infections, especially those of the skin, soft tissues, the respiratory and urinary tracts, and the middle ear. Produced in the form of capsules, and as a suspension (in three strengths) for dilution, Baxan is a preparation of the CEPHALOSPORIN cefadroxil monohydrate.
▲/✚ side-effects/warning: *see* CEFADROXIL.

Baypen (*Bayer*) is a proprietary broad-spectrum penicillin-type ANTIBIOTIC, used to treat various types of bacterial infections. Produced in the form of powder in vials for reconstitution as a medium for injection or infusion, Baypen is a preparation of mezlocillin.
▲/✚ side-effects/warning: *see* MEZLOCILLIN.

BCG vaccine (or *Bacillus Calmette-Guérin* vaccine) is a strain of the tuberculosis bacillus that does not cause the disease in humans, but does cause the formation in the body of the specific antibodies, and so can be used as the base for an ANTITUBERCULAR vaccine.

Becloforte (*Allen & Hanburys*) is a proprietary preparation of the CORTICOSTEROID drug beclomethasone dipropionate, available only on prescription, used to prevent the symptoms of asthma. It is produced in an aerosol for topical inhalation.
▲/✚ side-effects/warning: *see* BECLOMETHASONE DIPROPIONATE.

beclomethasone dipropionate is a CORTICOSTEROID used primarily to prevent the symptoms of asthma. It is thought to work by reducing inflammation in the mucous lining of the bronchial passages, and stemming allergic reactions. The drug is also used in the form of a cream or an ointment for topical application to treat serious non-infective inflammations on the skin, or as a nasal spray to treat conditions such as hay fever. For bronchial treatment, however, it is produced mostly in aerosols for inhalation, although it is available also as powder for insufflation or as a suspension for nebulization.
▲ side-effects: some patients undergoing bronchial treatment experience hoarseness; large doses increase a risk of fungal infection, such as oral thrush. The nasal spray may cause initial sneezing.
✚ warning: as with all corticosteroids, beclomethasone treats the symptoms and has no effect on any underlying infection.
Related articles: BECLOFORTE; BECOTIDE; VENTIDE.

Becodisks (*A&A*) is a proprietary preparation of the CORTICOSTEROID drug beclomethasone dipropionate available only on prescription. It is

B

used to prevent the symptoms of asthma, chronic bronchitis and emphysema. It is produced in the form of a powder for inhalation contained on disks with an inhaler, called a diskhaler, supplied.
▲/✚ side-effects/warning: *see* BECLOMETHASONE DIPROPIONATE.

Beconase (*Allen & Hanburys*) is a proprietary nasal spray, available only on prescription, used to treat conditions such as hay fever. Produced in both an aerosol and a nasal applicator, Beconase is a preparation of the CORTICOSTEROID beclomethasone dipropionate.
▲/✚ side-effects/warning: *see* BECLOMETHASONE DIPROPIONATE.

Becotide (*Allen & Hanburys*) is a proprietary preparation of the CORTICOSTEROID drug beclomethasone dipropionate, available only on prescription, used to prevent the symptoms of asthma. It is produced in an aerosol for inhalation (in two strengths, the stronger under the name Becotide 100), in inhalation cartridges (using the name Rotacaps), and as a suspension for nebulization.
▲/✚ side-effects/warning: *see* BECLOMETHASONE DIPROPIONATE.

Bedranol (*Lagap*) is a proprietary ANTIHYPERTENSIVE drug of the BETA-BLOCKER class, available only on prescription, used in adults to treat high blood pressure (hypertension), and also to relieve angina pectoris and to slow and/or regularize the heartbeat in order to prevent a recurrent heart attack. The drug may also be used to treat the effects of an excess of thyroid hormones in the bloodstream (thyrotoxicosis) or to try to prevent migraine attacks. Produced in the form of tablets (in four strengths), Bedranol is a preparation of the beta-blocker propranolol hydrochloride.
▲/✚ side-effects/warning: *see* PROPRANOLOL.

Beecham's Powders (*Beecham Health Care*) is a proprietary, non-prescription cold relief preparation. It contains paracetamol, caffeine and ascorbic acid.
▲/✚ side-effects/warning: *see* ASCORBIC ACID, CAFFEINE, PARACETAMOL.

bendrofluazide is a THIAZIDE DIURETIC that may be used to treat hypertension, either alone or in conjunction with other ANTIHYPERTENSIVE agents, because it has a slight lowering effect on blood pressure. Like the other thiazides, bendrofluazide is used in the treatment of oedema associated with congestive heart failure and renal and hepatic disorders. Blood potassium levels should be monitored in patients taking thiazide diuretics because they may deplete body reserves of potassium. However, potassium supplements or potassium-sparing diuretics should be added only when appropriate. Administration is oral in the form of tablets.
▲ side-effects: there may be tiredness, skin rashes, thirst, nausea and dizziness.
✚ warning: bendrofluazide should not be administered to patients with kidney failure or urinary retention, or who are lactating. It may aggravate conditions of diabetes or gout.
Related articles: APRINOX; CENTYL.

benethamine penicillin is a penicillin-type ANTIBIOTIC that is used to treat and prevent bactcrial infection.

▲ side-effects: there may be sensitivity reactions ranging from a minor rash to urticaria and joint pains, and (occasionally) to high temperature or anaphylactic shock.

✚ warning: benethamine penicillin should not be administered to patients who are known to be allergic to penicillins; it should be administered with caution to those who suffer from impaired kidney function.

Related article: TRIPLOPEN.

Benoxyl (*Stiefel*) is a proprietary preparation of the KERATOLYTIC drug benzoyl peroxide, which when applied topically in the form of a cream or an ointment removes hardened or dead skin while simultaneously treating bacterial infection. It is most used in the treatment of acne. In its standard form (under the name Benoxyl 5) it is produced as both a cream and an ointment, which are also available in a version that additionally contains sulphur (under the name Benoxyl 5 with Sulphur). There is also a stronger version of the standard (produced under the trade name Benoxyl 10) that appears as a lotion, and a corresponding cream that includes sulphur (produced under the name Benoxyl 10 with Sulphur).

▲/✚ side-effects/warning: *see* BENZOYL PEROXIDE

bentonite is an absorbent powder administered therapeutically in emergencies to absorb corrosive substances like paraquat (the toxic horticultural preparation) in cases of accidental poisoning, and to reduce further absorption by the body. The entire alimentary canâl has then to be evacuated, bathed, cleaned and soothed.

Benylin Decongestant (*Warner-Lambert*) is a proprietary nonprescription DECONGESTANT that is not available from the National Health Service. Produced in the form of a syrup for dilution (the potency of the syrup once dilute is retained for 14 days), it contains the ANTIHISTAMINE diphenhydramine hydrochloride, the SYMPATHOMIMETIC pseudoephedrine hydrochloride, and sodium citrate. It is not recommended for children aged under 12 months.

▲/✚ side-effects/warning: *see* DIPHENHYDRAMINE HYDROCHLORIDE; PSEUDOEPHEDRINE; SODIUM CITRATE.

Benylin Expectorant (*Warner-Lambert*) is a proprietary nonprescription EXPECTORANT that is not available from the National Health Service. Intended to promote the coughing up of bronchial secretions that might otherwise clog the air passages, it contains the expectorant ammonium chloride, the ANTIHISTAMINE diphenhydramine hydrochloride, sodium citrate and menthol. It is produced in the form of a syrup for dilution (the potency of the syrup once dilute is retained for 14 days), and is not recommended for children aged under 12 months. A version without ammonium chloride is also available (under the name Benylin Paediatric); and there is also a version that additionally includes the ANALGESIC codeine phosphate (under the name Benylin with Codeine).

▲/✚ side-effects/warning: *see* CODEINE PHOSPHATE; DIPHENHYDRAMINE HYDROCHLORIDE; SODIUM CITRATE.

B

Benzagel (*Bioglan*) is a proprietary preparation of the KERATOLYTIC drug benzoyl peroxide, which when applied topically in the form of a gel removes hardened or dead skin while simultaneously treating bacterial infection. It is most used in the treatment of acne, and is produced in two strengths (under the names Benzagel 5 and Benzagel 10, the figures representing the percentage of benzyl peroxide).
▲/✚ side-effects/warning: *see* BENZOYL PEROXIDE.

benzalkonium chloride is an astringent ANTISEPTIC that also has some KERATOLYTIC properties and may be used in topical application to remove hard, dead skin from around wounds or ulcers, or to dissolve warts. It is also used on minor abrasions and burns, and (in the form of lozenges to be sucked) on mouth ulcers or gum disease, simply as a disinfectant. For other than oral purposes, administration is topical in the form of a cream or, combined with bromine, as a paint.
✚warning: in topical application, keep benzalkonium chloride off normal skin.
Related articles: CALLUSOLVE; DRAPOLENE; EMULSIDERM.

benzathine penicillin is a penicillin-type ANTIBIOTIC that is used to treat many bacterial infections. Administration is oral in the form of a suspension or drops, or by injection.
▲ side-effects: there may be sensitivity reactions ranging from a minor rash to urticaria and joint pains, and (occasionally) to high temperature or anaphylactic shock.
✚warning: benzathine penicillin should not be administered to patients who are known to be allergic to penicillins; it should be administered with caution to those with impaired kidney function.
Related article: PENIDURAL.

benzocaine is a mild local ANAESTHETIC used in topical application for the relief of pain in the skin surface or mucous membranes, particularly in or around the mouth and throat, or (in combination with other drugs) in the ears. Administration is in various forms: as lozenges, as a cream, as anal suppositories, as an ointment, and as ear-drops.
✚warning: prolonged use should be avoided, some patients experience sensitivity reactions.
Related articles: AUDICORT; DEQUACAINE; MEDILAVE.

benzodiazepines are a large group of drugs that have a marked effect upon the central nervous system. That effect varies with different members of the group, however, and some are used primarily as SEDATIVES or HYPNOTICS, whereas others are used more as ANXIOLYTICS, MUSCLE RELAXANTS or ANTICONVULSANTS. Those that are used as hypnotics have virtually replaced the barbiturates, for the benzodiazepines are just as effective but are much safer − although some caution is necessary in treating patients who suffer from respiratory depression. However, it is now realized that dependence may result from continued usage. Best known and most used benzodiazepines include diazepam (used particularly to control the convulsions of epilepsy or drug poisoning), nitrazepam (a widely used

B

hypnotic), lorazepam (an anxiolytic) and loprazolam (a tranquillizer used to treat insomnia).

▲/✚ side-effects/warning: *see* CLONAZEPAM; DIAZEPAM; LORAZEPAM; NITRAZEPAM.

benzoic acid ointment is a non-proprietary compound ANTIFUNGAL formulation (known also as Whitfield's ointment) used most commonly to treat patches of the fungal infection ringworm. It contains the ANTIFUNGAL substances benzoic acid and SALICYLIC ACID in an emulsifying ointment base.

benzoyl peroxide is a KERATOLYTIC agent used in combination with other drugs or with sulphur in the treatment of skin conditions such as acne, or skin infections such as athlete's foot (which is a fungal infection). Administration is topical in the form of a cream, lotion or gel.

▲ side-effects: some patients experience skin irritation.

✚ warning: benzoyl peroxide should not be used to treat the skin disease of the facial blood vessels, rosacea. Topical application must avoid the eyes, mouth, and mucous membranes. (The drug may bleach fabrics.)

Related articles: ACETOXYL; ACNEGEL; ACNIDAZIL; BENOXYL; BENZAGEL; PANOXYL 2.5; QUINODERM; QUINOPED; THERADERM.

benzyl benzoate is a transparent liquid with an aromatic smell, used to treat infestation of the skin of the trunk and limbs by itch-mites (scabies) or by lice (pediculosis). A skin irritant, it is not suitable for use on the head, face and neck, and treatment of children should be in diluted form (or by another preparation altogether). Administration is in the form of a from-the-neck-down application two days consecutively, without washing in the interval.

▲ side-effects: there is usually skin irritation; there may also be a temporary burning sensation and it may cause a rash.

✚ warning: keep away from the eyes and avoid taking in by mouth.

Related article: ASCABIOL.

benzylpenicillin is the chemical name for the first of the penicillins to be discovered. It remains an important ANTIBIOTIC, widely used to counter bacterial infections, and especially the more serious systemic forms. Because it is inactivated by digestive acids in the stomach, poorly absorbed in the intestine, and rapidly excreted by the kidneys, it is difficult to maintain an effective concentration, so benzylpenicillin is most commonly administered by injection.

▲ side-effects: there may be sensitivity reactions ranging from a minor rash to urticaria and joint pains, and (occasionally) to high temperature or anaphylactic shock. Excessive dosage may cause convulsions.

✚ warning: benzylpenicillin should not be administered to patients known to be allergic to penicillins; it should be administered with caution to those with impaired kidney function.

Related article: CRYSTAPEN

bephenium is an ANTHELMINTIC drug used specifically to treat infestation of the small intestine by hookworms, which draw blood from the point of their attachment to the intestinal wall and may thus cause iron-deficiency anaemia. Administration is oral in the form of a solution.
▲ side-effects: there may be occasional nausea and vomiting; some patients experience diarrhoea, headache and vertigo.
Related article: ALCOPAR.

Berkmycen (*Berk*) is a proprietary ANTIBIOTIC, available only on prescription, used to treat infections of the soft tissues and respiratory tract. Produced in the form of tablets, Berkmycen is a preparation of the TETRACYCLINE oxytetracycline dihydrate. It is not recommended for children aged under 12 years.
▲/✚ side-effects/warning: *see* OXYTETRACYCLINE.

Berotec (*Boehringer Ingelheim*) is a proprietary BRONCHODILATOR, available only on prescription, used to treat asthma. Produced in the form of an aerosol inhalant (with metered inhalation) and a solution for nebulization, Berotec is a preparation of fenoterol hydrobromide.
▲/✚ side-effects/warning: *see* FENOTEROL.

*beta-blockers (or beta-adrenoceptor blockers) are drugs that inhibit the action of the hormonal and neurotransmitter substances ADRENALINE and noradrenaline (catecholamines) in the body. These catecholamines are involved in bodily response to stress: among other actions they speed the heart, constrict some blood vessels (so increasing blood pressure), suppress digestion and generally prepare the body for emergency action. In patients with heart conditions, with diseases of the blood vessels or with high blood pressure (hypertension), stresses that release catecholamines may quickly lead to angina pectoris (heart pain) and an inability of the heart to pump blood sufficiently. Beta-blockers are administered so that some receptor sites that would normally react to the presence of the catecholamines remain comparatively inactivated. Beta-blockers are thus used in the treatment of cardiac arrhythmias (heartbeat irregularities) and as ANTIHYPERTENSIVES. However, some of them have additional effects on catecholamine-sensitive receptor sites elsewhere in the body, particularly in the bronchial passages, and care must thus be taken in prescribing for patients with disorders of the respiratory tract, because their use may induce asthma attacks. These drugs are also used to treat the symptoms of over-active thyroid glands (hyperthyroidism). Best known and most used beta-blockers include propranolol and acebutolol.
▲/✚ side-effects/warning: *see* ACEBUTOLOL; LABETALOL HYDROCHLORIDE; PROPRANOLOL.

Betadine (*Napp*) is a proprietary non-prescription group of preparations of the ANTISEPTIC povidone-iodine. A dilute solution may be used as a mouthwash and gargle for inflammations in the mouth and throat. For the treatment of skin infections it is produced in solutions of differing concentrations as an aerosol spray, an antiseptic

B

B

paint, an alcoholic lotion, a scalp and skin cleanser, a shampoo, a skin cleanser solution, and a surgical scrub; it is also produced as a dry powder for insufflation. In the form of a water-miscible ointment it is used to dress leg ulcers.

▲/✚ side-effects/warning: *see* POVIDONE-IODINE.

betamethasone is a powerful synthetic CORTICOSTEROID, used for its ANTI-INFLAMMATORY effect to treat many kinds of inflammation, and especially those caused by allergic disorders. Unlike most corticosteroids, it does not cause salt or fluid retention in the body, and is thus particularly useful in treating conditions such as cerebral oedema (fluid retention in the brain). Administration is oral in the form of tablets, or by injection.

▲ side-effects: systemic treatment of susceptible patients may engender a euphoria − or a state of confusion or depression. Rarely, it causes peptic ulceration.

✚ warning: betamethasone should be administered with great caution to patients with infectious diseases, chronic renal failure, and uraemia. In children, prolonged administration of betamethasone may lead to stunting of growth. As with all corticosteroids, betamethasone treats only inflammatory symptoms; an undetected and potentially serious infection may have its effects masked by the drug until it is well established.
Related articles: BETNELAN; BETNESOL.

betamethasone dipropionate is a synthetic CORTICOSTEROID used in topical application to treat severe non-infective skin inflammations (such as eczema), particularly in cases where less powerful steroids have failed. Administration is in the form of a cream or ointment, or as a lotion for the scalp.

▲ side-effects: as with all corticosteroids, betamethasone dipropionate treats only the external symptoms; an undetected and potentially serious infection may have its effects masked by the drug until it has become well established. There may be local thinning of the skin, with increased hair growth. Younger patients, especially girls, may experience a local outbreak of acne.

✚ warning: betamethasone dipropionate is a powerful topical steroid and can be absorbed through the skin. Therefore its use as an ointment is not common with children.
Related articles: DIPROSALIC; DIPROSONE.

betamethasone sodium phosphate is a synthetic CORTICOSTEROID used in topical application to treat mild, local forms of inflammation (particularly of the eyes, ears or nose), and occasionally to assist in the treatment of more severe non-infective skin inflammations, such as eczema. Administration is in the form of drops (for eye, ear or nose) and as an ointment.

▲ side-effects: as with all corticosteroids, betamethasone sodium phosphate treats only the external symptoms; an undetected and potentially serious infection may have its effects masked by the drug until it has become well established. There may be local thinning of the skin, with increased hair growth. Younger patients,

especially girls, may experience a local outbreak of acne.
➕ warning: betamethasone sodium phosphate is a powerful topical steroid and can be absorbed through the skin. Therefore its use is not common in children.
Related articles: BETNESOL; VISTA-METHASONE.

betamethasone valerate is a synthetic CORTICOSTEROID used in topical application to treat severe non-infective skin inflammations such as eczema, particularly in cases where less powerful steroids have failed. Administration is in the form of a cream or ointment, or as a lotion.
▲ side-effects: as with all corticosteroids, betamethasone valerate treats only the external symptoms; an undetected and potentially serious infection may have its effects masked by the drug until it has become well established. There may be local thinning of the skin, with increased hair growth. Younger patients, especially girls, may experience a local outbreak of acne.
➕ warning: betamethasone valerate is a powerful topical steroid and can be absorbed through the skin. Therefore its use is not common with children.
Related articles: BETNOVATE; BETNOVATE-C; BETNOVATE-N; BETNOVATE-RD; BEXTASOL; FUCIBET.

*beta-receptor stimulants (or beta-adrenoceptor stimulants; or beta-agonists) are a class of drugs that act at sites, called beta-receptors, that "recognise" the natural neurotransmitters or hormones of the sympathetic nervous system. Drugs that act at such sites are regarded as SYMPATHOMIMETICS. Notable actions of beta-receptor stimulants include bronchodilation, speeding and strengthening of the heart beat and inhibition of contraction of the uterus. Importantly, differences in receptors at different sites allow, for example, beta-receptor stimulant drugs that give bronchodilation in asthma sufferers without overstimulation of the heart (in this case known as selective beta$_2$-receptor stimulants). The BETA-BLOCKERS have roughly the reverse of the actions of beta-receptor stimulants.
▲/➕ side-effects/warning: *see* ADRENALINE; FENOTEROL; ISOPRENALINE; PIRBUTEROL; REPROTEROL HYDROCHLORIDE; RIMITEROL; SALBUTAMOL; TERBUTALINE.

Betnelan (*Glaxo*) is a proprietary CORTICOSTEROID preparation, available only on prescription, used to treat inflammation, especially in rheumatic or allergic conditions, and particularly in severe asthma. Produced in the form of tablets, Betnelan is a preparation of the glucocorticoid, betamethasone. It is not recommended for babies and is rarely used in childhood.
▲/➕ side-effects/warning: *see* BETAMETHASONE.

Betnesol (*Glaxo*) is a proprietary CORTICOSTEROID preparation, available only on prescription, used to treat local inflammations as well as more widespread rheumatic or allergic conditions, particularly severe asthma. Produced in the form of tablets and in ampules for injection, Betnesol is a preparation of the glucocorticoid, betamethasone. The tablets are not recommended for children aged under 12 months.

B

Betnesol ear-, eye- and nose-drops and eye ointment are used for local inflammations, and are an alternative preparation of betamethasone sodium phosphate. A preparation is also available that additionally contains the ANTIBIOTIC neomycin sulphate; it too is produced in the form of ear-, eye- and nose-drops and eye ointment (under the trade name Betnesol-N).

▲/✚ side-effects/warning: *see* BETAMETHASONE; BETAMETHASONE SODIUM PHOSPHATE; NEOMYCIN.

Betnovate (*Glaxo*) is a proprietary group of CORTICOSTEROID preparations, available only on prescription, used to treat severe non-infective skin inflammations such as eczema, especially in patients who are not responding to less powerful corticosteroids. Produced in the form of a water-miscible cream, an ointment in an anhydrous paraffin base, a lotion, and a scalp application in an alcohol base, Betnovate is a preparation of betamethasone valerate.

▲/✚ side-effects/warning: *see* BETAMETHASONE VALERATE; LIGNOCAINE; PHENYLEPHRINE.

Betnovate-C (*Glaxo*) is a proprietary CORTICOSTEROID, available only on prescription, used to treat severe on-infective skin inflammations such as eczema. Produced in the form of a water-miscible cream and an ointment in a paraffin base, Betnovate-C is a compound preparation of the steroid betamethasone valerate and the ANTIMICROBIAL clioquinol.

▲/✚ side-effects/warning: *see* BETAMETHASONE VALERATE; CLIOQUINOL.

Betnovate-N (*Glaxo*) is a proprietary CORTICOSTEROID, available only on prescription, used to treat severe non-infective skin inflammations such as eczema. Produced in the form of a water-miscible cream, an ointment in a paraffin-base, and as a lotion, Betnovate-N is a compound preparation of the steroid betamethasone valerate and the ANTIBIOTIC neomycin sulphate.

▲/✚ side-effects/warning: *see* BETAMETHASONE VALERATE; NEOMYCIN.

Betnovate-RD (*Glaxo*) is a proprietary CORTICOSTEROID, available only on prescription, used as the basis for maintenance therapy in the treatment of severe non-infective skin inflammation (such as eczema) once control has initially been achieved with BETNOVATE. Produced in the form of a water-miscible cream and as an ointment in an anhydrous paraffin base, Betnovate-RD is a preparation of betamethasone valerate.

▲✚ side-effects/warning: *see* BETAMETHASONE VALERATE.

Bextasol (*Glaxo*) is a proprietary CORTICOSTEROID, available only on prescription, used to prevent asthma. Produced in an aerosol that emits individually metered doses, Bextasol is a preparation of the CORTICOSTEROID betamethasone valerate.

▲/✚ side-effects/warning: *see* BETAMETHASONE VALERATE.

Bi-Aglut (*Ultrapharm*) is a brand of non-prescription gluten-free biscuits. Gluten-, lactose-, and milk-protein-free cracker toast is also available for the dietary needs of patients who are unable to tolerate those substances, such as in coeliac disease.

B

Biophylline (*Delandale*) is a proprietary non-prescription BRONCHODILATOR, used to treat restrictions in the bronchial passages, as occur in asthma. Produced in the form of a sugar-free syrup, Biophylline is a preparation of theophylline hydrate. It is not recommended for children aged under two years.
▲/✚ side-effects/warning: *see* THEOPHYLLINE.

Bioral (*Winthrop*) is a proprietary non-prescription preparation, used to treat mouth ulcers and other sores in and around the mouth. Produced in the form of a gel, Bioral is a preparation of the drug carbenoxolone sodium.

bisacodyl is a stimulant LAXATIVE used not only to promote defecation and relieve constipation, but also to evacuate the colon prior to rectal examination or surgery. It probably works by stimulating the walls of the intestine. Administration is either oral in the form of tablets (full effects are achieved after ten hours), or topical as anal suppositories (effects achieved within one hour).
▲ side-effects: there may be abdominal pain, nausea, or vomiting. Suppositories sometimes cause rectal irritation.
✚ warning: bisacodyl should not be administered to patients with intestinal obstruction.

BJ6 (*Macarthys; Thornton & Ross*) is a proprietary non-prescription ophthalmic preparation, used to treat sore eyes caused by chronically reduced tear secretion. Produced in the form of eye-drops, BJ6 is a preparation of the water-soluble cellulose derivative hypromellose.

bleomycin is an ANTIBIOTIC that also has CYTOTOXIC properties. Unlike most ANTICANCER drugs, however, it has virtually no depressant effect on the blood-producing capacity of the bone-marrow. Sensitivity reactions are not uncommon, the symptoms of which are chills and fever a few hours after administration; these can be dealt with by the simultaneous administration of a CORTICOSTEROID (such as hydrocortisone). Bleomycin is administered by injection. The proprietary preparation of the same name is produced by Lundbeck and is available only on prescription.
▲ side-effects: there is generally nausea and vomiting (for which additional medications may be prescribed). Increased pigmentation of the skin and some hair loss is common. Some patients experience inflammation of the mucous membranes.
✚ warning: high dosage increases a risk of pulmonary fibrosis, a lung disease that is potentially very serious. Regular monitoring of lung function is essential.

Bocasan (*Cooper*) is a proprietary non-prescription ANTISEPTIC, used to cleanse and disinfect the mouth. Produced in the form of sealed sachets to be emptied into water to produce a mouth-wash, Bocasin is a preparation of sodium perborate.

B

Bonjela (*Reckitt & Colman*) is a proprietary non-prescription oral gel, used to treat mouth ulcers and to relieve pain during teething. Bonjela is a preparation of the mild ANALGESIC and local ANAESTHETIC, choline salicylate (and is sugar-free).

botulism antitoxin is a preparation that neutralizes the toxins produced by the botulism bacteria (rather than acting to counter the presence of the bacteria, as would a vaccine). In this way, it may be administered not only to people at risk from the disease following exposure to an infected patient, but also to the infected patient as a means of treatment. However, there are some strains of botulism in relation to which the antitoxin is not effective. Moreover, hypersensitivity reactions are common (and it is essential that an administering doctor has all relevant details of a patient's medical history, with regard especially to allergies). Administration is by injection or infusion, depending on whether it is for the purpose of prophylaxis or treatment.

Bradosol (*Ciba*) is a proprietary non-prescription DISINFECTANT, used to treat infections in the mouth and throat. Produced in the form of lozenges, Bradosol is a preparation of the detergent antiseptic, domiphen bromide.

Bradosol Plus (*Ciba*) is a proprietary, non-prescription DISINFECTANT used to treat infections in the mouth and throat. Produced in the form of lozenges, Bradosol Plus is a compound preparation of the detergent, domiphen bromide, and the local ANAESTHETIC, ANTISEPTIC, LIGNOCAINE HYDROCHLORIDE.

bran is perhaps the best-known natural bulking agent used to keep people "regular" or, if necessary, as a LAXATIVE to treat constipation. In either case it works by increasing the overall mass of faeces, so stimulating bowel movement (although in fact the full effect may not be achieved for more than 36 hours). As an excellent form of dietary fibre, bran may be said to reduce the risk of diverticular disease while actively assisting digestion.
▲ side-effects: some patients cannot tolerate bran (particularly patients sensitive to the compound gluten).
✚ warning: bran should not be consumed if there is any possibility of intestinal blockage: adequate fluid intake must be maintained to avoid faecal impaction. It should be avoided in children aged under two years.
Related article: PROCTOFIBE.

Brasivol (*Steifel*) is a proprietary non-prescription abrasive preparation, used to cleanse skin that suffers from acne. It is produced in the form of a paste containing particles of aluminium oxide in three grades (fine, medium and coarse) within a soap base. Treatment ordinarily begins with the fine grade and progresses to the medium and the coarse in more severe cases.

Bricanyl (*Astra*) is a proprietary form of the BRONCHODILATOR terbutaline sulphate, available only on prescription, which acts as a

selective BETA-RECEPTOR STIMULANT and SMOOTH MUSCLE RELAXANT and so relieves the bronchial spasms associated with such conditions as asthma and bronchitis. Bricanyl is produced in a variety of forms; as tablets (including sustained release tablets), as a sugar free syrup, in ampoules for injection, as a metered dose aerosol inhaler, as a respirator solution for use with a nebulizer, and as a dry powder inhaler (Turbohaler). The metered dose aerosol inhaler can be given to young children using a nebuhaler, and helps in overcoming problems resulting from poor inhaler technique. A spacer device (a collapsible extended mouthpiece) is also available for this purpose.
▲/✚ side-effects/warning: *see* TERBUTALINE.

Brietal Sodium (*Lilly*) is a proprietary preparation of the short-acting general ANAESTHETIC methohexitone, in the form of methohexitone sodium. It is used mainly for the initial induction of anaesthesia or for short, minor operations. Brietal Sodium is produced in vials for intravenous injection (in three strengths).
▲/✚ side-effects/warning: *see* METHOHEXITONE SODIUM.

Britcin (*DDSA Pharmaceuticals*) is a proprietary ANTIBIOTIC, available only on prescription, used to treat systemic bacterial infections and infections of the upper respiratory tract, of the ear, nose and throat, and of the urogenital tracts. Produced in the form of capsules (in two strengths), Britcin is a preparation of the broad-spectrum PENICILLIN ampicillin.
▲/✚ side-effects/warning: *see* AMPICILLIN.

brompheniramine maleate is an ANTIHISTAMINE, used to treat the symptoms of allergic conditions like hay fever and urticaria; it is also used, in combination with other drugs, in expectorants to loosen a dry cough. Administration is oral in the form of tablets, sustained-release tablets and a dilute elixir.
▲ side-effects: sedation may affect the patient's capacity for speed of thought and movement; there may be nausea, headaches and/or weight gain, dry mouth, gastrointestinal disturbances and visual problems.
Related articles: DIMOTANE; DIMOTANE EXPECTORANT; DIMOTANE PLUS; DIMOTANE WITH CODEINE; DIMOTAPP.

Bronchodil (*Degussa*) is a proprietary BRONCHODILATOR, available only on prescription, used to treat bronchospasm in asthma. Produced in the form of tablets, as a sugar-free elixir for dilution (the potency of the elixir once dilute is retained for 14 days), in a metered-dose aerosol, and as a respirator solution, Bronchodil is a preparation of the SYMPATHOMIMETIC reproterol hydrochloride.
▲/✚ side-effects/warning: *see* REPROTEROL HYDROCHLORIDE.

*bronchodilators are agents that relax the smooth muscle of the bronchial passages, so allowing more air to flow in or out, and treat bronchospasm (as in asthma). The type of drug most commonly used is the SYMPATHOMIMETIC. Best-known and most used sympathomimetic bronchodilators include SALBUTAMOL and TERBUTALINE. Other

B

bronchodilator medications include IPRATROPIUM and the THEOPHYLLINE. Many bronchodilators are available in the form of aerosols, ventilator sprays or nebulizing mists. In high dosage, some can affect the heart rate. There may also be fine muscular tremor, headaches and nervous tension.

Broxil (*Beecham*) is a proprietary ANTIBIOTIC, available only on prescription, used to treat many forms of infection. Produced in the form of capsules, and as a syrup for dilution (the potency of the syrup once dilute is retained for seven days), Broxil is a preparation of the PENICILLIN derivative phenethicillin.
▲/✚ side-effects/warning: *see* PHENETHICILLIN.

Brufen (*Boots*) is a proprietary non-narcotic ANALGESIC that has valuable additional anti-inflammatory properties. Available only on prescription, Brufen is used to relieve pain – particularly the pain of rheumatic disease and other musculo-skeletal disorders – and is produced in the form of tablets (in three strengths) and as a syrup for dilution (the potency of the syrup once dilute is retained for 14 days). It is a preparation of ibuprofen.
▲/✚ side-effects/warning: *see* IBUPROFEN.

budesonide is a CORTICOSTEROID drug used primarily to prevent the symptoms of asthma. It is thought to work by reducing inflammation in the mucous lining of the bronchial passages, and stemming allergic reactions. The drug is also used to treat the symptoms of nasal allergies such as hay fever. In both cases, administration is by inhaler (either from an aerosol or from a nasal spray); a nebuhaler may be useful for young children to overcome problems with inhalation technique.
▲ side-effects: some patients undergoing bronchial treatment experience hoarseness. Large doses may increase the risk of fungal infection, such as oral thrush.
Related articles: PULMICORT; RHINOCORT.

bumetanide is a quick-acting powerful DIURETIC with relatively short duration of action, which works by inhibiting reabsorption of ions in part of the kidney known as the loop of Henle. It is used to treat fluid retention in the tissues (oedema) and high blood pressure (*see* ANTIHYPERTENSIVE), and to assist a diseased kidney by promoting the excretion of urine. Administration is oral in the form of tablets or a sugar-free liquid, or by injection.
▲ side-effects: diuretic effect corresponds to dosage; large doses may cause deafness or ringing in the ears (tinnitus). There may be a skin rash.

bupivacaine hydrochloride is a long-acting local ANAESTHETIC that is related to lignocaine but is more powerful and has greater duration of action. Because of this, it is often administered by injection epidurally via the spinal membranes (particularly during labour).
▲ side-effects: there may be slow heart rate and low blood pressure (hypotension) that may with high dosage tend towards cardiac

B

arrest. Some patients enter states of euphoria, agitation of respiratory depression.

✚warning: bupivacaine hydrochloride should not be administered to patients who suffer from the neural disorder myasthenia gravis or from heart block, or who are suffering from an insufficient supply of blood (as in shock); it should be administered with caution to those with impaired heart or liver function, or epilepsy. Facilities for emergency cardio-respiratory resuscitation should be on hand during treatment.

Related article: MARCAIN.

buprenorphine is a narcotic ANALGESIC that is long-acting and is used to treat moderate to severe levels of pain. Although it is thought not to be seriously addictive, it may be dangerous to use in combination with other narcotic analgesics. Administration is oral in the form of tablets (which should be placed under the tongue), or by injection.

▲side-effects: nausea, vomiting, dizziness, sweating and drowsiness are fairly common. Rarely, there may be shallow breathing.

✚warning: buprenorphine should not be administered to patients who suffer from head injury or intracranial pressure; it should be administered with caution to those with impaired kidney or liver function, asthma, depressed respiration, insufficient secretion of thyroid hormones (hypothyroidism) or low blood pressure (hypotension).

Related article: TEMGESIC.

Burinex (*Leo*) is a proprietary DIURETIC drug, available only on prescription, used to treat the accumulation of fluids in the tissues (oedema) associated with congestive heart failure, and to assist a diseased kidney by promoting the excretion of urine. Produced in the form of tablets (in two strengths), as a sugar-free liquid, and in ampoules for injection, Burinex is a preparation of bumetanide. A compound preparation of bumetanide together with the potassium supplement POTASSIUM CHLORIDE is also available (under the name Burinex K).

▲/✚ side-effects/warning: *see* BUMETANIDE.

Buscopan (*Boehringer Ingelheim*) is a proprietary ANTICHOLINERGIC antispasmodic drug, available only on prescription, used to treat overactivity or spasm of the smooth muscle of the stomach or intestinal walls (causing colic pain) or of the muscles of the vagina (causing painful menstruation). Produced in the form of tablets (not recommended for children aged under six years) and in ampoules for injection (not recommended for children), Buscopan is a preparation of the SMOOTH MUSCLE RELAXANT hyoscine butylbromide.

▲/✚ side-effects/warning: *see* HYOSCINE.

Butacote (*Geigy*) is a proprietary ANTI-INFLAMMATORY non-narcotic ANALGESIC, available only on prescription (and now generally used only in hospitals), used to treat rheumatic disease of the type that causes bone fusion or deformity, especially in the backbone. Produced in the form of tablets (in two strengths), Butacote is a preparation of phenylbutazone.

▲/✚ side-effects/warning: *see* PHENYLBUTAZONE.

B

Butazolidin (*Geigy*) is a proprietary ANTI-INFLAMMATORY non-narcotic ANALGESIC, available only on prescription (and now generally used only in hospitals), used to treat rheumatic disease of the type that causes bone fusion or deformity, especially the backbone. Produced in the form of tablets (in two strengths), Butazolidin is a preparation of phenylbutzone.
▲/✚ side-effects/warning: *see* PHENYLBUTAZONE.

Butazone (*DDSA Pharmaceuticals*) is a proprietary ANTI-INFLAMMATORY non-narcotic ANALGESIC drug, available only on prescription in hospitals, used to treat rheumatic disease involving especially the backbone. Produced in the form of tablets (in two strengths), Butazone is a preparation of phenylbutazone.
▲/✚ side-effects/warning: *see* PHENYLBUTAZONE.

C

Cafadol (*Typharm*) is a proprietary non-prescription compound ANALGESIC that is not available from the National Health Service. Used for mild pain, it is produced in the form of tablets. Cafadol is a compound of paracetamol and caffeine.
▲/✚ side-effects/warning: *see* CAFFEINE; PARACETAMOL.

Cafergot (*Sandoz*) is a proprietary ANALGESIC, available only on prescription, used to treat migraine. Produced in the form of tablets and suppositories, Cafergot is a compound of caffeine and ergotamine tartrate.
▲/✚ side-effects/warning: *see* CAFFEINE; ERGOTAMINE TARTRATE.

caffeine is a weak STIMULANT. Present in both tea and coffee, it is included in many ANALGESIC preparations, often to increase absorption.

Calaband (*Seton*) is a proprietary non-prescription form of bandaging impregnated with ZINC OXIDE, CALAMINE, glycerol and other soothing substances. (Further bandaging is required to hold it in place.)

Caladryl (*Warner-Lambert*) is a proprietary non-prescription ANTIHISTAMINE, used to treat skin irritations, stings and bites, and sunburn. Produced in the form of a cream or lotion, Caladryl contains CALAMINE, diphenhydramine hydrochloride and camphor in solution.
▲/✚ side-effects/warning: *see* DIPHENHYDRAMINE HYDROCHLORIDE.

calamine is a preparation that cools and soothes itching skin. Produced in the form of a lotion, cream or ointment, it is a suspension of mainly zinc carbonate.

calamine and coal tar ointment is a preparation combining the soothing effects of CALAMINE (zinc carbonate) and the ANTISEPTIC properties of COAL TAR, which also relieves itching and softens hard skin.

calciferol is the chemical name for the fat-soluble VITAMIN D. It occurs in four main forms (D_1 to D_4) which are formed in plants or in human skin by the action of sunlight. Vitamin D promotes the absorption of calcium and, to a lesser extent, phosphorus into the bones; a deficiency of vitamin D therefore results in bone deficiency disorders, such as rickets in children. Good food sources in normal diets include eggs, milk and cheese; fish liver oil is particularly rich as a dietary supplement. However, as with most other vitamins, large doses are toxic.

calcitonin is a hormone produced and secreted by the thyroid gland at the base of the neck. Its function is to lower the levels of calcium and phosphate in the blood, and so, together with the correspondingly opposite action of a parathyroid hormone, to regulate the levels of these minerals.

calcium is a metallic element essential in compound form for the normal growth and development of the body, and especially (in the

C

form of calcium phosphate) of the bones and the teeth. It is also a
constituent of blood, its level regulated by the opposing actions of the
hormones CALCITONIN and parathyroid hormone (parathormone). Its
uptake from food ingested involves CALCIFEROL (vitamin D). Good food
sources are all dairy products.

✚ warning: deficiency of vitamin D leads to calcium deficiency, and
corresponding bone, blood and nerve disorders. Excess calcium in
the body may cause the formation of stones (calculi, generally
composed of calcium oxalate), particularly in the kidney or gall
bladder.
see CALCIUM GLUCONATE; CALCIUM LACTATE.

calcium gluconate is one of several common forms in which CALCIUM
is administered as a supplement to patients who suffer from calcium
deficiency (through dietary insufficiency or disease) or who
temporarily need more, with or without the simultaneous
administration of CALCIFEROL (vitamin D). Administration is oral in the
form of tablets (which may be chewed) or (in solution) by injection or
infusion.

▲ side-effects: following treatment by injection or infusion there may
be a slowing of the heart rate together with heartbeat irregularity.
There may be irritation at the site of injection.

✚ warning: calcium gluconate should be administered with caution to
patients who suffer from heart disease.
Related article: SANDOCAL.

calcium lactate is one of several common forms in which CALCIUM is
administered as a supplement to patients who suffer from calcium
deficiency (through dietary insufficiency or disease) or who
temporarily need more, with or without the simultaneous
administration of CALCIFEROL (vitamin D). Administration is oral in the
form of tablets (which may be chewed) or (in solution) by injection or
infusion.

▲ side-effects: following treatment by injection or infusion there
may be a slowing of the heart rate together with heartbeat
irregularity. There may be irritation at the site of
injection.

✚ warning: calcium lactate should be administered with caution to
patients who suffer from heart disease.
Related article: SANDOCAL.

Calcium Resonium (*Winthrop*) is a proprietary non-prescription
preparation used to treat high blood POTASSIUM levels, particularly
in patients who suffer from impaired kidney function or kidney
failure. It is produced in the form of a powdered resin, as a
calcium polystyrene salt.

Calcium-Sandoz (*Sandoz*) is a proprietary CALCIUM supplement, used
to treat patients with the neuro-muscular symptoms of calcium
deficiency. Produced in the form of a syrup (non-prescription) and in
ampoules for injection (available only on prescription), Calcium-
Sandoz contains several calcium salts.

Callusolve (*Dermal*) is a proprietary non-prescription preparation, used to treat warts and remove hard, dead skin. Produced in the form of a solute paint, Callusolve is a preparation of the keratolytic, benzalkonium chloride (as a bromine adduct). It should not come into contact with normal skin.
➕ warning: see BENZALKONIUM CHLORIDE.

Calpol (*Calmic*) is a proprietary form of the non-narcotic ANALGESIC paracetamol. It is produced in the form of a suspension in two strengths: the weaker (non-prescription) is produced under the name Calpol Infant; the stronger (not available from the National Health Service) under the name Calpol Six Plus.
▲/➕ side-effects/warning: see PARACETAMOL.

Calpol Sugar Free (*Calmic*) is a proprietary form of the non-narcotic ANALGESIC paracetamol. It is produced in the form of a suspension which contains no sugar.
▲/➕ side-effects/warning: see PARACETAMOL.

Calthor (*Ayerst*) is a proprietary penicillin-type ANTIBIOTIC, available only on prescription, used to treat bronchitis and infections in the skin and urinary tract. Produced in the form of tablets (in two strengths) and as a syrup for dilution, Calthor is a preparation of ciclacillin. Calthor is not recommended for children aged under two months.
▲/➕ side-effects/warning: see CICLACILLIN.

CAM (*Rybar*) is a proprietary non-prescription SYMPATHOMIMETIC, a BRONCHODILATOR used to treat patients suffering from asthma and other conditions involving bronchial spasm. Produced in the form of a syrup, CAM's active constituent is ephedrine hydrochloride. CAM is not recommended for children aged under 18 months, and is now generally little used.
▲/➕ side-effects/warning: see EPHEDRINE HYDROCHLORIDE.

Canesten (*Bayer*) is a proprietary non-prescription ANTIFUNGAL preparation, used to treat infections and particularly ones that cause inflammation. Treatment is topical, as a solution, as a spray, as a cream and as a dusting-powder. Canesten is a preparation of clotrimazole.
▲/➕ side-effects/warning: see CLOTRIMAZOLE.

Canesten-HC (*Bayer*) is a proprietary ANTIFUNGAL steroid preparation, available only on prescription, used to treat fungal infections, particularly those that cause inflammation. Produced in the form of a cream for topical application, Canesten-HC consists of a combination of clotrimazole and hydrocortisone.
▲/➕ side-effects/warning: see CLOTRIMAZOLE; HYDROCORTISONE.

Capastat (*Dista*) is a proprietary ANTITUBERCULAR drug, used to treat tuberculosis resistant to other drugs. Produced in the form of powder for reconstitution as intramuscular injections, Capastat is a

C

preparation of the ANTIBIOTIC capreomycin sulphate. It is not normally used in children.

▲/✚ side-effects/warning: *see* CAPREOMYCIN.

Capitol (*Dermal*) is a proprietary non-prescription ANTIBACTERIAL preparation, used to treat dandruff and other scalp conditions. Produced in the form of a gel applied as a shampoo, Capitol is a preparation of the antiseptic BENZALKONIUM CHLORIDE.

Capoten (*Squibb*) is a proprietary ANTIHYPERTENSIVE drug, available only on prescription, used accordingly to treat high blood pressure (hypertension). It is occasionally used to treat resistant heart failure when diuretics alone have failed. Capoten is a preparation of the drug captopril.

▲/✚ side-effects/warning: *see* CAPTOPRIL.

capreomycin is an ANTIBIOTIC drug used specifically in the treatment of tuberculosis that proves to be resistant to the drugs ordinarily used first, or in cases where those drugs are not tolerated. Administration is by intra-muscular injection. It is not normally used in children.

▲ side-effects: there may be kidney toxicity and impaired hearing with or without ringing in the ears (tinnitus) or vertigo; sometimes there are sensitivity reactions such as rashes or urticaria.

✚ warning: capreomycin should not be administered to patients who are pregnant, and should be administered with caution to those who have impaired function of the liver, kidney or sense of hearing (functions that should be monitored during treatment), or who are already taking other powerful antibiotics, or who are lactating.

Related article: CAPASTAT.

captopril is a powerful vasodilator used in the treatment of high blood pressure (hypertension). It may also be used to treat heart failure, although a supplementary DIURETIC is then commonly administered. Captopril works by inhibiting enzymes involved in producing vasoactive hormones in the blood thus dilating the smaller arteries. Administration of captopril is oral in the form of tablets.

▲ side-effects: there may be marked low blood pressure (hypotension); thereafter there may be a loss of the sense of taste and a dry cough; sometimes there is abdominal pain and/or a rash. In patients with impaired kidney function (or who are given a high dosage) there may be changes in the composition of the blood, and protein in the urine.

✚ warning: the first dose may cause very rapid reduction in blood pressure, especially if a diuretic is given simultaneously; dosage thereafter may be adjusted for optimum effect. Monitoring of kidney function, white blood cell count and urinary contents during treatment is essential.

Related article: CAPOTEN.

carbamazepine is an ANTICONVULSANT drug used to treat major convulsions. It may cause drowsiness when first taken, but this soon wears off.

C

▲ side-effects: there may be blurring of vision and unsteadiness; high dosage may cause severe dizziness.
Sometimes there are gastrointestinal disturbances; occasionally there is a rash.
✚ warning: dosage should begin at a minimum level and be adjusted upwards for optimum effect. Blood monitoring is essential if high doses are administered.
Related article: TEGRETOL.

carbaryl is an insecticide used in the treatment of scalp or pubic lice. Administration is (in aqueous or alcohol solution) in the form of a lotion, or shampoo which is applied to wet hair, allowed to dry, and then rinsed after a specified time (usually about 12 hours). The procedure may need to be repeated after a week.
✚ warning: keep away from the eyes.
Related articles: CARYLDERM; CLINICIDE; DERBAC-C; SULEO-C.

carbenicillin is a penicillin-like ANTIBIOTIC used to treat bacterial infections, particularly of the urinary tract. Administration is by injection or infusion in the case of systemic infections, or by intramuscular injections for urinary tract infections.
▲ side-effects: there may be sensitivity reactions – serious ones in hypersensitive patients. Body temperature may rise, and there may be pains in the joints and skin rashes or urticaria; potassium and platelet levels in the blood may decline.
✚ warning: carbenicillin should not be administered to patients known to be sensitive to penicillins, and should be administered with caution to those who suffer from impaired kidney function.
Related article: PYOPEN.

carbimazole prevents the production or secretion of the hormone thyroxine by the thyroid gland, so treating an excess in the blood of thyroid HORMONES and the symptoms that it causes (thyrotoxicosis). Treatment may be on a maintenance basis over a long period (dosage adjusted to optimum effect), or may be merely preliminary to surgical removal of the thyroid gland. Administration is oral in the form of tablets.
▲ side-effects: an itching rash is common, but may indicate a need for alternative treatment. There may also be nausea and headache; occasionally there is jaundice or hair loss (alopecia). Also on rare occasions carbimazole can be associated with a marked lowering of the white cell count in the blood. This can predispose the patient to infection, but the effect disappears on stopping treatment.
Related article: NEO-MERCAZOLE.

Carbo-Cort (*Lagap*) is a proprietary ANTISEPTIC and CORTICOSTEROID preparation available only on prescription, used to treat serious non-infective skin diseases such as psoriasis and eczema. Produced in the form of a water-miscible cream, Carbo-Cort contains the powerful steroid hydrocortisone together with COAL TAR. In this formulation it is suitable for the face, unlike many other formulations of coal tar.
▲/✚ side-effects/warning: *see* HYDROCORTISONE.

C

Carbo-Dome (*Lagap*) is a proprietary non-prescription ANTISEPTIC used to treat non-infective skin conditions like psoriasis. Produced in the form of a water-miscible cream, Carbo-Dome's active constituent is COAL TAR.

Carbomix (*Penn*) is a proprietary non-prescription adsorbent preparation, used to treat patients suffering from poisoning or a drug overdose. Produced in the form of granulated powder to be mixed with water, Carbomix's active constituent is CHARCOAL.

carboplatin is a CYTOTOXIC drug derived from the ANTICANCER drug cisplatin. Side-effects of nausea and vomiting are less than those caused by cisplatin. Administration is by injection.
▲ side-effects: there may be nausea and vomiting, progressive deafness and symptoms of kidney dysfunction. The blood-forming capacity of the bone-marrow may be suppressed (and treatment should not be repeated within four weeks).
✚ warning: an anti-emetic may be administered simultaneously to lessen the risk of nausea and vomiting. Monitoring of kidney function and of hearing is advisable.
Related article: PARAPLATIN.

cardiac glycosides are a class of drugs that have a pronounced effect on the heart, increasing the force of contraction of cardiac muscle. They therefore have an important use in the treatment of congestive heart failure. they also have an important role in slowing the heart rate to prevent arrhythmia. Examples include ouabain and DIGOXIN.

carfecillin sodium is a penicillin-like ANTIBIOTIC used to treat bacillary infections, particularly of the urinary tract. Administration is oral in the form of tablets.
▲ side-effects: there may be sensitivity reactions – serious ones in hypersensitive patients. Body temperature may rise, and there may be pains in the joints and skin rashes or urticaria.
✚ warning: carfecillin sodium should not be administered to patients known to be sensitive to penicillin, and should be administered with caution to those with impaired kidney function.
Related article: UTICILLIN.

carmellose sodium is a substance used as the basis for a paste and a powder that is spread or sprinkled over lesions in or around the mouth in order to protect them while they heal. Both paste and powder also contain soft animal and vegetable proteins.
Related articles: ORABASE; ORAHESIVE.

Carobel, Instant (*Cow & Gate*) is a proprietary non-prescription powder, used to thicken liquid and semi-liquid diets in the treatment of vomiting, especially in infants. Carobel is a preparation of carob seed flour.

Carylderm (*Napp*) is a proprietary non-prescription drug used to treat infestations of the scalp and pubic hair by lice. Produced in the form

of a lotion and a shampoo, Carylderm is a preparation of the PEDICULICIDE carbaryl.
+ warning: see CARBARYL.

cascara is a slightly old-fashioned but powerful stimulant LAXATIVE which acts by increasing the muscular activity of the intestinal walls. It is now used less commonly, not just because of its cumulatively detrimental side-effects but because it may take up to eight hours to have any relieving effect on constipation. Administration is oral in the form of tablets.
▲ side-effects: the urine may be coloured red. Prolonged use of such a stimulant can eventually fatigue the muscles on which it works, thus causing severe intestinal problems in terms of motility and absorption.

castor oil is a slightly old-fashioned stimulant LAXATIVE which probably acts by increasing the muscular activity of the intestinal walls. It is now used less commonly because of its cumulatively detrimental side-effects, although its use in hospitals and clinics before surgical examinations and procedures is still well attested. Yet it may take up to eight hours to relieve constipation. Administration is oral.
▲ side-effects: there may be nausea and vomiting. Prolonged use of such a stimulant can eventually fatigue the muscles on which it works, thus causing severe intestinal problems in terms of motility and absorption.
+ warning: castor oil should not be taken by any patient who suffers from intestinal obstruction.

cefaclor is a broad-spectrum ANTIBIOTIC, one of the cephalosporins, used to treat a wide range of bacterial infections, particularly of the skin and soft tissues, the urinary tract, the upper respiratory tract, and the middle ear. Administration is oral in the form of capsules or a dilute suspension.
▲ side-effects: there may be sensitivity reactions – some of which may be serious. Sometimes there is nausea and vomiting, with diarrhoea.
+ warning: cefaclor should be administered with caution to patients who might be sensitive to penicillins; it should not be given to patients allergic to cephalosporins. It should be administered with caution to those with impaired kidney function.
Related article: DISTACLOR.

cefadroxil is a broad-spectrum ANTIBIOTIC, one of the cephalosporins, used to treat a wide range of bacterial infections, particularly of the skin and soft tissues, the urinary tract, and the middle ear. Administration is oral in the form of capsules or a dilute suspension.
▲ side-effects: there may be sensitivity reactions – some of which may be serious. Sometimes there is nausea and vomiting, with diarrhoea.
+ warning: cefadroxil should be administered with caution to patients who might be sensitive to penicillins; it should not be given to

C

patients allergic to cephalosporins. It should be administered with caution to those who suffer from impaired kidney function.
Related article: BAXAN.

Cefizox (*Wellcome*) is a proprietary ANTIBIOTIC, available only on prescription, used to treat infections in the upper respiratory tract and urinary tract. Produced in the form of powder for reconstitution as injections, Cefizox is a preparation of ceftizoxime as a salt of sodium. It is not recommended for children aged under three months.
▲/✚ side-effects/warning: *see* CEFTIZOXIME.

cefotaxime is a broad-spectrum ANTIBIOTIC, one of the cephalosporins, used to treat a wide range of bacterial infections, particularly of the skin and soft tissues, the urinary tract, the meninges (meningitis) and the blood (septicaemia). It is also used to prevent infection during surgery. Administration is by intravenous or intramuscular injection.
▲ side-effects: there may be sensitivity reactions − some of which may be serious. Sometimes there is nausea and vomiting, with diarrhoea.
✚ warning: cefotaxime should be administered with caution to patients who might be sensitive to penicillins; it should not be given to patients allergic to cephalosporins. It should be administered with caution to those with impaired kidney function, or who are pregnant or lactating.
Related article: CLAFORAN.

cefoxitin is a broad-spectrum ANTIBIOTIC, one of the cephalosporins, used to treat a wide range of bacterial infections, particularly of the skin and soft tissues, the urinary tract, the upper respiratory tract, the peritoneum (peritonitis) and the blood (septicaemia). Administration is by intravenous or intramuscular injection.
▲ side-effects: there may be sensitivity reactions − some of which may be serious. Sometimes there is nausea and vomiting, with diarrhoea.
✚ warning: cefoxitin should be administered with caution to patients who might be sensitive to penicillins; it should not be given to patients allergic to cephalosporins. It should be administered with caution to those with impaired kidney function.
Related article: MEFOXIN.

cefsulodin is a broad-spectrum ANTIBIOTIC, one of the cephalosporins, used to treat a wide range of bacterial infections, particularly of the skin and soft tissues, the urinary tract, and the upper respiratory tract. Administration is by intravenous or intramuscular injection.
▲ side-effects: there may be sensitivity reactions − some of which may be serious. Sometimes there is nausea and vomiting, with diarrhoea.
✚ warning: cefsulodin should be administered with caution to patients who might be sensitive to penicillins; it should not be given to patients allergic to cephalosporins. It should be administered with caution to those with impaired kidney function, or who are pregnant.
Related article: MONASPOR.

C

ceftazidime is a broad-spectrum ANTIBIOTIC, one of the cephalosporins, used to treat a wide range of bacterial infections, particularly of the skin and soft tissues, the urinary tract, the upper respiratory tract, the ear, nose and throat, the bones and joints, the gastrointestinal tract (stomach and intestines), the meninges (meningitis) and the blood (septicaemia). It is also used to treat infection in patients whose immune systems are defective. Administration is by intravenous or intramuscular injection.

▲ side-effects: there may be sensitivity reactions – some of which may be serious. Alternatively, sometimes there is nausea and vomiting, with diarrhoea.

✚ warning: ceftazidime should be administered with caution to patients who might be sensitive to penicillins; it should not be given to patients allergic to cephalosporins, or to patients who are already taking certain diuretic drugs. It should be administered with caution to those who suffer from impaired kidney function. *Related article:* FORTUM.

ceftizoxime is a broad-spectrum ANTIBIOTIC, one of the cephalosporins, used to treat a wide range of bacterial infections, particularly of the skin and soft tissues, the urinary tract, the genital organs, the lower respiratory tract, and the blood (septicaemia). It is also used to treat infection in patients whose immune systems are defective. Administration is by intravenous or intramuscular injection.

▲ side-effects: there may be sensitivity reactions – some of which may be serious. Alternatively, sometimes there is nausea and vomiting, with diarrhoea.

✚ warning: ceftizoxime should be administered with caution to patients who might be sensitive to penicillins; it should not be given to patients allergic to cephalosporins. It should be administered with caution to those who suffer from impaired kidney function. *Related article:* CEFIZOX.

cefuroxime is a broad-spectrum ANTIBIOTIC, one of the cephalosporins, used to treat a wide range of bacterial infections, particularly of the skin and soft tissues, the urinary tract, the upper respiratory tract, the genital organs, and the meninges (meningitis). It is also used to prevent infection during surgery. Administration is by intravenous or intramuscular injection.

▲ side-effects: there may be sensitivity reactions – some of which may be serious. Alternatively, sometimes there is nausea and vomiting, with diarrhoea.

✚ warning: cefuroxime should be administered with caution to patients who might be sensitive to penicillins; it should not be given to patients allergic to cephalosporins, or to patients who are already taking certain diuretic drugs. It should be administered with caution to those who suffer from impaired kidney function. *Related article:* ZINACEF.

Celevac (*Boehringer Ingelheim*) is a proprietary non-prescription form of the type of LAXATIVE known as a bulking agent, which works by

C

increasing the overall mass of faeces within the rectum, so stimulating bowel movement. It can thus be used to treat either constipation or diarrhoea, to control the consistency of faeces for patients with a colostomy, and to reduce appetite in the medical treatment of obesity. Produced in the form of tablets and as granules for solution, Celevac is a preparation of methylcellulose.

▲/✚ side-effects/warning: *see* METHYLCELLULOSE.

Centyl (*Burgess*) is a proprietary DIURETIC, available only on prescription, used – particularly in combination with ANTIHYPERTENSIVE drugs – to treat an accumulation of fluid in the tissues (oedema) and high blood pressure (hypertension). Produced in the form of tablets (in two strengths), Centyl is a preparation of bendrofluazide.

▲/✚ side-effects/warning: *see* BENDROFLUAZIDE.

Centyl-K (*Burgess*) is a proprietary DIURETIC, available only on prescription, used to treat an accumulation of fluid in the tissues (oedema) and high blood pressure (hypertension). Produced in the form of tablets, Centyl-K is a preparation of bendrofluazide with a potassium supplement for sustained release.

▲/✚ side-effects/warning: *see* BENDROFLUAZIDE.

cephalexin is a broad-spectrum ANTIBIOTIC, one of the cephalosporins, used to treat a wide range of bacterial infections, particularly of the skin and soft tissues, urinary tract, upper respiratory tract, and middle ear. Administration is oral in the form of capsules, tablets and liquids.

▲ side-effects: there may be sensitivity reactions – some of which may be serious. Sometimes there is nausea and vomiting, with diarrhoea.

✚ warning: cephalexin should be administered with caution to patients who might be sensitive to penicillins; it should not be given to patients allergic to cephalosporins. It should be administered with caution to those with impaired kidney function. *Related articles:* CEPOREX; KEFLEX.

cephalosporins are broad-spectrum ANTIBIOTICS that act against both gram-positive and gram-negative bacteria. They bear a strong resemblance in chemical structure to the penicillins, both contain a beta lactam ring, hence their classification as beta lactam antibiotics. The similarity in structure extends to mechanism of action; both inhibit the synthesis of the bacterial cell wall so killing growing bacteria. Many cephalosporins are actively excreted by the kidney, therefore reaching considerably higher concentrations in the urine than in the blood. For this reason they may be used to treat infections of the urinary tract during their own excretion. In general cephalosporins are rarely the drug of first choice, but provide a useful alternative or reserve option for particular situations. The currently used cephalosporins are relatively non-toxic, with only occasional blood clotting problems, superinfections and hypersensitivity reactions (only 10% of patients allergic to penicillin show sensitivity to cephalosporins).

cephalothin is a broad-spectrum ANTIBIOTIC, one of the cephalosporins, used to treat a wide range of bacterial infections, particularly of the skin and soft tissues, the urinary tract, upper respiratory tract, and middle ear. It is also used to prevent infection during surgery. Administration is by injection.

▲ side-effects: there may be sensitivity reactions − some of which may be serious. Sometimes there is nausea and vomiting, with diarrhoea.

✚ warning: cephalothin should be administered with caution to patients who might be sensitive to penicillins; it should not be given to patients allergic to cephalosporins, or to those with impaired kidney functions.
Related article: KEFLIN.

cephamandole is a broad-spectrum ANTIBIOTIC, one of the cephalosporins, used to treat a wide range of bacterial infections, particularly of the skin and soft tissues, the urinary tract, upper respiratory tract, and middle ear. It is also used to prevent infection during surgery. Administration is by injection.

▲ side-effects: there may be sensitivity reactions − some of which may be serious. Sometimes there is nausea and vomiting, with diarrhoea.

✚ warning: cephamandole should be administered with caution to patients who might be sensitive to penicillins; it should not be given to patients allergic to cephalosporins. It should be administered with caution to those with impaired kidney function.
Related article: KEFADOL.

cephazolin is a broad-spectrum ANTIBIOTIC, one of the cephalosporins, used to treat a wide range of bacterial infections, particularly of the skin and soft tissues, urinary tract, upper respiratory tract, and middle ear. It is also used to prevent infection during surgery. Administration is by injection.

▲ side-effects: there may be sensitivity reactions − some of which may be serious. Sometimes there is nausea and vomiting, with diarrhoea.

✚ warning: cephazolin should be administered with caution to patients who might be sensitive to penicillins; it should not be given to patients allergic to cephalosporins. It should be administered with caution to those with impaired kidney function.
Related article: KEFZOL.

cephradine is a broad-spectrum ANTIBIOTIC, one of the cephalosporins, used to treat a wide range of bacterial infections, particularly of the skin and soft tissues, the urinary tract, upper respiratory tract, and middle ear. It is also used to prevent infection during surgery. Administration is oral in the form of capsules or a dilute syrup, or by injection.

▲ side-effects: there may be sensitivity reactions – some of which may be serious. Sometimes there is nausea and vomiting, with diarrhoea.

✚ warning: cephradine should be administered with caution to patients who might be sensitive to penicillins; it should not be given to patients allergic to cephalosporins. It should be administered with caution to those with impaired kidney function. *Related article:* VELOSEF.

Ceporex (*Glaxo*) is a proprietary ANTIBIOTIC, available only on prescription, used to treat infections in the respiratory tract, urogenital area, soft tissues and middle ear. Produced in the form of capsules (in two strengths), as tablets (in two strengths), as drops for children, as a suspension (in two strengths), and as a syrup (in three strengths) for dilution (the potency of the syrup once diluted is retained for 7 days), Ceporex is a preparation of the CEPHALOSPORIN cephalexin.

▲/✚ side-effects/warning: *see* CEPHALEXIN.

Cerumol (*Laboratories for Applied Biology*) is a proprietary non-prescription preparation used to remove wax from the ear. Produced in the form of ear-drops, Cerumol's active constituent is the ANTIBACTERIAL, ANTIFUNGAL, astringent agent chlorbutol.

▲ side-effects: it may cause a sensitivity reaction.

Cesamet (*Lilly*) is a proprietary ANTI-EMETIC, available only on prescription, used to treat nausea in patients undergoing chemotherapy in the treatment of cancer. Produced in the form of capsules, Cesamet's active constituent is the synthetic drug nabilone.

▲/✚ side-effects/warning: *see* NABILONE.

Cetavlon (*ICI*) is a proprietary non-prescription DISINFECTANT, used to treat skin and scalp conditions, or in cleansing cuts and burns. Produced in the form of a solution, Cetavlon's active constituent is CETRIMIDE.

Cetavlon P.C. (*Care*) is a proprietary non-prescription DISINFECTANT, used to treat dandruff. Produced in the form of a solution to be used as a shampoo, Cetavlon P.C.'s active constituent is CETRIMIDE.

cetrimide is a detergent that has ANTISEPTIC properties; therapeutically, it is often combined with the antiseptic CHLORHEXIDINE. It is used in the form of a solution as a disinfectant for the skin and scalp, and in the form of a water-miscible cream as a soap substitute in the care of conditions such as acne and seborrhoea. In use, it should be kept away from the eyes and out of body cavities; some patients find it a mild skin irritant.

cetylpyridinium chloride in mild solution is used as a mouth-wash or gargle for oral hygiene.
Related article: MEROCET.

charcoal is an adsorbent material used medically for its absorbency in either of two ways. Its primary use is in soaking up poisons in the stomach or small intestine — especially drug overdoses in cases when only a small quantity of the drug may be extremely toxic. Powdered, it is taken in solution, repeated as necessary. Its secondary use is as a constituent in antidiarrhoeal preparations, in which it is effective in binding together faecal material. In this use it is also effective in relieving flatulence.

*chelating agents are chemical compounds which, when inside the body, bind to specific metallic ions before being excreted in the normal way. Chelating agents can thus be used to treat metal poisoning — poisoning by lead, for example. They may be incorporated in barrier creams for industrial protection.

Chemotrim Paed (*RP Drugs*) is a proprietary ANTIBIOTIC available only on prescription, used to treat many infections, such as of the respiratory and urinary tracts, and to assist in the treatment of skin infections. Produced in the form of a suspension specifically intended for children, Chemotrim Paed is a compound combination of the SULPHONAMIDE sulphamethoxazole with trimethoprim — a compound itself known as co-trimoxazole. It is not recommended for children aged under six weeks.
▲/✚ side-effects/warning: *see* SULPHAMETHOXAZOLE; TRIMETHOPRIM.

Chloractil (*DDSA Pharmaceuticals*) is a proprietary preparation of the powerful PHENOTHIAZINE drug chlorpromazine hydrochloride, used primarily as a major TRANQUILLIZER in patients who are undergoing behavioural disturbances, or who are psychotic (*see* ANTIPSYCHOTIC), particularly schizophrenic. More mundanely, it is used to treat severe anxiety, or as an anti-emetic sedative prior to surgery. Available only on prescription, Chloractil is produced in the form of tablets (in three strengths).
▲/✚ side-effects/warning: *see* CHLORPROMAZINE.

chloral hydrate is a water-soluble SEDATIVE and HYPNOTIC that is uncommonly rapid-acting. It is particularly useful for inducing sleep in children, although the drug must be administered in very dilute solution to minimize any gastric irritation. Administration is thus by the oral route.
▲ side-effects: concentration and speed of thought and movement are affected. There is often drowsiness and dizziness, with dry mouth. Susceptible patients may experience excitement or confusion.
✚ warning: chloral hydrate should be administered with caution to those with lung disease and respiratory depression. Contact with skin or mucous membranes should be avoided.

chloramphenicol is an ANTIBIOTIC that is produced both by derivation from a micro-organism and by synthetic means. It has the capacity to treat many forms of infection effectively, but the serious side-effects that very rarely accompany its systemic use demand that it is ordinarily restricted to the treatment of severe

C

infection (such as meningitis). In topical application to the eyes, ears or skin, however, the drug is useful in treating such conditions as bacterial conjunctivitis, otitis externa, or many types of skin infection. Topical administration is in the form of eye-drops, ear-drops or a cream. Systemic administration is in the form of capsules or a dilute suspension, or by injection or infusion.

▲ side-effects: systemic treatment may cause serious changes in the blood composition. Overdosage in the newborn can result in a condition called the "grey baby syndrome", which leads to shock.

✚ warning: when chloramphenicol is given to the newborn the dosage should be greatly reduced. Blood level tests can be performed to avoid toxic effects.

Related articles: CHLOROMYCETIN; KEMICETINE; MINIMS; OPULETS; SNO PHENICOL.

Chlorasol (*Schering-Prebbles*) is a proprietary non-prescription DISINFECTANT and cleanser, used to treat skin infections, and especially in cleansing wounds and ulcers. Produced in the form of a solution in sachets, Chlorasol is a preparation of SODIUM HYPOCHLORITE SOLUTION.

chlorhexidine is an ANTISEPTIC that is a constituent in many DISINFECTANT preparations, for use especially prior to surgery or in obstetrics, but that is primarily used (in the form of chlorhexidine gluconate, chlorhexidine acetate or chlorhexidine hydrochloride) either as a mouth wash for oral hygiene, or as a dressing for minor skin wounds and infections; it is also used for instillation in the bladder to relieve minor infections.

▲ side-effects: some patients experience sensitivity reactions.

✚ warning: caution should be exercised in assessing suitable solution concentration for bladder instillation: too high a concentration may lead to the appearance of blood in the urine. Avoid contact with mucous membranes.

Related articles: BACTICLENS; BACTIGRAS; CORSODYL; DISPRAY 1 QUICK PREP; ELUDRIL; HIBIDIL; HIBISCRUB; HIBISOL; HIBITANE; NASEPTIN; NYSTAFORM; pHISO-MED; SAVLOCLENS; SAVLODIL; SAVLON HOSPITAL CONCENTRATE; TRAVASEPT; UNISEPT; XYLOCAINE.

chlormethiazole is a HYPNOTIC drug that also has ANTICONVULSANT properties. In children it can be used by intravenous infusion to control convulsions which have failed to respond to simple measures.

▲ side-effects: there may be headache, sneezing and gastrointestinal disturbance. High dosage by intravenous infusion may cause depressed breathing and reduced heart rate, and presents a risk of thrombophlebitis.

Related article: HEMINEVRIN.

Chloromycetin (*Parke-Davis*) is a proprietary broad-spectrum ANTIBIOTIC, available only on prescription, used to treat potentially dangerous bacterial infections, such as meningitis. Produced in the form of capsules, as a suspension for dilution (the potency of the dilute suspension is retained for 14 days), as eye-ointment and

eye-drops, as a powder, and in vials for injection, Chloromycetin is a preparation of chloramphenicol.
▲/✚ side-effects/warning: *see* CHLORAMPHENICOL.

Chloromycetin Hydrocortisone (*Parke-Davis*) is a proprietary ANTIBIOTIC and CORTICOSTEROID preparation, available only on prescription, used to treat eye infections. Produced in the form of an eye ointment, Chloromycetin Hydrocortisone contains the antibiotic chloramphenicol and the steroid hydrocortisone.
▲/✚ side-effects/warning: *see* CHLORAMPHENICOL; HYDROCORTISONE.

chloroquine is the major ANTIMALARIAL drug in use, effective against most forms of the malarial organism, *Plasmodium*, and used both to treat and to prevent contraction of the disease. However, it does not kill those organisms which migrate to the liver, and thus cannot prevent relapses caused by any form of *Plasmodium* that does so. Moreover, several strains of *Plasmodium* have recently exhibited resistance to chloroquine in certain areas of the world, and in those areas alternative therapy is now advised. Chloroquine is sometimes also used to treat infection caused by amoebae, or to halt the progress of rheumatic disease. Administration is oral in the form of tablets or a dilute syrup, or by injection or infusion.
▲ side-effects: there may be nausea and vomiting, with headache and itching; gastrointestinal disturbance may be severe; some patients break out in a rash. Susceptible patients may undergo psychotic episodes. Prolonged high dosage may cause ringing in the ears (tinnitus) and damage to the cornea and retina of the eyes.
✚ warning: chloroquine should not be administered to patients with retinal disease, or who are allergic to quinine; it should be administered with caution to patients with porphyria, psoriasis, or who have impaired kidney or liver function; who are elderly; or who are children. Prolonged treatment should be punctuated by ophthalmic checks.
Related articles: AVLOCLOR; MALARIVON; NIVAQUINE.

chlorothiazide is a DIURETIC, one of the THIAZIDES, used to treat fluid retention in the tissues (oedema), high blood pressure (hypertension) and mild to moderate heart failure. Because all thiazides tend to deplete body reserves of potassium, chlorothiazide may be administered in combination either with potassium supplements or with diuretics that are complimentarily potassium-sparing. Administration is oral in the form of tablets.
▲ side-effects: there may be tiredness and a rash.
✚ warning: chlorothiazide should not be administered to patients with kidney failure or urinary retention. It may aggravate conditions of diabetes or gout.

chloroxylenol is an antiseptic effective in killing some bacteria but not others, and is an established constituent in at least one well-known skin disinfectant. A few patients experience mild skin irritation that may lead to sensitivity reactions, however.
Related article: DETTOL.

chlorpheniramine is an ANTIHISTAMINE, used to treat the symptoms of allergic conditions like hay fever and urticaria; it is also sometimes used in emergencies to treat anaphylactic shock. Administration (as chlorpheniramine maleate) is oral in the form of tablets, sustained-release tablets and a dilute syrup, or by injection.
▲ side-effects: concentration and speed of thought and movement may be affected. There may be nausea, headaches, and/or weight gain, dry mouth, gastrointestinal disturbances and visual problems. Treatment by injection may cause tissue irritation that leads to a temporary drop in blood pressure.
Related articles: ALUNEX; PIRITON.

chlorpromazine is an ANTIPSYCHOTIC drug used as a major TRANQUILLIZER for patients suffering from schizophrenia and other psychoses, particularly during behavioural disturbances. The drug may also be used in the short term to treat severe anxiety, to soothe patients who are dying, as a premedication prior to surgery, and to remedy an intractable hiccup. It may also be used to relieve nausea and vertigo caused by disorders in the middle or inner ear. It can also be used to potentiate the effect of a narcotic analgesic, such as PETHIDINE. Administration (as chlorpromazine hydrochloride) is oral in the form of tablets or an elixir, as anal suppositories, or by intramuscular injection.
▲ side-effects: concentration and speed of thought and movement are affected.
Related articles: CHLORACTIL; DOZINE; LARGACTIL.

chlortetracycline is a broad-spectrum ANTIBIOTIC used to treat many forms of infection caused by any of several types of micro-organism; conditions it is particularly used to treat include infections of the urinary tract, of the respiratory tract, in and around the eye, of the genital organs, and of the skin, including acne and impetigo. Administration (as chlortetracycline hydrochloride) is oral in the form of capsules or a solution, or topical in the form of a cream, an ointment, and an ophthalmic ointment.
▲ side-effects: there may be nausea and vomiting, with diarrhoea. Occasionally, there is sensitivity to light or some other sensitivity reaction. These side-effects may still occur even if the causative organism of the disorder proves to be resistant to the drug.
✚ warning: chlortetracycline should not be administered systemically to patients who are aged under 12 years, who are pregnant, or with impaired kidney function; it should be administered with caution to those who are lactating. The cream and the ointment may stain fabric.
Related article: AUREOMYCIN.

cholecalciferol is one of the natural forms of calciferol (vitamin D), formed in humans by the action of sunlight on the skin.
see CALCIFEROL.

Choledyl *(Parke-Davis)* is a proprietary non-prescription BRONCHODILATOR, used to treat the symptoms of asthma. Produced in the form of tablets (in two strengths) and as a syrup for dilution (the potency of the syrup once diluted is retained for 14 days), Choledyl is a preparation of choline theophyllinate.

▲/✚ side-effects/warning: *see* CHOLINE THEOPHYLLINATE.

cholera vaccine is a suspension containing non-infective versions of the bacteria that cause the dangerous intestinal epidemic disease cholera. Administration is initially by subcutaneous or intramuscular injection, followed two to four weeks later by a booster shot. The vaccine cannot guarantee total protection, and travellers should be warned still to take great care over the hygiene of the food and drink they consume. In any case, what protection is afforded lasts only for about six months.

cholestyramine is a resin which, when taken orally, binds to bile salts in the intestines that can then be excreted in the normal way. This is a useful property in the treatment of high blood fat, especially cholesterol levels (hyperlipidaemia), and of the itching associated with obstruction in the bile ducts. The property can also be utilized in the treatment of diarrhoea following intestinal disease or surgery. Administration is oral in the form of a powder taken with liquids.
▲ side-effects: there may be nausea, heartburn, flatulence with abdominal discomfort, constipation or diarrhoea, and a rash.
✚ warning: cholestyramine should not be administered to patients who suffer from complete blockage of the bile ducts. High dosage may require simultaneous administration of fat-soluble vitamins.
Related article: QUESTRAN.

choline theophyllinate is a modified form of the BRONCHODILATOR theophylline used to treat conditions such as asthma and bronchitis. It is thought to be slightly better tolerated than theophylline. Administration is oral in the form of tablets, sustained-release tablets, or a dilute syrup.
▲ side-effects: there may be nausea and gastrointestinal disturbances, and increase or irregularity in the heartbeat, and/or insomnia.
✚ warning: treatment should initially be gradually progressive in the quantity administered. Tests on its level in the blood may be performed to discover the optimum dosage.
Related article: CHOLEDYL.

Cicatrin (*Calmic*) is a proprietary ANTIBIOTIC drug, available only on prescription, used in topical application to treat skin infections. Produced in the form of a cream, as a dusting-powder and as an aerosol powder-spray, Cicatrin's major active constituents include neomycin sulphate and bacitracin zinc.
▲/✚ side-effects/warning: *see* NEOMYCIN.

ciclacillin is an ANTIBIOTIC, a PENICILLIN used to treat infections of the upper respiratory tract, of the urinary tract, and of the soft tissues. Administration is oral in the form of tablets or a dilute suspension.
▲ side-effects: the drug may cause diarrhoea if given in tablet form; there may be sensitivity reactions ranging from a minor rash to

urticaria and joint pains, and (occasionally) to high temperature and anaphylactic shock. High dosage may in any case cause convulsions.

+ warning: ciclacillin should not be administered to patients known to be allergic to penicillins; it should be administered with caution to those with impaired kidney function.
Related article: CALTHOR.

Cidomycin (*Roussel*) is a proprietary ANTIBIOTIC, available only on prescription, used to treat many forms of infection. Produced in ampoules for injection (in two strengths), in vials for the treatment of children, in ampoules for intrathecal injections, as a powder for reconstitution as a medium for injection, as ear- and eye-drops, as an eye ointment, and as a cream and an ointment for topical application, Cidomycin is a preparation of gentamicin sulphate.

▲/+ side-effects/warning: *see* GENTAMICIN.

Cidomycin Topical (*Roussel*) is a proprietary ANTIBIOTIC preparation, available only on prescription, used in topical application to treat skin infections. Produced in the form of a water-miscible cream and a paraffin-based ointment, Cidomycin Topical is a preparation of gentamicin sulphate.

▲/+ side-effects/warning: *see* GENTAMICIN.

cimetidine is an ulcer healing drug that reduces the secretion of gastric acids, and is thus used primarily to assist in the healing of peptic ulcers in the stomach and duodenum. It may also be helpful in reducing the symptoms of heartburn when these are severe. Cimetidine works by blocking histamine H_2 receptors, is well tolerated, and side-effects are comparatively rare. Administration is oral in the form of tablets or a dilute syrup, or by injection or infusion.

▲ side-effects: the drug may enhance the effects of benzodiazepines or beta-blockers taken simultaneously.

+ warning: cimetidine should be administered with caution to patients with impaired liver or kidney function. Treatment of undiagnosed dyspepsia may potentially mask the onset of stomach or duodenal cancer and is therefore undesirable.
Related article: TAGAMET.

cisplatin is an unusual CYTOTOXIC drug that contains an organic complex of platinum. It works by damaging the DNA of newly-forming cells, and is used to treat certain tumours in childhood. Side-effects may be severe. Administration is by injection.

▲ side-effects: there is severe nausea and vomiting. There may also be disturbances in hearing, loss of sensation at the fingertips, and reduced levels of many elements of the blood. Toxic effects may require withdrawal of treatment.

+ warning: cisplatin should be administered with caution to patients with impaired kidney function.
Related article: PLATOSIN.

C

Claforan (*Roussel*) is a proprietary ANTIBIOTIC preparation, available only on prescription, used to treat many forms of infection, including meningitis. Produced in vials as a powder for reconstitution as a medium for injection, Claforan is a preparation of the CEPHALOSPORIN cefotaxime.
▲/✚ side-effects/warning: *see* CEFOTAXIME.

clavulanic acid is a weakly antibiotic substance which has the effect of inhibiting resistance in bacteria that have become resistant to some penicillin-type antibiotics, notably amoxycillin and ticarcillin. It is a potent inhibitor of bacterial penicillinase enzymes that can inactivate many antibiotics of the penicillin family. It is therefore used in combination with amoxycillin or ticarcillin to treat infective conditions in which the penicillin alone might be unsuccessful, and has the additional effect of extending the activity of the antibiotic.
Related article: AUGMENTIN; TIMENTIN.

clemastine is an ANTIHISTAMINE used in the relief of allergic disorders such as hay fever, urticaria and some rashes. Administration is oral in the form of tablets or a dilute elixir.
▲/✚ side-effects/warning: concentration and speed of thought and movement may be affected; there may be nausea, headaches, and/or weight gain, dry mouth, gastrointestinal disturbances and visual problems.
Related articles: ALLER-EZE; TAVEGIL.

clindamycin is an ANTIBIOTIC used to treat infections of bones and joints, and to assist in the treatment of peritonitis (inflammation of the peritoneal lining of the abdominal cavity). Administration is oral in the form of capsules or a dilute suspension, or by injection.
▲ side-effects: there may be diarrhoea or other symptoms of colitis. There may also be nausea and vomiting.
✚ warning: clindamycin should not be administered to patients suffering from diarrhoea; and if diarrhoea or other symptoms of colitis appear during treatment, administration must be halted at once. This is because clindamycin may cause colitis, with potentially severe symptoms. It should be administered with caution to those with impaired liver or kidney function.
Related article: DALACIN C.

Clinicide (*De Witt*) is a proprietary non-prescription preparation used to treat scalp and pubic infestations of lice (pediculosis). Produced in the form of a lotion, Clinicide's active constituent is CARBARYL.

Clinifeed (*Roussel*) is a proprietary non-prescription nutritionally complete feed, used as a dietary supplement for patients whose metabolic processes are unable to break down protein. Produced in four formulations, Clinifeed contains protein, carbohydrate, fat and vitamins and minerals, but it is free of gluten. It is unsuitable for children aged under 12 months.

Clinitar Cream (*Smith & Nephew Pharmaceuticals*) is a proprietary non-prescription tar preparation, used in topical application to treat severe non-infective skin conditions such as eczema and psoriasis. Produced in the form of cream and a gel, Clinitar Cream's active constituent is COAL TAR.

clioquinol is an ANTISEPTIC compound that contains iodine and is effective against infections by amoebae and some other micro-organisms. Its primary use is to treat infections of the skin and the outer ear. Administration is topical (in the form of drops, creams, ointments and anal suppositories).

▲ side-effects: some patients experience sensitivity reactions. Systemic use of the drug has been associated with serious toxicity of the optic nerve, causing blindness.

✚ warning: prolonged or excessive use encourages the onset of fungal infection. The drug stains skin and fabric.
Related article: LOCORTEN-VIOFORM.

clobazam is an ANXIOLYTIC drug, one of the BENZODIAZEPINES, used to treat anxiety in the short term, and sometimes to assist in the treatment of some forms of epilepsy. Administration is oral in the form of capsules.

▲ side-effects: concentration and speed of thought and movement may be affected; the effects of alcohol consumption may be enhanced. There is often drowsiness and dry mouth; there may also be dizziness, headache, and shallow breathing, and sensitivity reactions may occur.

✚ warning: clobazam should be administered with caution to patients with depressed respiration, closed angle glaucoma, or impaired kidney or liver function. Prolonged use and abrupt withdrawal of treatment should be avoided.
Related article: FRISIUM.

clobetasol propionate is an extremely powerful CORTICOSTEROID, used in topical application on severe non-infective skin inflammations such as eczema, especially in cases where less powerful steroid treatments have failed. Administration is in the form of an aqueous cream, a paraffin-based ointment or an alcohol-based scalp lotion. Because clobetasol is such a powerful topical steroid it is rarely recommended for use in children.

▲ side-effects: topical application may result in local thinning of the skin, with possible whitening, and an increased local growth of hair. Some young patients experience the outbreak of a kind of inflammatory dermatitis on the face or at the site of application.

✚ warning: as with all corticosteroids, clobetasol propionate treats the symptoms of inflammation but has no effect on any underlying infection. Undetected infection may thus become worse because its effects are masked by the steroid. The steroid should not in any case be administered to patients with untreated skin lesions; use on the face is best avoided.
Related articles: DERMOVATE; DERMOVATE-NN.

clobetasone butyrate is a CORTICOSTEROID, used in topical application on severe non-infective skin inflammations such as eczema, especially in cases where less powerful steroid treatments have failed. Administration is in the form of a water-miscible cream, and a paraffin-based ointment.

▲ side-effects: topical application may result in local thinning of the skin, with possible whitening, and an increased local growth of hair. Some young patients experience the outbreak of a kind of inflammatory dermatitis on the face or at the site of application.

✚ warning: as with all corticosteroids, clobetasone butyrate treats the symptoms of inflammation but has no effect on any underlying infection. Undetected infection may thus become worse because its effects are masked by the steroid. The steroid should not in any case be administered to patients with untreated skin lesions; use on the face is best avoided.

Related articles: EUMOVATE; TRIMOVATE.

clomocycline sodium is a broad-spectrum ANTIBIOTIC, one of the tetracyclines, used to treat many forms of infection caused by any of several types of micro-organism. It is used particularly to treat infections of the urinary tract, respiratory tract and genital organs, and acne. Administration is oral in the form of capsules.

▲ side-effects: there may be nausea and vomiting, with diarrhoea. Occasionally there is sensitivity to light or other sensitivity reaction. These side-effects may still occur even if the causative organism of the disorder being treated proves to be resistant to the drug.

✚ warning: clomocycline sodium should not be administered to patients who are aged under 12 years, who are pregnant, or with impaired kidney function; it should be administered with caution to those who are lactating.

clonazepam is a drug related to DIAZEPAM and the BENZODIAZEPINES but is in effect an ANTICONVULSANT drug used to treat certain forms of epilepsy. Administration is oral in the form of tablets.

▲ side-effects: concentration and speed of thought and movement are affected; in susceptible patients the degree of sedation may be marked. There may also be dizziness, fatigue and muscular weakness. Again in susceptible patients, there may be mood changes.

✚ warning: clonazepam is more sedative than most drugs used to treat epilepsy.

Related article: RIVOTRIL.

clonidine hydrochloride is an ANTIHYPERTENSIVE drug used to treat moderate to severe high blood pressure (hypertension). Although controversial, use of the drug has also been extended to assisting in the prevention of migraine attacks. It is thought to work by reducing release of the neurotransmitter noradrenaline both in the brain and in blood vessels. Administration is oral in the form of tablets and sustained-release capsules, or by injection. Clonidine hydrochloride also increases the production of growth hormone by the body, and it is used in a test to rule out growth hormone deficiency.

clotrimazole is an ANTIFUNGAL drug used in topical application to treat fungal infection on the skin and mucous membranes (especially the vagina and the outer ear). Administration is in the form of a water-miscible cream, a dusting-powder, a spray and a lotion (solution).
▲ side-effects: rarely, there is a burning sensation or irritation; a very few patients experience sensitivity reactions.
Related article: CANESTEN.

cloxacillin is an ANTIBIOTIC of the penicillin family, used primarily to treat forms of infection which other penicillins are incapable of countering, because of the production of the enzyme penicillinase by the bacteria concerned. However, cloxacillin is not inactivated by the penicillinase enzymes produced, for example, by certain Staphylococci. It is therefore classed as a penicillinase-resistant penicillin. Administration is oral in the form of capsules and a dilute syrup, and by injection.
▲ side-effects: there may be sensitivity reactions ranging from a minor rash to urticaria and joint pains, fever or anaphylactic shock.
✚ warning: cloxacillin should not be administered to patients who are known to be allergic to penicillins; it should be administered with caution to those with impaired kidney function.
Related articles: AMPICLOX; ORBENIN.

coal tar is a black, viscous liquid obtained by the distillation of coal: it has both anti-itching and keratolytic properties, and works by speeding up the rate at which the surface scale of skin is lost naturally. Therapeutically employed primarily to treat psoriasis and eczema, coal tar is used in solution in which the concentration is decided by each individual patient's condition and response. It is a constituent in many non-proprietary and proprietary formulations, especially pastes, some of which are not suitable for the treatment of facial conditions.
▲ side-effects: some patients experience skin irritation and an acne-like rash. Rarely, there is sensitivity to light.
✚ warning: avoid contact with broken or inflamed skin. Coal tar stains skin, hair and fabric.
Related articles: ALPHOSYL; CARBO-CORT; CARBO-DOME; CLINITAR; COLTAPASTE; GELCOTAR; GENISOL; IONIL T; MEDITAR; POLYTAR EMOLLIENT; PRAGMATAR; PSORIDERM; PSORIGEL: TARBAND; TARCORTIN; T/GEL.

Cobadex (*Cox Pharmaceuticals*) is a proprietary CORTICOSTEROID preparation, available only on prescription, used to treat mild inflammatory skin conditions, and itching in the anal and vulval regions. Produced in the form of a water-miscible cream (in two strengths), Cobadex contains the steroid hydrocortisone and the antifoaming agent DIMETHICONE.
▲/✚ side-effects/warning: *see* HYDROCORTISONE.

Cobutolin (*Cox Pharmaceuticals*) is a proprietary BETA-RECEPTOR STIMULANT BRONCHODILATOR, available only on prescription, used to treat bronchial asthma. It is produced in the form of tablets (in two strengths) and in an aerosol that emits metered doses. Cobutolin is a preparation of the selective beta$_2$-adrenoceptor stimulant salbutamol.

▲/✚ side-effects/warning: *see* SALBUTAMOL.

co-codamol is a compound ANALGESIC combining the OPIATE codeine phosphate with paracetamol in a ratio of 2:125. As a compound it forms a constituent in a number of proprietary analgesic preparations, but although it has the advantages of both drugs, it also has the disadvantages.

▲/✚ side-effects/warning: *see* CODEINE PHOSPHATE; PARACETAMOL.

Codanin (*Whitehall Laboratories*) is a proprietary, non-prescription ANALGESIC produced in the form of tablets and as a powder. It is a preparation of codeine phosphate and paracetamol.

▲/✚ side-effects/warning: *see* CODEINE PHOSPHATE; PARACETAMOL.

codeine phosphate is an OPIATE, a narcotic ANALGESIC that also has the properties of a cough suppressant. As an analgesic, codeine is a common, but often minor, constituent in non-proprietary and proprietary preparations to relieve pain (a majority of which are not available from the National Health Service), although some authorities dislike any combined form that contains codeine. Even more authorities disapprove of the drug's use as a cough suppressant. The drug also has the capacity to reduce intestinal motility (and so treat diarrhoea). Administration is oral or by injection.

▲ side-effects: tolerance occurs readily, although dependence (addiction) is relatively unusual. Constipation is common. There may be sedation and dizziness, especially following injection. The effects of alcohol consumption may be enhanced.

✚ warning: codeine phosphate should not be administered to patients who suffer from depressed breathing, or who are aged under 12 months.

Related articles: ANTOIN; BENYLIN EXPECTORANT; DIARREST; DIMOTANE WITH CODEINE; GALCODINE; KAODENE; MEDOCODENE; MIGRALEVE; PANADEINE; PARACODOL; PARADEINE; PARAHYPON; SOLPADEINE; TERCODA; TERCOLIX.

co-dydramol is a compound ANALGESIC combining the OPIATE dihydrocodeine tartrate together with paracetamol in a ratio of 1:50. As a compound it forms a constituent in a number of proprietary analgesic preparations, but although it has the advantages of both drugs, it also has the disadvantages.

▲/✚ side-effects/warning: *see* DIHYDROCODEINE TARTRATE; PARACETAMOL.

Coldrex (*Sterling Health*) is a proprietary, non-prescription cold relief preparation produced in the form of tablets and as a powder. It contains paracetamol, phenylephrine and ascorbic acid. The tablet formulation also contains caffeine.

▲/✚ side-effects/warning: *see* ASCORBIC ACID; CAFFEINE; PARACETAMOL; PHENYLEPHRINE.

Colofac (*Duphar*) is a proprietary ANTICHOLINERGIC drug available only on prescription, used to treat gastrointestinal disturbance caused by spasm

of the muscles of the intestinal walls (irritable bowel syndrome).
Produced in the form of tablets and as a sugar-free suspension,
Colofac is a preparation of the antispasmodic drug mebeverine
hydrochloride. It is not recommended for children aged under ten
years.

Cologel (*Lilly*) is a proprietary non-prescription LAXATIVE that is not
available from the National Health Service. Used to treat
constipation that results from inadequate fibre intake, it acts as a
bulking agent to form a mass of faecal material that stimulates bowel
movement. Produced in the form of sugar-free syrup for dilution (the
potency of the syrup once diluted is retained for 14 days), Cologel is a
preparation of METHYLCELLULOSE.

Colpermin (*Tillotts*) is a proprietary non-prescription SMOOTH MUSCLE
RELAXANT, used to treat gastrointestinal disturbance caused by spasm
of the muscles of the intestinal walls. Produced in the form of
capsules, Colpermin is a preparation of peppermint oil. It is not
usually recommended for children.
▲/✚ side-effects/warning: *see* PEPPERMINT OIL.

Coltapaste (*Smith & Nephew*) is a proprietary non-prescription form
of impregnated bandaging, used to dress and treat serious non-
infective skin diseases (such as eczema and psoriasis). The bandaging
is impregnated with COAL TAR and ZINC paste.

Colven (*Reckitt & Colman*) is a proprietary ANTICHOLINERGIC smooth
muscle relaxant, available only on prescription, used to treat
gastrointestinal disturbance caused by spasm of the muscles of the
intestinal walls. Produced in the form of effervescent granules in
sachets, Colven is a preparation of the antispasmodic drug
mebeverine hydrochloride with the ANTIDIARRHOEAL bulking agent
ispaghula husk. It is not usually recommended for children.
▲/✚ side-effects/warning: *see* ISPAGHULA HUSK.

Combantrin (*Pfizer*) is a proprietary ANTHELMINTIC preparation,
available only on prescription, used to treat infestations by
roundworm, threadworm, hookworm and whipworm. Produced in the
form of tablets, Combantrin is a preparation of pyrantel embonate. It
is not recommended for children aged under six months.

Comox (*Norton*) is a proprietary broad-spectrum ANTIBIOTIC drug,
available only on prescription, used to treat infections of the urinary
tract, the sinuses or the middle ear, and diseases such as typhoid
fever. Produced in the form of tablets (in two strengths, the stronger
under the name Comox Forte), as soluble (dispersible) tablets, and as
a suspension for children, Comox is a compound of the SULPHONAMIDE
sulphamethoxazole and trimethoprim – a compound itself known as
CO-TRIMOXAZOLE.
▲/✚ side-effects/warning: *see* SULPHAMETHOXAZOLE; TRIMETHOPRIM.

Congesteze is a proprietary non-prescription oral preparation
intended to clear a stuffed nose. It contains the SYMPATHOMIMETIC

VASOCONSTRICTOR ophedrine and the ANTIHISTAMINE azatadine maleate. It is produced in the form of tablets as a syrup (in two strengths, the weaker labelled for children).

▲/✚ side-effects/warning: *see* EPHEDRINE HYDROCHLORIDE; AZATADINE MALEATE.

Contac 400 (*Menley & James*) is a proprietary, non-prescription cold relief preparation. It contains the ANTIHISTAMINE chlorpheniramine and the DECONGESTANT propanolamine.

▲/✚ side-effects/warning: *see* CHLORPHENIRAMINE.

co-proxamol is a compound ANALGESIC combining the narcotic dextropropoxyphene with paracetamol in a ratio of 1:10. As a compound it forms a constituent in a number of proprietary analgesic preparations, but although it has the advantages of both drugs, it also has the disadvantages.

▲/✚ side-effects/warning: *see* DEXTROPROPOXYPHENE; PARACETAMOL.

Corlan (*Glaxo*) is a proprietary CORTICOSTEROID, available only on prescription, used in topical application to treat ulcers and sores in the mouth. Produced in the form of lozenges, Corlan's active constituent is the steroid hydrocortisone.

▲/✚ side-effects/warning: *see* HYDROCORTISONE.

Corsodyl (*ICI*) is a proprietary non-prescription ANTISEPTIC preparation, used in topical application to treat inflammations and infections of the mouth. Produced in the form of a gel and as a mouth-wash, Corsodyl is a preparation of chlorhexidine gluconate.

Cortacream (*Smith & Nephew*) is a proprietary brand of dressings, available only on prescription, used to treat mild inflammatory skin conditions. Produced in the form of an impregnated bandage, it requires additional bandaging to keep it in place. It should be applied only to the affected area. Cortacream's active constituent is the CORTICOSTEROID hydrocortisone acetate.

▲/✚ side-effects/warning: *see* HYDROCORTISONE.

Cortelan (*Glaxo*) is a proprietary preparation of the CORTICOSTEROID hormone cortisone acetate, available only on prescription, used less commonly now in replacement therapy to make up hormonal deficiency following surgical removal of one or both of the adrenal glands. It is produced in the form of tablets.

▲/✚ side-effects/warning: *see* CORTISONE ACETATE

*corticosteroids are STEROID HORMONES produced and secreted by the cortex (the outer portion) of the adrenal glands, or substances produced synthetically that resemble them. There are two main types: glucocorticoids and mineralocorticoids. The glucocorticoids assist in the metabolism of fats, carbohydrate and protein in the body, and contribute to the neuromuscular and tissue processes that convey the body's reaction to stress. The mineralocorticoids assist in maintaining the balance of salt and water in the body. Therapeutically, the

glucocorticoids are far more important, used particularly for their anti-inflammatory properties – it is they that are the basis of almost all therapy with corticosteroids. Best known are HYDROCORTISONE (cortisol), CORTISONE ACETATE, TRIAMCINOLONE, BETAMETHASONE, PREDNISONE, PREDNISOLONE and DEXAMETHASONE. Mineralocorticoids include FLUDROCORTISONE ACETATE.
▲ side-effects: with prolonged use corticosteroids cause excessive weight gain and stunting of growth can occur.

corticotrophin (or adrenocorticotrophic hormone; ACTH) is a hormone produced and secreted by the pituitary gland in order to control the production and secretion of other hormones – CORTICOSTEROIDS – in the adrenal glands, generally as a response to stress. Therapeutically, corticotrophin may be administered to make up for hormonal deficiency in the pituitary gland, to cause the production of extra corticosteroids in the treatment of inflammatory conditions such as rheumatism and asthma, or to test the function of the adrenal glands. However, it is now rarely used for this purpose. ACTH is used in the treatment of a rare form of epilepsy, called infantile spasms.

cortisol is another name for the CORTICOSTEROID hormone hydrocortisone.
see HYDROCORTISONE.

cortisone acetate is a CORTICOSTEROID hormone that has the properties both of glucocorticoids and of mineralocorticoids. It can thus theoretically be used both to treat inflammatory conditions caused, for instance, by allergy or rheumatism, and to make up for hormonal deficiency (especially relating to the salt and water balance of the body) following surgical removal of the adrenal glands. In practice, however, it is not generally used for the suppression of inflammation because it has a tendency to cause fluid retention. Administration is oral in the form of tablets.
▲ side-effects: treatment of susceptible patients may engender euphoria, or a state of confusion or depression. Rarely, there is peptic ulcer.
✚ warning: in children, prolonged administration of cortisone acetate may lead to stunting of growth. The effects of potentially serious infections may be masked by the drug during treatment. Withdrawal of treatment must be gradual.
Related articles: CORTELAN; CORTISTAB; CORTISYL.

Cortistab (*Boots*) is a proprietary preparation of the CORTICOSTEROID hormone cortisone acetate, available only on prescription, used less commonly now in replacement therapy to make up hormonal deficiency following surgical removal of one or both of the adrenal glands; it is even less commonly used to treat allergic and rheumatic inflammation. It is produced in the form of tablets (in two strengths).
▲/✚ side-effects/warning: *see* CORTISONE ACETATE.

Cortisyl (*Roussel*) is a proprietary preparation of the CORTICOSTEROID hormone cortisone acetate, available only on prescription, used less

commonly now in replacement therapy to make up hormonal deficiency following surgical removal of one or both of the adrenal glands. It is produced in the form of tablets; administration is by the oral route.
▲/✚ side-effects/warning: *see* CORTISONE ACETATE.

Cosmegen Lyovac (*Merck, Sharp & Dohme*) is a proprietary CYTOTOXIC drug that also has ANTIBIOTIC PROPERTIES. AVAILABLE ONLY ON PRESCRIPTION, IT IS USED MAINLY TO TREAT CANCERS IN CHILDREN, AND IS PRODUCED IN THE FORM OF A POWDER FOR RECONSTITUTION AS A MEDIUM FOR INJECTION. COSMEGEN LYOVAC IS A PREPARATION OF ACTINOMYCIN D.
▲/✚ side-effects/warning: *see* ACTINOMYCIN D.

Cosuric (*DDSA Pharmaceuticals*) is a proprietary form of the xanthine-oxidase inhibitor allopurinol, used to treat high levels of uric acid in the bloodstream. Available only on prescription, Cosuric is produced in the form of tablets (in two strengths).
▲/✚ side-effects/warning: *see* ALLOPURINOL.

Cotazym (*Organon*) is a proprietary non-prescription preparation of digestive enzymes, used to make up a deficiency of digestive juices normally supplied by the pancreas, such as in cystic fibrosis. It is produced in the form of capsules to be sprinkled on food.

co-trimoxazole is the name for an ANTIBIOTIC combination of the SULPHONAMIDE sulphamethoxazole and the similar but not related trimethoprim (a folic acid inhibitor). At one time it was thought that each agent enhanced the action of the other giving a combined effect greater than the sum of the two. While there is in fact little evidence to support this, the combination remains a very useful antibiotic preparation. It is used to treat and to prevent the spread of infections of the urinary tract, the nasal passages and upper respiratory tract, and the bones and joints, and such diseases as typhoid fever or gonorrhoea (particularly in patients allergic to penicillin); it is the active constituent of many proprietary antibiotic preparations. Administration is oral in the form of tablets or a suspension, or by injection or infusion. Side-effects are largely due to the sulphonamide.
▲ side-effects: there may be nausea and vomiting; rashes are not uncommon. Blood disorders may occur.
✚ warning: co-trimoxazole should not be administered to patients with blood disorders, jaundice, or impaired liver or kidney function. It should be administered with caution to infants under six weeks old. Adequate fluid intake must be maintained. Prolonged treatment requires regular blood counts.
Related articles: BACTRIM; CHEMOTRIM PAED; COMOX; FECTRIM; LARATRIM; SEPTRIN.

Cradocap (*Napp*) is a proprietary non-prescription ANTISEPTIC, used to treat the infants' skin conditions cradle cap or scurf cap. Produced in the form of a shampoo, Cradocap is a 10% solution of CETRIMIDE.

Creon (*Duphar*) is a proprietary non-prescription preparation of digestive enzymes, used to make up a deficiency of digestive juices normally supplied by the pancreas. This preparation is particularly useful in conditions such as cystic fibrosis because the enzymes are in a slow-release preparation. They therefore tend to be protected from the acid in the patient's stomach, and a greater amount is released in the small bowel where they help in digestion.

crotamiton is a drug used both to relieve itching and to kill parasitic mites on the skin (as in scabies). It is applied to the skin in the form of a lotion or a cream, usually following a bath; the application should be left in position for as long as possible — ideally 24 hours for treatment of parasitic mites — before being washed off.

✚ warning: crotamiton should not be used on broken skin or near the eyes.

crystal violet is another name for gentian violet.
see GENTIAN VIOLET.

Crystapen (*Glaxo*) is a proprietary ANTIBIOTIC, available only on prescription, used to treat infections of the skin, of the middle ear, and of the respiratory tract (such as tonsillitis), and certain severe systemic infections (such as meningitis). Produced as a powder for reconstitution in any of three forms suited to specific sites of injection, Crystapen is a preparation of benzylpenicillin sodium.
▲/✚ side-effects/warning: *see* BENZYLPENICILLIN.

Crystapen V (*Glaxo*) is a proprietary ANTIBIOTIC, available only on prescripton, used to treat many forms of infection, and to prevent rheumatic fever. Produced in the form of a syrup (in two strengths) for dilution (the potency of the syrup once dilute is retained for 7 days), Crystapen V is a preparation of phenoxymethylpenicillin.
▲/✚ side-effects/warning: *see* PHENOXYMETHYLPENICILLIN.

Cuplex (*Smith & Nephew*) is a proprietary non-prescription preparation used to remove warts and hard skin (a keratolytic). Produced in the form of a gel, Cuplex's active constituents are salicylic acid and lactic acid.

Cyclimorph (*Calmic*) is a proprietary form of the narcotic ANALGESIC morphine tartrate together with the anti-emetic ANTIHISTAMINE cyclizine tartrate, and is on the controlled drugs list. Used to treat moderate to severe pain, it is produced in ampoules (in two strengths, under the names Cyclimorph-10 and Cyclimorph-15) for injection.
▲/✚ side-effects/warning: *see* CYCLIZINE; MORPHINE.

cyclizine is an ANTIHISTAMINE used primarily as an ANTI-EMETIC in the treatment or prevention of motion sickness and vomiting caused either by chemotherapy for cancer or by infection of the middle or inner ear. Administration (as cyclizine hydrochloride, cyclizine lactate or cyclizine tartrate) is oral in the form of tablets, or by injection.
Related article: VALOID.

cyclopentolate hydrochloride is an ANTICHOLINERGIC drug that is used in eye-drops to dilate the pupil and paralyse the ciliary muscle (which

C

alters the curvature of the lens). Used to prepare a patient for ophthalmic examination and, less commonly, to assist in the treatment of eye inflammations, cyclopentolate's action may last for up to 24 hours.

▲ side-effects: vision may be affected to some degree for the duration of the drug's action. Susceptible patients may experience raised pressure within the eye.

✚ warning: cyclopentolate hydrochloride should be administered with caution to patients with raised pressure within the eyeball (glaucoma). Contact dermatitis may appear where the drug touches the skin.

Related articles: MINIMS CYCLOPENTOLATE; MYDRILATE; OPULETS.

cyclophosphamide is a CYTOTOXIC drug that is widely used in the treatment of some forms of leukaemia and lymphoma, and some solid tumours. It works by interfering with the DNA of new cells, so preventing normal cell replication, but it remains inactive until metabolised by the liver. On rare occasions it has been used to treat "resistant" nephrotic syndrome in children. Administration is oral in the form of tablets, or by injection, and should be accompanied by increased fluid intake.

▲ side-effects: there is commonly nausea and vomiting; there is often also hair loss.

✚ warning: cyclophosphamide should be administered with caution to patients with impaired kidney function. It may in susceptible patients cause an unpleasant form of cystitis (inflammation of the bladder); greatly increased fluid intake or the simultaneous administration of the synthetic drug MESNA may help to avoid the problem.

Related article: ENDOXANA.

cyclopropane is a gas used as an inhalant general ANAESTHETIC for both induction and maintenance of general anaesthesia. It has some MUSCLE RELAXANT properties too, although in practice a muscle relaxant drug is usually administered simultaneously. However, it has the great disadvantage of being potentially explosive in air, and must be used via closed-circuit systems.

▲ side-effects: although recovery afterwards is rapid, there may be vomiting and agitation.

✚ warning: cyclopropane causes respiratory depression, and some form of assisted pulmonary ventilation may be necessary during anaesthesia.

cycloserine is an ANTIBIOTIC drug used specifically in the treatment of tuberculosis that proves to be resistant to the powerful drugs ordinarily used first, or in cases where those drugs are not tolerated. Administration is oral in the form of capsules.

▲ side-effects: there may be headache, dizziness, and drowsiness; possible sensitivity reactions include a rash or, rarely, convulsions.

✚ cycloserine should not be administered to patients with epilepsy, depressive illness, anxiety or psychosis; it should be administered with caution to those with impaired kidney function.

cyclosporin is a powerful IMMUNOSUPPRESSANT that is particularly used to limit tissue rejection during and following transplant surgery. Unusually, it has very little effect on the blood-cell producing capacity of the bone-marrow. Administration is oral in the form of an oily solution, or by dilute intravenous infusion. Treatment can be monitored by measuring the amount of the drug in the bloodstream.
▲ side-effects: treatment may result in impaired liver and kidney function, with gastrointestinal disturbances; some patients experience tremor or excessive hair growth.
✚ warning: treatment with cyclosporin inevitably leaves the body much more open to infection because part of the immune system – its defence mechanism against microbial invasion – is rendered non-functional.
Related article: SANDIMMUN.

cyproheptadine hydrochloride is a powerful ANTIHISTAMINE that has the unusual distinction of inhibiting not only allergic responses resulting from the release of histamine in the body, but also those allergic responses resulting from the similar release of serotonin. Cyproheptadine is thus capable of treating a much wider range of allergic symptoms than almost any other antihistamine. Moreover, it is sometimes also used to treat migraine and – under medical supervision – to stimulate the appetite (especially in children). Administration is oral in the form of tablets or a dilute syrup.
▲ side-effects: there may be a sedative effect (or, in susceptible patients – especially children – excitement), a headache, and/or weight gain; some patients experience dry mouth, blurred vision, gastrointestinal disturbances and/or urinary retention.
✚ warning: cyproheptadine hydrochloride should be administered with caution to patients with epilepsy, glaucoma, liver disease or enlargement of the prostate gland.
Related article: PERIACTIN.

cytarabine is an ANTICANCER drug used primarily in the treatment of leukaemia. It works by combining with newly forming cells in a way that prevents normal cell replication (it is cytostatic rather than cytotoxic). Administration is by injection.
▲ side-effects: there is commonly nausea and vomiting; there is often also hair loss.
✚ warning: cytarabine has a severely depressive effect upon the blood-cell forming capacity of the bone-marrow: constant blood counts are essential. Leakage of the drug into the tissues at the site of the injection my cause tissue damage.
Related article: CYTOSAR.

Cytosar (*Upjohn*) is a proprietary ANTICANCER drug, available only on prescription, used to treat acute forms of leukaemia. Produced in the form of a powder for reconstitution as a medium for injection (in vials in two strengths, with or without diluent), Cytosar is a preparation of the cytostatic drug cytarabine.
▲/✚ side-effects/warning: *see* CYTARABINE

*cytotoxic drugs are used mainly in the treatment of cancer (and thus form a major group of the ANTICANCER drugs). They have the essential property of preventing normal cell replication, and so inhibiting the growth of tumours or of excess cells in body fluids. There are several mechanisms by which they do this. However, in every case they inevitably also affect the growth of normal healthy cells and cause toxic side-effects, generally in the form of nausea and vomiting, with hair loss. Most used cytotoxic drugs are the alkylating agents, which work by interfering with the action of DNA in cell replication; they include CYCLOPHOSPHAMIDE and CISPLATIN. The VINCA ALKALOIDS damage part of the metabolic features of newly forming cells; they too are effective cytotoxic drugs but tend to have severely limiting neural side-effects. Some cytotoxic drugs have additional antibiotic properties: such drugs include DOXORUBICIN HYDROCHLORIDE, ACTINOMYCIN D and BLEOMYCIN. Not all cytotoxic drugs are used in cancer treatment; some, for example AZATHIOPRINE, are used as immunosuppressants to limit tissue rejection during and following transplant surgery.

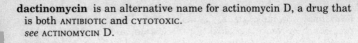

dactinomycin is an alternative name for actinomycin D, a drug that is both ANTIBIOTIC and CYTOTOXIC.
see ACTINOMYCIN D.

Daktacort (*Janssen*) is a proprietary cream for topical application, available only on prescription, that contains the CORTICOSTEROID hydrocortisone and the ANTIFUNGAL agent miconazole nitrate in a water-miscible base. It is used to treat skin inflammation in which fungal infection is also present.
▲/✚ side-effects/warning: *see* HYDROCORTISONE; MICONAZOLE.

Daktarin (*Janssen*) is a proprietary ANTIFUNGAL drug, available only on prescription, used to treat both systemic and skin-surface fungal infections. Produced in the form of tablets and as a solution for infusion (after dilution), Daktarin is a preparation of the IMIDAZOLE miconazole. Three other versions are available without prescription, in the form of a sugar-free gel for oral treatment, and a water-miscible cream and a spray powder in an aerosol for topical application.
▲/✚ side-effects/warning: *see* MICONAZOLE.

Dalacin C (*Upjohn*) is a proprietary ANTIBIOTIC, available only on prescription, used to treat staphylococcal infections of bones and joints, and peritonitis (inflammation of the peritoneal lining of the abdominal cavity). Produced in the form of capsules (in two strengths), as a pediatric suspension for dilution (the potency of the suspension once dilute is retained for 14 days), and in ampoules for injection, Dalacin C is a preparation of the drug clindamycin. Side-effects are potentially severe.
▲/✚ side-effects/warning: *see* CLINDAMYCIN.

Dalacin T (*Upjohn*) is a proprietary ANTIBIOTIC available only on prescription, used to treat acne. Produced in the form of a solution for topical application, it is a preparation of the antibiotic clindamycin phosphate; not recommended for children. The serious colitis, which affects a small percentage of patients who take clindamycin orally, is not a problem with the topical use of this product.
▲/✚ side-effects/warning: *see* CLINDAMYCIN.

Dalivit (*Paines & Byrne*) is a proprietary non-prescription MULTIVITAMIN compound for use as a dietary supplement that is not available from the National Health Service. Produced in the form of tablets, as oral drops, and as a syrup, Dalivit contains retinol (vitamin A), many forms of vitamin B (thiamine, riboflavine, PYRIDOXINE, nicotinamide and pantothenic acid), ASCORBIC ACID (vitamin C), and CALCIFEROL (vitamin D).

Daneral SA (*Hoechst*) is a proprietary non-prescription ANTIHISTAMINE used to treat the symptoms of allergy, such as hay fever or urticaria. Produced in the form of sustained-release tablets, Daneral SA is a preparation of pheniramine maleate.
▲/✚ side-effects/warning: *see* PHENIRAMINE MALEATE.

D

dapsone is an ANTIBIOTIC compound used specifically to treat leprosy (in both lepromatous and tuberculoid forms); it is also sometimes used to treat severe forms of dermatitis or, in combination with the enzyme-inhibitor pyrimethamine (under the trade name Maloprim), to prevent tropical travellers from contracting malaria. Administration is oral in the form of tablets, or by injection.
▲ side-effects: side-effects are rare at low doses (as for leprosy), but with higher dosage there may be nausea, vomiting and headache, insomnia and increased heart rate, severe weight loss, anaemia and/or hepatitis.
✚ warning: dapsone should be administered with caution to patients with heart or lung disease.
Related article: MALOPRIM.

Daraprim (*Wellcome*) is a proprietary non-prescription ANTIMALARIAL drug used to prevent tropical travellers from contracting malaria. It works by interfering with the cellular composition of the parasitic organism that causes malaria, but treatment must be continued for four weeks after leaving the area of exposure. A preparation of pyrimethamine, Daraprim is not recommended for children aged under five years.
▲/✚ side-effects/warning: *see* PYRIMETHAMINE.

Day Nurse (*Beecham Health Care*) is a proprietary, non-prescription cold relief preparation produced in the form of tablets and as a syrup. It contains paracetamol, the DECONGESTANT phenylpropanolamine and the ANTITUSSIVE dextromethorphan.
▲/✚ side-effects/warning: *see* PARACETAMOL; DEXTROMETHORPHAN.

DDAVP (*Ferring*) is a proprietary preparation of the antidiuretic hormone vasopressin in the form of its analog DESMOPRESSIN. Available only on prescription, it is administered primarily to diagnose or to treat pituitary-originated diabetes insipidus. DDAVP is also used to treat bed wetting, which has not responded to simpler measures in older children. It is produced in ampoules for injection but is most commonly given by the intranasal route.
▲/✚ side-effects/warning: *see* VASOPRESSIN.

Decadron (*Merck, Sharp & Dohme*) is a proprietary CORTICOSTEROID preparation, available only on prescription, used to treat inflammation especially in rheumatic or allergic conditions. Produced in the form of tablets, it comprises the glucocorticoid steroid dexamethasone. Because Decadron is such a powerful corticosteroid it is rarely used in childhood.
▲/✚ side-effects/warning: *see* DEXAMETHASONE.

Decadron Injection (*Merck, Sharp & Dohme*) is a proprietary CORTICOSTEROID preparation (produced in vials), available only on prescription, used primarily in emergencies to replace steroid loss; but the injection − comprising dexamethasone sodium phosphate − can also be used to treat inflammation in the joints or in soft tissues.
▲/✚ side-effects/warning: *see* DEXAMETHASONE.

Decadron Shock-pak (*Merck, Sharp & Dohme*) is a proprietary CORTICOSTEROID preparation of dexamethasone sodium phosphate (produced in greater concentration and larger vials than Decadron Injection), available only on prescription, used in emergencies to replace steroid loss and thus to assist in the treatment of shock. Administered by intravenous injection, it is not recommended for children.
▲/✚ side-effects/warning: *see* DEXAMETHASONE.

*decongestants are drugs administered to relieve or reduce nasal congestion. Generally applied in the form of nose-drops or as a nasal spray − although some are administered orally − most decongestants are SYMPATHOMIMETIC drugs, which work by constricting the blood vessels within the mucous membranes of the nasal cavity, so reducing the membranes' thickness and creating more room for drainage and ventilation. Nasal congestion caused by allergy, as in hay fever, however, is usually dealt with by using ANTIHISTAMINES, which inhibit the allergic response, or CORTICOSTEROIDS, which inhibit the allergic response and reduce any inflammation. If used for too long, nasal decongestants can result in rebound congestion of the nose on stopping of their use. Therefore saline nose drops (consisting of water with a little salt) are often preferred.

Decortisyl (*Roussel*) is a proprietary CORTICOSTEROID preparation, available only on prescription, used to treat inflammation especially in rheumatic or allergic conditions. Produced in the form of tablets, it contains the glucocorticoid steroid prednisone. It is not recommended for children aged under 12 months.
▲/✚ side-effects/warning: *see* PREDNISONE.

Deltacortril (*Pfizer*) is a proprietary CORTICOSTEROID preparation, available only on prescription, used to treat allergic conditions, such as asthma, requiring systemic treatment with corticosteroids. Produced in the form of tablets in two strengths, (also under the name Deltacortril Enteric), it contains the glucocorticoid steroid prednisolone.
▲/✚ side-effects/warning: *see* PREDNISOLONE.

Deltalone (*DDSA Pharmaceuticals*) is a proprietary CORTICOSTEROID preparation, available only on prescription, used to treat inflammation and allergic conditions such as asthma. Produced in the form of tablets (in two strengths), it contains the glucocorticoid steroid prednisolone.
▲/✚ side-effects/warning: *see* PREDNISOLONE.

Delta-Phoricol (*Wallace*) is a proprietary CORTICOSTEROID preparation, available only on prescription, used to treat inflammation especially in rheumatic and allergic conditions such as asthma. Produced in the form of tablets, it contains the glucocorticoid steroid prednisolone.
▲/✚ side-effects/warning: *see* PREDNISOLONE.

Deltastab (*Boots*) is a proprietary CORTICOSTEROID preparation, available only on prescription, used to treat inflammation especially in allergic conditions such as asthma. It may also be used for systemic corticosteroid therapy. Produced in the form of tablets (in two strengths), and in vials for injection (as an aqueous solution), it contains the glucocorticoid steroid prednisolone.

▲/✚ side-effects/warning: *see* PREDNISOLONE.

demeclocycline hydrochloride is a broad-spectrum ANTIBIOTIC, one of the TETRACYCLINES, used to treat infections of many kinds. Administration is oral in the form of tablets and capsules.

▲ side-effects: there may be nausea and vomiting, with diarrhoea. Some patients experience a sensitivity to light. Rarely, there are allergic reactions.

✚ warning: demeclocycline hydrochloride should not be administered to patients with kidney failure, or who are aged under 12 years. It should be administered with caution to patients with impaired liver function.

Related articles: DETECLO; LEDERMYCIN.

Depo-Medrone (*Upjohn*) is a proprietary CORTICOSTEROID preparation, available only on prescription, used to treat inflammation and sometimes used additionally to treat shock. Produced in vials and pre-prepared syringes for intramuscular depot injection, Depo-Medrone is a preparation of the steroid methylprednisolone acetate (in aqueous solution).

▲/✚ side-effects/warning: *see* METHYLPREDNISOLONE.

Dequacaine (*Farley*) is the name of a proprietary non-prescription lozenge containing the local ANAESTHETIC benzocaine together with the ANTIFUNGAL agent dequalinium chloride, to be sucked slowly until it dissolves, so affording relief from the pain of mouth ulcers or other oral lesions.

✚ warning: *see* BENZOCAINE.

Dequadin (*Farley*) is the name of a proprietary non-prescription lozenge containing the ANTIFUNGAL agent dequalinium chloride, to be sucked slowly until it dissolves, so treating oral infections.

Derbac-C (*International Labs*) is a proprietary non-prescription antiparasitic drug used to treat infestations of the scalp and pubic hair by lice (pediculosis). Produced in the form of a shampoo, Derbac-C (also called Derbac Shampoo) is a preparation of the pediculicide carbaryl.

▲/✚ side-effects/warning: *see* CARBARYL.

Derbac-M (*International Labs*) is a proprietary non-prescription antiparasitic drug used to treat infestations of the scalp and pubic hair by lice (pediculosis), or of the skin by the itch-mite (scabies). Produced in the form of a lotion, Derbac-M is a preparation of the insecticide malathion.

✚ warning: see MALATHION.

Derbac Shampoo is another name for Derbac-C.
see DERBAC-C.

D

Dermalex (*Labaz*) is a proprietary non-prescription skin lotion and emollient (soother and softener), used to treat nappy rash and to prevent bedsores. Its major active constituent is the ANTISEPTIC hexachlorophane. It is not recommended for children aged under two years.
▲/✚ side-effects/warning: *see* HEXACHLOROPHANE.

Dermonistat (*Ortho-Cilag*) is a proprietary non-prescription ANTIFUNGAL cream used to treat infections of the skin and the nails. Dermonistat is a preparation of the IMIDAZOLE miconazole nitrate.
▲/✚ side-effects/warning: *see* MICONAZOLE.

Dermovate (*Glaxo*) is an extremely powerful CORTICOSTEROID preparation for topical application, available only on prescription, used (in the short term only) to treat severe exacerbations in serious inflammatory skin disorders such as discoid lupus erythematosus. Produced in the form of a water-miscible cream for dilution (the potency of the cream once dilute is retained for 14 days), and as a scalp application in an alcohol base, Dermovate is in all forms a preparation of the steroid clobetasol propionate. It is rarely used in children.
▲/✚ side-effects/warning: *see* CLOBETASOL PROPIONATE.

Dermovate-NN (*Glaxo*) is a combined ANTIBIOTIC, ANTIFUNGAL and CORTICOSTEROID preparation for topical application, available only on prescription, used (in the short term only) to treat severe exacerbations in serious inflammatory skin disorders such as discoid lupus erythematosus. Produced in the form of a cream, and as an ointment in an anhydrous base for dilution with white soft paraffin (the potency of the ointment once dilute is retained for 14 days), Dermovate-NN is in both forms a preparation of the steroid clobetasol propionate with the broad-spectrum ANTIBIOTIC neomycin sulphate and the ANTIFUNGAL agent nystatin. It is rarely used in children.
▲/✚ side-effects/warning: *see* CLOBETASOL PROPIONATE; NEOMYCIN; NYSTATIN.

Deseril (*Sandoz*) is a proprietary preparation of the potentially dangerous drug methysergide, available only on prescription (and generally only in hospitals under strict medical supervision). It is used primarily to prevent severe recurrent migraine and similar headaches in patients for whom other forms of treatment have failed. Deseril is produced in the form of tablets.
▲/✚ side-effects/warning: *see* METHYSERGIDE.

Desferal (*Ciba*) is a proprietary form of the CHELATING AGENT desferrioxamine mesylate, available only on prescription, used to treat iron poisoning. It is also used in an effort to reduce iron levels in children who require frequent blood transfusions (as in thalassaemia).
▲/✚ side-effects/warning: *see* DESFERRIOXAMINE MESYLATE.

desferrioxamine mesylate is a CHELATING AGENT used to treat iron poisoning. It is also used in an effort to reduce iron levels in children who require frequent blood transfusions (as in thalassaemia). In cases of poisoning
administration can be oral (in water) following initial emptying of the stomach either by induction of vomiting or by stomach pump. Iron can also be chelated by an intramuscular injection of desferrioxamine mesylate or subcutaneous infusion.
▲ side-effects: there may be pain at the site of injection.
✚ warning: over-rapid injection of the drug can lead to sensitivity reactions and low blood pressure (hypotension).
Related article: DESFERAL.

desmopressin is one of two major forms of the antidiuretic hormone vasopressin, which reduces urine production. It is used primarily to diagnose or to treat pituitary-originated diabetes insipidus. Desmopressin is also used to treat bed wetting, which has not responded to simpler measures, in older children. It is produced in ampoules for injection but is usually given by way of the nose.
▲/✚ side-effects/warning: *see* VASOPRESSIN.

desonide is a powerful CORTICOSTEROID, used in topical application on severe skin inflammations (such as eczema), especially in cases where less powerful steroid treatments have failed. Administration is in the form of a dilute aqueous cream or a dilute paraffin-based ointment. It is not usually used in children.
▲ side-effects: topical application may result in the thinning of skin, with possible whitening, and an increased local growth of hair. Some young patients experience the outbreak of a kind of inflammatory dermatitis on the face or at the site of application.
✚ warning: as with all corticosteroids, desonide treats the symptoms of inflammation but has no effect on any underlying infection; undetected infection may thus become worse because its effects are masked by the steroid. Desonide should not in any case be administered to patients who suffer from infected skin lesions; use on the face should also be avoided; caution is advised in treatment of children.
Related article: TRIDESILON.

desoxymethasone is a CORTICOSTEROID drug used to treat acute inflammatory conditions resulting from skin disorders and allergic reactions. Administration is topical in the form of an oily cream. It is not usually used in children.
▲ side-effects: topical application may result in the thinning of skin, with possible whitening, and an increased local growth of hair. Some young patients experience the outbreak of a kind of inflammatory dermatitis on the face or at the site of application when they use desoxymethasone.
✚ warning: as with all corticosteroids, desoxymethasone treats the symptoms of inflammation but has no effect on any underlying infection; undetected infection may thus become worse because its effects are masked by the steroid. Desoxymethasone should not in

D

any case be administered to patients with untreated skin lesions; use on the face should also be avoided; caution is advised in treatment of children.
Related article: STIEDEX.

Deteclo (*Lederle*) is a proprietary compound ANTIBIOTIC preparation, available only on prescription, used to treat many kinds of infection, but especially those of the respiratory tract, the ear, nose and throat, the gastrointestinal tract and the urinary tract, and the soft tissues. Deteclo consists of a combination of TETRACYCLINES − chlortetracycline hydrochloride, tetracycline hydrochloride and demeclocycline hydrochloride − is produced in the form of tablets, and is not recommended for children under 12 years.
▲/✚ side-effects/warning: *see* CHLORTETRACYCLINE; DEMECLOCYCLINE HYDROCHLORIDE; TETRACYCLINE.

Dettol (*Reckitt & Colman*) is a well-known proprietary non-prescription ANTISEPTIC lotion, used for ordinary disinfectant purposes or in treating abrasions and minor wounds. It is a preparation of chloroxylenol (in mild solution).

dexamethasone is a synthesized powerful CORTICOSTEROID used, as are most corticosteroids, in the treatment of non-infective inflammation. It is sometimes also used in the treatment of swelling of the brain (raised intracranial pressure), but, apart from this use, it is rarely used in children.
▲ side-effects: systemic treatment of susceptible patients may engender a euphoria − or a state of confusion or depression. Rarely, there is peptic ulceration.
    Treatment of eye inflammations may, in susceptible patients, lead to a form of glaucoma (and should therefore be carried out under careful supervision).
✚ warning: in children, prolonged administration of dexamethasone may lead to stunting of growth. As with all corticosteroids, dexamethasone treats only inflammatory symptoms; an undetected and potentially serious infection may have its effects masked by the drug until it is well established.
Related articles: DECADRON; DECADRON SHOCK-PAK; DEXA-RHINASPRAY; MAXIDEX; MAXITROL; SOFRADEX.

Dexa-Rhinaspray (*Boehringer Ingelheim*) is a proprietary nasal inhalation, available only on prescription, used to treat hay fever (allergic rhinitis). Produced in a metered-dose aerosol, it is a preparation of the CORTICOSTEROID dexamethasone isonicotinate together with the ANTIBIOTIC neomycin sulphate and the SYMPATHOMIMETIC tramazoline hydrochloride. It is not recommended for children aged under five years.
▲/✚ side-effects/warning: *see* DEXAMETHASONE; NEOMYCIN.

dextran is a carbohydrate, chemically consisting of glucose units, used in solution as a plasma substitute − that is, as a substitute for the fluid in which blood cells are normally suspended. It is most used in infusion to increase a patient's overall volume of blood following drastic haemorrhage or other forms of shock (such as burns or septicaemia). Generally, administration is on an emergency basis only, until properly tissue-matched blood can be infused. Even so, dextran in a patient's circulation may interfere with the cross-matching process and such tissue-typing should ideally take place first. There are two major preparations of dextran: dextran 40 and dextran 70. Dextran 40 is a 10% concentration in glucose or saline solution, and is used mostly to improve blood flow in the limbs and extremities (so treating ischaemic conditions and preventing thrombosis or embolism). Dextran 70 is a 6% concentration in glucose or saline solution, and is used mostly as outlined initially above to expand a patient's overall blood volume. There is also a proprietary form of dextran 110 which is to all intents and purposes very much the same as dextran 70.

⚠ side-effects: rarely, there are hypersensitivity reactions.

✚ warning: dextran should not be administered to patients with severe congestive heart failure or kidney failure, or who may experience blood clotting difficulties.

Related articles: DEXTRAVEN 110; GENTRAN; MACRODEX; RHEOMACRODEX.

Dextraven 110 (*CP Pharmaceuticals*) is a proprietary preparation of dextran 110, available only on prescription, used in infusion to boost the overall volume of a patient's blood circulation in emergency circumstances. It is produced in flasks (bottles).

⚠/✚ side-effects/warning: *see* DEXTRAN.

Dextrolyte (*Cow & Gate*) is a proprietary non-prescription oral rehydration solution, used the management of gastroenteritis. Dextrolyte is produced in the form of an oral solution containing SODIUM CHLORIDE (salt), POTASSIUM CHLORIDE, GLUCOSE and sodium lactate.

dextromethorphan is an ANTITUSSIVE, an opiate that is used singly or in combination with other drugs in linctuses, syrups and lozenges to relieve dry or painful coughs.

⚠ side-effects: constipation is a comparatively common side-effect.

✚ warning: dextromethorphan should not be administered to patients who suffer from liver disease. Used as a linctus, it may cause sputum retention which may be injurious to patients with asthma, chronic bronchitis or bronchiectasis (two conditions for which linctuses are commonly prescribed). Its use should be avoided in babies.

Related articles: ACTIFED COMPOUND LINCTUS.

dextromoramide is a synthesized derivative of morphine, and like morphine is used as a narcotic ANALGESIC to counter severe and intractable pain, particularly in the final stages of terminal illness. Proprietary forms are on the controlled drugs list because, also like morphine, dextromoramide is potentially addictive.

⚠ side-effects: shallow breathing, urinary retention, constipation, and nausea are all common; tolerance and dependence (addiction) occur fairly readily. There may also be drowsiness, and pain at the site of injection (where there may also be tissue damage).

D

✚warning: dextromoramide should not be administered to patients who suffer from a head injury or intracranial pressure; it should be administered with caution to those with impaired kidney or liver function, asthma, depressed respiration, insufficient secretion of thyroid hormones (hypothyroidism) or low blood pressure (hypotension).
Related article: PALFIUM.

dextropropoxyphene is a weak ANALGESIC that is nevertheless similar to a narcotic, used to treat pain anywhere in the body. It is usually combined with other analgesics (especially paracetamol or aspirin) for compound effect. Administration of the drug alone is oral in the form of capsules.
▲side-effects: shallow breathing, urinary retention, constipation, and nausea are all common; in high overdosage, tolerance and dependence (addiction) occur fairly readily, leading possibly to psychoses and convulsions.
✚warning: dextropropoxyphene should not be administered to patients who suffer from head injury or intracranial pressure; it should be administered with caution to those with impaired kidney or liver function, asthma, depressed respiration, insufficient secretion of thyroid hormones (hypothyroidism) or low blood pressure (hypotension).

dextrose (or dextrose monohydrate) is another term for glucose.
see GLUCOSE.

DF118 (*Duncan, Flockhart*) is a proprietary narcotic ANALGESIC available on prescription only to private patients, used to treat moderate to severe pain anywhere in the body. Produced in the form of tablets and as an elixir for dilution (the potency of the elixir once dilute is retained for 14 days) and in ampoules (as a controlled drug) for injection, DF118 is a preparation of the narcotic dihydrocodeine tartrate.
▲/✚ side-effects/warning: *see* DIHYDROCODEINE TARTRATE.

Dialamine (*Scientific Hospital Supplies*) is a proprietary non-prescription nutritional supplement for patients who need extra amino acids (perhaps following kidney failure). Produced in the form of a powder for reconstitution as an orange-flavoured liquid, Dialamine contains essential amino acids, carbohydrate, ascorbic acid (vitamin C), minerals and trace elements.

diamorphine is the chemical name of heroin, a white crystalline powder that is a derivative of morphine. Like morphine, it is a powerful narcotic ANALGESIC useful in the treatment of moderate to severe pain, although it has a shorter duration of effect. Again like morphine, its use quickly leads to tolerance and then dependence (addiction). Administration is oral in the form of tablets or an elixir, or by injection.
▲side-effects: there may be euphoria, depending on dosage. There may also be constipation and low blood pressure. In some patients

there is respiratory depression with high dosage.
+ warning: diamorphine should not be administered to patients with
renal or liver disease; it should be administered with caution to
those with asthma (because it tends to cause sputum retention).

Diarrest (*Galen*) is a proprietary antidiarrhoeal drug, available only
on prescription, that is a preparation of the OPIATE codeine phosphate
together with sodium and potassium salts as supplements to replace
minerals lost through vomiting and diarrhoea. (The opiate has the
capacity to reduce intestinal motility). Diarrest is produced in the
form of a liquid (for swallowing); prolonged use must be avoided.
Treatment of diarrhoea in childhood is best carried out using oral
rehydration therapy. Medication should rarely, if ever, be used.
▲/+ side-effects/warning: *see* CODEINE PHOSPHATE.

Diatensec (*Gold Cross*) is a proprietary DIURETIC, available only on
prescription, used to treat the symptoms of cirrhosis of the liver or of
kidney disease, and to assist in the treatment of heart failure.
Produced in the form of tablets, it is a preparation of the mild
potassium-sparing diuretic spironolactone.
▲/+ side-effects/warning: *see* SPIRONOLACTONE.

Diazemuls (*KabiVitrum*) is a proprietary ANXIOLYTIC drug, available
only on prescription, used to treat anxiety. Its most common use in
children is to stop convulsions, when it is given by intravenous
injection. It may be used additionally to provide sedation for very
minor surgery or as a premedication prior to surgical procedures.
Produced as an emulsion in ampoules for injection, Diazemuls is a
preparation of the BENZODIAZEPINE diazepam.
▲/+ side-effects/warning: *see* DIAZEPAM.

diazepam is an ANXIOLYTIC drug, one of the BENZODIAZEPINES, used to
treat anxiety. Its most common use in children is to stop convulsions,
when it is given by intravenous injection and rectally. It may be used
additionally to provide sedation for very minor surgery or as a
premedication prior to surgical procedures. Diazepam also has
properties as a muscle relaxant, which may be useful in the treament
of spasticity. Administration is oral in the form of tablets, capsules or
a dilute elixir, topical as suppositories, or by injection.
▲ side-effects: there may be drowsiness, dizziness, headache, dry
mouth, urinary retention, and shallow breathing; hypersensitivity
reactions may occur.
+ warning: concentration and speed of thought and movement are
often affected. Diazepam should be administered with caution to
patients with respiratory difficulties.
Related articles: ALUPRAM; ATENSINE; DIAZEMULS; STESOLID; VALIUM.

diazoxide is used to treat chronic conditions involving a deficit of
glucose in the bloodstream (as occurs, for example, if a pancreatic
tumour causes excessive secretion of insulin). It is given by mouth. It
is also useful in treating an acute hypertensive crisis (apoplexy).
Administration is then by injection.

▲ side-effects: there may be nausea and vomiting, an increased heart rate with low blood pressure (hypotension), loss of appetite, accumulation of fluid in the tissues (oedema), arrhythmias, and hyperglycaemia.

✚ warning: diazoxide should be administered with caution to patients with reduced blood supply to the heart or impaired kidney function. During prolonged treatment, regular monitoring of blood constituents and pressure is essential.

Related article: EUDEMINE.

Dibenyline (*Smith, Kline & French*) is a proprietary vasodilator used (in combination with a BETA-BLOCKER) in the treatment of the high blood pressure (*see* ANTIHYPERTENSIVE) caused by tumours in the adrenal glands and the resulting secretion of the hormones adrenaline and noradrenaline. Produced in the form of capsules and in ampoules for injection, Dibenyline is a preparation of phenoxybenzamine hydrochloride.

dichloralphenazone is a HYPNOTIC drug used to treat insomnia, particularly in children. Prolonged use leads to tolerance and dependence (addiction). Administration is oral in the form of tablets or a dilute elixir.

▲ side-effects: there is commonly drowsiness, dizziness, headache and dry mouth. More rarely there may be gastrointestinal disturbances or a rash.

✚ warning: concentration and speed of movement and thought are affected. Dichloralphenazone should be administered with caution to patients with lung disease. Keep the drug off the skin and the mucous membranes.

Related article: WELLDORM.

diclofenac sodium is a non-steroidal ANTI-INFLAMMATORY non-narcotic ANALGESIC drug used to treat pain and inflammation in rheumatic disease and other muscular-skeletal disorders (such as arthritis and gout). Administration is oral in the form of tablets, topical in the form of anal suppositories, or by injection.

▲ side-effects: there may be nausea and gastrointestinal disturbance (to avoid which a patient may be advised to take the drug with food or milk), headache and ringing in the ears (tinnitus). Some patients experience sensitivity reactions (such as a rash or the symptoms of asthma). Fluid retention and/or blood disorders may occur.

✚ warning: diclofenac sodium should be administered with caution to patients with gastric ulcers, impaired kidney or liver function, or allergic disorders (particularly if induced by aspirin or anti-inflammatory drugs).

Related article: VOLTAROL.

dicyclomine hydrochloride is a synthetic ANTICHOLINERGIC antispasmodic used primarily to assist in the treatment of gastrointestinal disorders caused by spasm (rigidity) in the muscular walls of the stomach or intestines. Administration is oral in the form of tablets, gel, or dilute syrup. It is not recommended for use on infants under the age of six months.

▲ side-effects: there is commonly dry mouth and thirst; there may also be visual disturbances, flushing, irregular heartbeat and constipation. Rarely there may be high temperature accompanied by delirium.
Related article: MERBENTYL.

Dicynene (*Delandale*) is a proprietary haemostatic drug, available only on prescription, used to treat haemorrhage blood vessels or to relieve excessive menstrual flow. Produced in the form of tablets (in two strengths) and in ampoules for injection (in two strengths), Dicynene is a preparation of ethamsylate. It is occasionally used to try to prevent haemorrhage in the brains of very premature babies.
▲/✚ side-effects/warning: *see* ETHAMSYLATE.

diethyl ether is the now old-fashioned "ether" used as a general ANAESTHETIC. Powerful as it is, it is now unpopular both because it is flammable and explosive in the presence of oxygen, and because it tends to cause nausea and vomiting in the patient. All the same, it is an effective anaesthetic under the influence of which body processes – in particular the heart rhythm – are generally well maintained.

Digibind (*Wellcome*) is an antidote to an overdose of the heart stimulant digoxin, and consists of digoxin-specific antibody fragments for emergency injection.
see DIGOXIN.

digoxin is a heart stimulant derived from the leaf of the digitalis plant, and is a CARDIAC GLYCOSIDE. The effect is to regularize and strengthen a heartbeat that is either too fast or too slow. Useful as it is, however, the drug has common toxic side-effects, the severity of which depend on each individual patient's specific condition. Monitoring of kidney function is particularly advisable. (Overdosage can be corrected by the administration of an antidote called DIGIBIND.) Digoxin is administered orally in the form of tablets or an elixir, or by injection. It is possible to perform blood level tests to decide on the correct dosage and this also helps prevent overdosage.
▲ side-effects: there is commonly a loss of appetite, nausea and vomiting, with a consequent weight loss (resulting in some cases in anorexia). There may also be visual disturbances. Overdosage may lead to heart irregularities.
✚ warning: digoxin should be administered with caution to patients who suffer from under-secretion of thyroid hormones (hypothyroidism). Regular monitoring of the blood potassium level is also recommended.
Related article: LANOXIN.

Dihydergot (*Sandoz*) is a proprietary preparation, available only on prescription, that is used specifically to treat migraine attacks. It also has ANTINAUSEANT properties. Produced in the form of tablets, as an oral solution, and in ampoules for injection, Dihydergot is a preparation of the ergotamine derivative dihydroergotamine mesylate.

D

▲/✚ side-effects/warning: *see* DIHYDROERGOTOMINE MESYLATE.

dihydrocodeine tartrate is a narcotic ANALGESIC that is similar to codeine. It is used to relieve pain, especially in cases where continued mobility is required, although it may cause some degree of dizziness and constipation. It is commonly used before and after surgery. Administration is oral in the form of tablets or a dilute elixir, or by injection.

▲ side-effects: there is dizziness, headache, and sedation; often there is also nausea and constipation. The effects of alcohol consumption may be increased.

✚ warning: dihydrocodeine tartrate should not be administered to patients with respiratory depression, obstructive airways disease, or to children aged under 12 months. Tolerance and dependence (addiction) readily occur.
Related article: DF118.

dihydroergotomine mesylate is an anti-migraine drug, a derivative of ergotamine that also has ANTINAUSEANT properties. It is used to treat migraine attacks, and is administered orally in the form of tablets or a solution, or by injection.

▲ side-effects: there may be nausea and vomiting, with headache, and paraesthesia, and possibly vascular spasm; if these develop the medication should be stopped.

✚ warning: dihydroergotamine mesylate should not be administered to patients with any infection or circulatory disorders of the limbs; it should be administered with caution to those with heart, liver or kidney disease, or an excess of thyroid hormones in the bloodstream (thryotoxicosis).
Related article: DIHYDERGOT.

dihydrotachysterol is a synthetic form of CALCIFEROL (vitamin D), used to make up body deficiencies. Calcium levels in the body should be regularly monitored during treatment. Administration is oral in the form of tablets and a solution.

✚ warning: overdosage may cause kidney damage. Although an increased amount of vitamin D is necessary during pregnancy, high body levels while lactating may also cause high levels of calcium in the breast-fed infant.
Related article: A.T. 10.

dimenhydrinate is an ANTIHISTAMINE that is effective in quelling nausea, and useful in preventing vomiting caused by travelling in a moving vehicle, by chemotherapy or radiation sickness. It is also used to assist in the treatment of the vertigo and loss of balance that accompanies infections of the middle or inner ear. Administration is oral in the form of tablets.

▲ side-effects: there may be dry mouth, drowsiness and headache, with blurred vision. Some patients experience gastrointestinal disturbances.

✚ warning: dimenhydrinate should be administered with caution to

patients who suffer from liver disease or epilepsy. Concentration and speed of thought and movement are affected.
Related article: DRAMAMINE.

dimercaprol is a CHELATING AGENT used as an antidote to poisoning with antimony, arsenic, bismuth, gold, mercury or thallium. Administration is by injection.
▲ side-effects: there is an increase in heart rate and blood pressure, sweating, weeping and agitation, nausea and vomiting, constriction of the throat and chest, and a burning sensation — all temporary unless too high a dosage is administered.

dimethicone is a water-repellent silicone used as an antifoaming agent and, when taken orally, thought to reduce flatulence while protecting mucous membranes. It is also a constituent in many barrier creams intended to protect against irritation or chapping (as in nappy rash). Not for use on acutely inflamed or weeping skin.
Related articles: ALTACITE PLUS; ASILONE; SIOPEL; VASOGEN.

dimethindene maleate is an ANTIHISTAMINE, used to treat the symptoms of allergic conditions such as hay fever and urticaria; it is also used, in combination with other drugs, in expectorants to loosen a dry cough. Administration is oral in the form of sustained-release tablets.
▲ side-effects: sedation may affect speed of thought and movement; there may be nausea, headaches and/or weight gain, dry mouth, gastrointestinal disturbances and visual problems.
Related articles: FENOSTIL RETARD.

Dimotane (*Robins*) is a proprietary non-prescription ANTIHISTAMINE, used to treat the symptoms of allergic conditions such as hay fever and urticaria. Produced as tablets, as sustained-release tablets (under the name Dimotane LA), and as an elixir for dilution (the potency of the elixir once dilute is retained for 14 days), Dimotane is a preparation of brompheniramine maleate.
▲/✚ side-effects/warning: *see* BROMPHENIRAMINE MALEATE.

Dimotane Expectorant (*Robins*) is a proprietary non-prescription EXPECTORANT that is not available from the National Health Service. Intended to promote the expulsion of excess bronchial secretions, it contains the ANTIHISTAMINE brompheniramine maleate and the VASOCONSTRICTOR phenylephrine hydrochloride, and is produced as a sugar-free elixir for dilution (the potency of the elixir once diluted is retained for 14 days).
▲/✚ side-effects/warning: *see* BROMPHENIRAMINE MALEATE; PHENYLEPHRINE.

Dimotane Plus (*Robins*) is a proprietary non-prescription oral preparation intended to clear a stuffed nose. It is a combination of the ANTIHISTAMINE brompheniramine maleate and the SYMPATHOMIMETIC pseudoephedrine hydrochloride, and is produced as a sugar-free liquid (in two strengths, the weaker labelled for children) for dilution with glycerol (the potency of the liquid once diluted is retained for 14 days).

D

▲/✚ side-effects/warning: *see* BROMPHENIRAMINE MALEATE; EPHEDRINE HYDROCHLORIDE.

Dimotane with Codeine (*Robins*) is a proprietary non-prescription cough linctus that is not available from the National Health Service. Intended both to promote the expulsion of excess bronchial secretions and to suppress a cough, it contains the OPIATE codeine phosphate, the ANTIHISTAMINE brompheniramine maleate and the SYMPATHOMIMETIC pseudoephedrine hydrochloride, and is produced as a sugar-free elixir (in two strengths, the weaker labelled for children) for dilution with glycerol (the potency of the elixir once diluted is retained for 14 days).
▲/✚ side-effects/warning: *see* BROMPHENIRAMINE MALEATE; CODEINE PHOSPHATE; EPHEDRINE HYDROCHLORIDE.

Dimotapp (*Robins*) is a proprietary non-prescription oral preparation intended to clear a stuffed nose; it is not available from the National Health Service. It contains the ANTIHISTAMINE brompheniramine maleate, the SYMPATHOMIMETIC VASOCONSTRICTOR phenylephrine hydrochloride, and the SYMPATHOMIMETIC phenylpropanolamine, and is produced as a sugar-free elixir (in two strengths, the weaker labelled for children) for dilution (the potency of the elixir once diluted is retained for 14 days), and in the form of sustained-release tablets (under the trade name Dimotapp LA).
▲/✚ side-effects/warning: *see* BROMPHENIRAMINE MALEATE; PHENYLEPHRINE.

Dinneford's (*Beecham Health Care*) is a proprietary, non-prescription magnesia gripe mixture. It contains citric acid, sucrose, ALCOHOL and the ANTACIDS sodium bicarbonate and magnesium carbonate.
▲/✚ side-effects/warning: *see* SODIUM BICARBONATE; MAGNESIUM CARBONATE.

Diocalm (*Beecham Health Care*) is a proprietary, non-prescription ANTIDIARRHOEAL preparation, containing the OPIATE morphine and attapulgite (magnesium aluminium silicate).
▲/✚ side-effects/warning: *see* MORPHINE.

Dioctyl (*Medo*) is a proprietary non-prescription LAXATIVE used to relieve constipation and also to evacuate the rectum prior to abdominal X-ray procedures. Produced in the form of tablets, and as a syrup (in two strengths, the weaker for children) for dilution (the potency of the syrup once diluted is retained for 14 days), Dioctyl is a preparation of DIOCTYL SODIUM SULPHOSUCCINATE (also called docusaste sodium).

Dioctyl Ear Drops (*Medo*) is a proprietary non-prescription preparation of DIOCTYL in the form of ear-drops, used for the dissolution and removal of ear wax. It is not for use in patients with perforated ear drum. Dioctyl Ear Drops is a preparation of DIOCTYL SODIUM SULPHOSUCCINATE (also called docusate sodium).

dioctyl sodium sulphosuccinate (or docusate sodium) is primarily a LAXATIVE that is used not only to relieve constipation but also to

evacuate the rectum prior to abdominal X-rays. It is a constituent of many proprietary compound laxatives because it appears to have few, if any, side-effects. It works as a surfactant, applying a very thin film of low surface tension (like a detergent) over the intestinal wall surface. Dioctyl sodium sulphosuccinate is also used in the form of ear-drops to dissolve and remove ear wax; again it is a constituent in many proprietary ear-drop preparations.
Related articles: DIOCTYL; DIOCTYL EAR DROPS; FLETCHER'S ENEMETTE; MOLCER; SOLIWAX; WAXSOL.

Dioderm (*Dermal*) is a proprietary, water-miscible, CORTICOSTEROID cream for topical application, used to treat mild inflammation of the skin. Available only on prescription, its major active constituent is the steroid hydrocortisone.
▲/✚ side-effects/warning: *see* HYDROCORTISONE.

Dioralyte (*Armour*) is a proprietary non-prescription oral rehydration solution used to treat gastroenteritis. Dioralyte is produced in the form of sachets containing a powder for solution, consisting of a compound of SODIUM CHLORIDE, POTASSIUM CHLORIDE, SODIUM BICARBONATE and GLUCOSE; flavours are plain, cherry or pineapple. It is also available in the form of effervescent tablets which dissolve in water. This latter preparation is not suitable for babies and very young children as it is fizzy.

Diovol (*Pharmax*) is a proprietary non-prescription ANTACID used to relieve acid stomach and flatulence, and to assist digestion in patients with peptic ulcers or hiatus hernia. Produced in the form of tablets for chewing or sucking, and as a mint- or fruit-flavoured suspension, Diovol is a compound preparation of aluminium hydroxide together with the antifoaming agent DIMETHICONE. It is not recommended for children aged under six years.

diphenhydramine hydrochloride is an ANTIHISTAMINE, one of the first to be discovered, used to treat allergic conditions such as hay fever and urticaria, some forms of dermatitis, and some sensitivity reactions to drugs. Its additional sedative properties are useful in the treatment of some allergic conditions, but the fact that it is also an ANTINAUSEANT makes it useful in the treatment or prevention of travel sickness, vertigo, and infections of the inner and middle ears. Administration is oral in the form of capsules.
▲ side-effects: the sedation that is caused by the drug may affect speed of thought and movement; there may be headache and/or weight gain, dry mouth, gastrointestinal disturbances and visual problems.
Related articles: BENYLIN DECONGESTANT; BENYLIN EXPECTORANT; HISTALIX.

diphenoxylate hydrochloride is a powerful ANTIDIARRHOEAL drug, an OPIATE used to treat chronic diarrhoea. It works by reducing the rate at which material travels along the intestines. Overdosage is uncommon but does occur, particularly in young children − however, the symptoms of overdosage (chiefly sedation) may not appear until some 48 hours after treatment, so monitoring of patients for at least that time is necessary. Because long-term treatment with diphenoxylate hydrochloride is liable to induce dependence (addiction), the drug is usually administered in combination with the belladonna alkaloid ATROPINE, which makes this less likely. Administration is oral in the form of tablets or as a sugar-free dilute liquid.

✚ warning: fluid intake must be maintained during treatment. The drug should not be used in patients with gastrointestinal obstruction or jaundice. Care should be taken in patients with ulcerative colitis, or hepatic disorders.

▲ side-effects: overdosage causes sedation. Prolonged usage may lead to impaired gastrointestinal function and eventual dependence. The presence of atropine, if added, may cause dry mouth, thirst and some visual disturbance in susceptible patients.
Related article: LOMOTIL.

diphenylpyraline hydrochloride is an ANTIHISTAMINE used to treat allergic conditions such as hay fever and urticaria, some forms of dermatitis, and some sensitivity reactions to drugs. Its additional sedative properties are useful in the treatment of some allergic conditions. Administration of the drug is oral in the form of sustained-release capsules (spansules) or tablets.

▲ side-effects: sedation may affect speed of thought and movement; there may be nausea, headache and/or weight gain, dry mouth, gastrointestinal disturbances and visual problems.
Related article: HISTRYL.

diphtheria vaccine is a VACCINE preparation of an antitoxin – that is, an antibody produced in response to the presence of the toxin of the diphtheria bacterium, rather than to the presence of the bacterium itself – prepared in horses, and adsorbed on to a mineral carrier (almost always aluminium hydroxide). Available only on prescription, the vaccine is produced in ampoules for injection. However, far more commonly, it is administered as one constituent in a triple vaccine (additionally against whooping cough – known as pertussis – and tetanus, often called the DPT vaccine) or in a double vaccine (with TETANUS VACCINE). Administered singly or in combination, diphtheria vaccine often causes allergic reactions.

diphtheria-pertussis-tetanus (DPT) vaccine is a combination of VACCINES against diphtheria, whooping cough and tetanus used for the routine immunization of infants.

▲/✚ side-effects/warning: *see* DIPHTHERIA VACCINE; PERTUSSIS VACCINE; TETANUS VACCINE.

diphtheria-tetanus vaccine is a combination of VACCINES against diphtheria and tetanus used for the routine immunization of infants, where for some reason it is thought best to avoid the pertussis (whooping cough) vaccine. This double vaccine is also used as a booster shot for children at the age of school entry.

▲/✚ side-effects/warning: *see* DIPHTHERIA VACCINE; TETANUS VACCINE.

Diprivan *(ICI)* is a proprietary form of the general ANAESTHETIC propofol, used primarily for the induction of anaesthesia at the start of a surgical operation, but sometimes also for its maintenance thereafter. Available only on prescription, it is produced as an emulsion in ampoules for injection.
▲/✚ side-effects/warning: *see* PROPOFOL.

Diprobase *(Kirby-Warrick)* is a proprietary non-prescription form of OINTMENT used as a base for medications; it is a combination of paraffins (and is intended for particular use with DIPROSONE).

Diprosalic *(Kirby-Warrick)* is a proprietary CORTICOSTEROID preparation, available only on prescription, used to treat severe non-infective skin inflammations such as eczema, particularly in patients who are not responding to less powerful steroids. Produced in the form of an ointment and an alcohol-based lotion for topical application, Diprosalic is a compound preparation of the steroid betamethasone dipropionate together with the ANTIBACTERIAL/ANTIFUNGAL drug salicylic acid. It is not usually used in children.
▲/✚ side-effects/warning: *see* BETAMETHASONE DIPROPIONATE; SALICYLIC ACID.

Diprosone *(Kirby-Warrick)* is a proprietary CORTICOSTEROID preparation, available only on prescription, used to treat severe non-infective skin inflammation such as eczema, particularly in patients who are not responding to less powerful steroids. Produced in the form of a water-miscible cream, as an ointment and as an alcohol-based lotion for topical application, Diprosone is a preparation of the steroid betamethasone dipropionate. It is not usually used in children.
▲/✚ side-effects/warning: *see* BETAMETHASONE DIPROPIONATE.

Disadine DP *(Stuart)* is a proprietary non-prescription form of the compound DISINFECTANT povidone-IODINE, prepared as a powder within an aerosol. For topical application, it is used to treat or prevent infection of the skin following injury or surgery, or to cleanse bedsores.

*disinfectants are agents that destroy micro-organisms, or inhibit their activity to a level such that they are less or no longer harmful to health. The term is applied to agents used on inanimate objects as well as to those used to treat the skin and living tissue, and in the latter case the term is often used synonymously with ANTISEPTIC.

Diskhaler *(A&H)* is a dry powder inhaler for asthma, used to deliver either VENTOLIN or BECOTIDE. The device is loaded with a disc containing eight doses. This form of inhaler is easier for children to use than a standard meter dosed aerosol inhaler.

Dispray 1 Quick Prep *(Stuart)* is a proprietary non-prescription DISINFECTANT used primarily to cleanse the skin prior to surgery or

D

injection. Produced in an aerosol for immediate topical application, it is a solution of CHLORHEXIDINE gluconate.

Disprol (*Reckitt & Colman*) is a proprietary non-prescription non-narcotic ANALGESIC for children that also helps to reduce high body temperature. Produced in the form of a sugar-free suspension, it is a preparation of paracetamol. Even as a paediatric preparation, however, it is not recommended for children aged under three months.
▲/✚ side-effects/warning: *see* PARACETAMOL.

Distaclor (*Dista*) is a proprietary broad-spectrum ANTIBIOTIC, available only on prescription, used to treat a wide range of bacterial infections, particularly of the skin and soft tissues, urinary tract, upper respiratory tract, and middle ear. Produced in the form of capsules and as a suspension (in two strengths) for dilution (the potency of the suspension once dilute is retained for 14 days), Distaclor is a preparation of the cephalosporin cefaclor.
▲/✚ side-effects/warning: *see* CEFACLOR.

Distamine (*Dista*) is a proprietary preparation, available only on prescription, used specifically to relieve the pain of rheumatoid arthritis, and potentially to halt the progress of the disease. Patients should be warned that treatment may take up to 12 weeks for any improvement to be manifest, and up to a year before full effect is achieved. The drug may also be used as a long-term CHELATING AGENT to treat poisoning by the metals copper (as in Wilson's disease) or lead. Produced in the form of tablets (in three strengths), Distamine is a preparation of the penicillin derivative penicillamine.
▲/✚ side-effects/warning: *see* PENICILLAMINE.

Distaquaine V-K (*Dista*) is a proprietary preparation of the penicillin-type ANTIBIOTIC phenoxymethylpenicillin, used mainly to treat infections of the head and throat, and some skin conditions; it may also be used to reduce high body temperature. Available only on prescription, it is produced in the form of tablets (in two strengths) or as an elixir (in three strengths) for dilution (the potency of the elixir once dilute is retained for seven days).
▲/✚ side-effects/warning: *see* PHENOXYMETHYLPENICILLIN.

dithranol is the most powerful drug presently used to treat chronic or milder forms of psoriasis in topical application. For about an hour at a time, lesions are covered with a dressing on which there is a preparation of the drug in mild solution. Concentration is adjusted not only to suit individual response but also in relation to each patient's tolerance of the associated skin irritation. Healthy skin (and the eyes) must be avoided. The drug may be used in combination with others that have a moisturizing effect.
▲ side-effects: irritation and a local sensation of burning are common.
✚ warning: dithranol is not suitable for the treatment of acute forms of psoriasis. The drug stains skin, hair and fabrics.
Related articles: ANTHRANOL; ANTRADERM; DITHROCREAM; DITHROLAN; PSORIN.

dithranol triacetate is a salt of dithranol and is used for the same purpose – the treatment of psoriasis – but is less effective and may be compared in this respect with COAL TAR.
▲/✚ side-effects/warning: *see* DITHRANOL.
    Related article: EXOLAN.

Dithrocream (*Dermal*) is a proprietary non-prescription preparation of the powerful drug dithranol, in dilute solution, used in topical application on dressings to treat chronic and mild forms of psoriasis. It is produced in the form of a water-miscible cream (in four strengths).
▲/✚ side-effects/warning: *see* DITHRANOL.

Dithrolan (*Dermal*) is a proprietary non-prescription preparation of the powerful drug dithranol, in dilute solution, together with the ANTIBACTERIAL/ANTIFUNGAL drug salicylic acid, and is used in topical application on dressings to treat chronic and mild forms of psoriasis. It is produced in the form of a paraffin-based ointment for dilution (the potency of the ointment once dilute is retained for 14 days).
▲/✚ side-effects/warning: *see* DITHRANOL; SALICYLIC ACID.

Diuresal (*Lagap*) is a proprietary DIURETIC, available only on prescription, used to treat the accumulation of fluid in the tissues (oedema) associated with heart, liver or kidney disorders. Produced in the form of tablets, and in ampoules for injection, Diuresal is a preparation of frusemide.
▲/✚ side-effects/warning: *see* FRUSEMIDE.

*diuretics are drugs that rid the body of fluids, generally by promoting their excretion in the form of urine. Accumulation of fluid in the tissues (oedema) is a common symptom of many disorders, particularly chronic disorders of the heart, liver, kidneys or lungs. Treatment with diuretics can thus assist in remedying such disorders. Salt and water retention also occurs in high blood pressure (hypertension), and diuretics are particularly used to treat that condition (as ANTIHYPERTENSIVE therapy), often in combination with a potassium supplement. Some diuretics are also useful in reducing the aqueous content of the eyeballs, so relieving internal pressure (as in glaucoma). Best known and most used diuretics are the THIAZIDES; other non-thiazide diuretics include ACETAZOLAMIDE, FRUSEMIDE, SPIRONOLACTONE and triamterene.

Dixarit (*WB Pharmaceuticals*) is a proprietary preparation of the ANTIHYPERTENSIVE drug clonidine hydrochloride, used in low dosage sometimes to try to prevent recurrent migraine and similar headaches. It is produced in the form of tablets, and administration is by the oral route.
▲/✚ side-effects/warning: *see* CLONIDINE HYDROCHLORIDE.

dobutamine hydrochloride is a SYMPATHOMIMETIC drug used to treat cardiogenic shock and other serious heart disorders. It works by increasing the heart's force of contraction without affecting the heart rate. Administration is by injection or infusion.

▲ side-effects: the heart rate following treatment may increase too rapidly and result in high blood pressure (hypertension).

✚ warning: dobutamine hydrochloride should be administered with caution to patients with severe low blood pressure (hypotension). *Related article:* DOBUTREX.

Dobutrex (*Lilly*) is a proprietary preparation of the SYMPATHOMIMETIC drug dobutamine hydrochloride, used to treat cardiogenic shock and other serious heart disorders. It is a available only on prescription as a medium for intravenous infusion.

▲/✚ side-effects/warning: *see* DOBUTAMINE HYDROCHLORIDE.

docusaste sodium is an alternative term for dioctyl sodium sulphosuccinate, a constituent in many LAXATIVES.
see DIOCTYL SODIUM SULPHOSUCCINATE

Dome-Cort (*Lagap*) is a proprietary, water-miscible, CORTICOSTEROID cream for topical application, used to treat mild inflammations of the skin. Available only on prescription, its major active constituent is the steroid hydrocortisone.

▲/✚ side-effects/warning: *see* HYDROCORTISONE.

domperidone is an ANTINAUSEANT drug that works by inhibiting the action of the substance dopamine on the vomiting centre of the brain; this can be useful in patients undergoing treatment with CYTOTOXIC drugs. It also has the effect of stimulating the emptying of the stomach and promoting the passage of nutritional debris through the small intestine. Administration is oral in the form of tablets or in suspension, or as anal suppositories.

▲ side-effects: there may be muscle spasms in the face and other voluntary muscles. Occasionally, spontaneous lactation in females or the development of feminine breasts in males may occur. *Related article:* MOTILIUM.

dopamine is a neurotransmitter substance (a catecholamine) that is an intermediate in the synthesis of noradrenaline, acts as a neurotransmitter (relaying nerve "messages"), and is particularly concentrated in the brain and in the adrenal glands. It is possible that some psychoses may in part be caused by abnormalities in the metabolism of dopamine because drugs that antagonize its activity as a neurotransmitter (such as chlorpromazine) tend to relieve schizophrenic symptoms. Dopamine may be administered to seriously ill patients suffering cardiogenic shock to improve the blood pressure and circulation. Administration is by injection or infusion.

▲ side-effects: there may be nausea and vomiting, with changes in heart rate and blood pressure – the fingertips and toes may become cold.

✚ warning: dopamine hydrochloride should not be administered to patients who suffer from certain disorders of the adrenal glands (such as phaeochromocytoma) or from heartbeat irregularities

involving very rapid heart rate. Dosage to treat shock after a heart attack need only be low.
Related articles: I<small>NTROPIN</small>; S<small>ELECT</small>-A-J<small>ET</small> D<small>OPAMINE</small>.

doxorubicin hydrochloride is a powerful and widely used C<small>YTOTOXIC</small> drug that also has A<small>NTIBIOTIC</small> properties, used to treat leukaemia, lymphomas and some solid tumours. Administration is by fast-running infusion (usually at intervals of 21 days, although a low dose weekly may result in fewer toxic side-effects).
▲ side-effects: nausea and vomiting, hair loss and reduction in the blood-forming capacity of the bone marrow are all fairly common side-effects. Rarely, there is also an increased heart rate.
✚ warning: doxorubicin hydrochloride should be administered with caution to patients with heart disease, or who are receiving radiotherapy in the cardiac region. Heart monitoring is essential throughout treatment: high doses tend to cause eventual heart dysfunction. Leakage of the drug from the site of infusion into the tissues may cause tissue damage.

doxycycline is a broad-spectrum A<small>NTIBIOTIC</small>, one of the tetracyclines, used to treat severe infections of many kinds. Administration is oral in the form of tablets and capsules, soluble (dispersible) tablets for solution, and as a dilute syrup.
▲ side-effects: there may be nausea and vomiting, with diarrhoea. Some patients experience a sensitivity to light. Rarely, there are allergic reactions.
✚ warning: doxycycline should not be administered to patients with kidney failure, or who are aged under 12 years.
Related articles: D<small>OXATET</small>; D<small>OXYLAR</small>; N<small>ORDOX</small>; V<small>IBRAMYCIN</small>.

Doxylar (*Lagap*) is a proprietary broad-spectrum A<small>NTIBIOTIC</small>, available only on prescription, used to treat infections of many kinds. Produced in the form of capsules, Doxylar is a preparation of the tetracycline doxycycline hydrochloride. It is not suitable for children under 12 years.
▲/✚ side-effects/warning: *see* D<small>OXYCYCLINE</small>.

Dozic (*RP Drugs*) is a proprietary A<small>NTIPSYCHOTIC</small> drug, available only on prescription, used to treat psychosis (especially schizophrenia or the hyperactive, euphoric condition, mania) and to tranquilize patients undergoing behavioural disturbance. It may also be used in the short term to treat severe anxiety. Produced in the form of a sugar-free liquid (for swallowing, in two strengths), Dozic is a preparation of the powerful drug haloperidol.

Dozine (*RP Drugs*) is a proprietary A<small>NTIPSYCHOTIC</small> drug available only on prescription, used to treat psychosis (especially schizophrenia) and to tranquillize patients undergoing behavioural disturbance. It may also be used in the short term to treat severe anxiety (especially in the case of terminal disease) or to treat an intractable hiccup. Produced in the form of an elixir for dilution (the potency of the elixir

D

once dilute is retained for 14 days), Dozine is a preparation of the powerful drug chlorpromazine hydrochloride.

▲/✚ side-effects/warning: *see* CHLORPROMAZINE.

Dramamine (*Searle*) is a proprietary non-prescription ANTI-EMETIC, used to treat nausea and vomiting, to prevent forms of motion sickness, and to relieve the loss of balance and vertigo experienced by patients with infections of the middle or inner ear or who have radiation sickness. Produced in the form of tablets, Dramamine is a preparation of dimenhydrinate. It is not recommended for children aged under 12 months.

▲/✚ side-effects/warning: *see* DIMENHYDRINATE.

Drapolene (*Wellcome*) is a proprietary non-prescription ANTISEPTIC cream used primarily to treat nappy rash, although it can also be used to dress abrasions and minor wounds. It contains the ANTISEPTICS benzalkonium chloride and cetrimide in very dilute solution.

Dryptal (*Berk*) is a proprietary DIURETIC, available only on prescription, used to treat fluid retention in the tissues (oedema) and mild to moderate high blood pressure (*see* ANTIHYPERTENSIVE). In high dosage it may also be used to assist a failing kidney. Produced in the form of tablets (in two strengths, the stronger for hospital use only), Dryptal is a preparation of the powerful but short-acting diuretic frusemide.

▲/✚ side-effects/warning: *see* FRUSEMIDE.

Duo-autohaler (*Riker*) is a proprietary SYMPATHOMIMETIC compound bronchodilator, available only on prescription, used to treat bronchospasm in asthma. Produced in a metered-dose aerosol, it is a combination of the BETA-RECEPTOR STIMULANT isoprenaline hydrochloride together with the VASOCONSTRICTOR phenylephrine bitartrate. It is rarely, if ever, used nowadays having been replaced by the more selective B_2-receptor stimulants, such as SALBUTAMOL or TERBUTALINE.

▲/✚ side-effects/warning: *see* ISOPRENALINE; PHENYLEPHRINE.

Duofilm (*Stiefel*) is a proprietary non-prescription liquid preparation intended to remove warts, particularly verrucas (on the soles of the feet). For daily topical application, avoiding normal skin surfaces, it is a compound in which the major active constituent is salicylic acid.

Duovent (*Boehringer Ingelheim*) is a proprietary compound BRONCHODILATOR, available only on prescription, used to treat bronchospasm in asthma. Produced in a metered-dose aerosol with mouthpiece, it is a combination of the SYMPATHOMIMETIC fenoterol hydrobromide together with the ANTICHOLINERGIC drug ipratropium bromide. It is not recommended for children aged under six years and is rarely used in children.

▲/✚ side-effects/warning: *see* FENOTEROL; IPRATROPIUM.

Duphalac (*Duphar*) is a proprietary non-prescription LAXATIVE that is not available from the National Health Service. It works by maintaining a volume of fluid within the intestines through osmosis, so lubricating the faeces and reducing levels of ammonia-producing organisms. Produced in the form of a syrup, Duphalac is a preparation of the semi-synthetic disasccharide lactulose.

▲/✚ side-effects/warning: *see* LACTULOSE.

E45 Cream (*Crookes*) is a proprietary non-prescription skin emollient (softener and soother) containing a mixture of paraffins and fats, including wool fat.

✚ warning: wool fat causes sensitivity reactions in some patients.

Ebufac (*DDSA Pharmaceuticals*) is a proprietary non-narcotic ANALGESIC that has additional ANTI-INFLAMMATORY properties. Available only on prescription, Ebufac is used to relieve pain – particularly the pain of rheumatic disease and other musculo-skeletal disorders – and is produced in the form of tablets consisting of a preparation of ibuprofen.

▲/✚ side-effects/warning: *see* IBUPROFEN.

Econacort (*Squibb*) is a proprietary preparation that combines the CORTICOSTEROID hydrocortisone with the ANTIFUNGAL econazole nitrate. Available only on prescription and produced in the form of a cream for topical application, Econacort is used to treat inflammation in which infection is also diagnosed. The cream, applied sparingly, should be massaged into the skin; prolonged use should be avoided.

▲/✚ side-effects/warning: *see* ECONAZOLE NITRATE; HYDROCORTISONE.

econazole nitrate is an ANTIBACTERIAL and ANTIFUNGAL agent, one of the IMIDAZOLES used particularly in topical applications to treat fungal infections of the skin or mucous membranes. Administration is in the form of creams or ointments,

▲ side-effects: there may be local skin irritation, even to the extent of a burning sensation and redness.

Related articles: ECOSTATIN; PEVARYL.

Econocil VK (*DDSA Pharmaceuticals*) is a proprietary preparation of the penicillin-type ANTIBIOTIC phenoxymethylpenicillin, used mainly to treat infections of the head and throat, and some skin conditions. Available only on prescription, it is produced in the form of capsules and tablets (in two strengths).

▲/✚ side-effects/warning: *see* PHENOXYMETHYLPENICILLIN.

Economycin (*DDSA Pharmaceuticals*) is a proprietary ANTIBIOTIC, available only on prescription, used to treat many kinds of infection, but especially those of the respiratory tract, ear, nose and throat, urinary tract, and soft tissues. Produced in the form of capsules and tablets, Economycin is a preparation of the TETRACYCLINE tetracycline hydrochloride. It is not suitable for children aged under 12 years.

▲/✚ side-effects/warning: *see* TETRACYCLINE.

Econosone (*DDSA Pharmaceuticals*) is a proprietary CORTICOSTEROID preparation, available only on prescription, used to treat inflammation especially in cases where it is caused by allergy. Produced in the form of tablets (in two strengths), it is a form of the steroid prednisone.

▲/✚ side-effects/warning: *see* PREDNISONE.

Ecostatin (*Squibb*) is a proprietary non-prescription ANTIFUNGAL preparation of econazole nitrate, used primarily to treat yeast

infections of the skin and mucous membranes, especially in the urogenital areas. It is produced (in solution) in the form of a water-miscible cream, as a lotion, as a spray for topical application, as a dusting-powder, and as a talc-based powder in a spray container.
▲ side-effects: see ECONAZOLE NITRATE.

Eczederm (*Quinoderm*) is a proprietary non-prescription skin emollient (softener and soother) in the form of a cream that contains CALAMINE (zinc carbonate) and starch, of use in the treatment of eczematous dermatotes.

Eczederm with Hydrocortisone (*Quinoderm*) is a proprietary form of the emollient skin cream ECZEDERM that also contains the CORTICOSTEROID hydrocortisone.
    Available only on prescription, it is used to soften and soothe dry or cracked skin and to treat local inflammation. Prolonged use should be avoided.
▲/✚ side-effects/warning: *see* HYDROCORTISONE.

edrophonium chloride is a drug that has the effect of enhancing the transmission of neural impulses between the nerves and the muscles they serve. However, its effect is of only very brief duration, and so it is used mainly for the diagnosis of a rare condition called myastenia gravis (which is a condition characterized by muscular weakness). Administration is by injection.
▲ side-effects: there may be nausea and vomiting with an excess of saliva in the mouth, diarrhoea and abdominal cramps. High dosage may cause gastrointestinal disturbance and sweating; and overdosage may result in urinary and faecal incontinence, loss of coordination in vision, nervous agitation and weakness amounting to paralysis.
✚ warning: edrophonium chloride should not be administered to patients who suffer from intestinal or urinary blockage. It should be administered only with caution to those with asthma, epilepsy, parkinsonism, slow heart rate or low blood pressure (hypotension), or who have respiratory depression. Some doctors administer atropine (or a similar drug) simultaneously to forestall some side-effects.
    Related article: TENSILON.

Efcortelan (*Glaxo*) is a proprietary preparation of the CORTICOSTEROID hydrocortisone, available only on prescription, used to treat inflammation especially where it is caused by allergy. It is produced in the form of a cream, as an ointment, and as a lotion for topical application (undiluted).
▲/✚ side-effects/warning: *see* HYDROCORTISONE.

Efcortelan Soluble (*Glaxo*) is a proprietary preparation of the CORTICOSTEROID hydrocortisone, available only on prescription, used to treat inflammation especially where it is caused by allergy, to treat shock, or to make up a deficiency of steroid hormones in a patient. It is produced in the form of a powder for reconstitution (in water) as a medium for injection.

▲/➕ side-effects/warning: *see* HYDROCORTISONE.

Efcortesol (*Glaxo*) is a proprietary preparation of the CORTICOSTEROID hydrocortisone, available only on prescription, used to treat inflammation especially where it is caused by allergy, to treat shock, or to make up a deficiency of steroid hormones in a patient. It is produced in ampoules for injection.

▲/➕ side-effects/warning: *see* HYDROCORTISONE.

Elavil (*DDSA Pharmaceuticals*) is a proprietary ANTIDEPRESSANT drug, available only on prescription, administered to treat depressive illness (and especially in cases where some degree of sedation is deemed necessary). Like many such drugs, it has also been used to treat bed wetting by children at night although this use is now becoming less common. Produced in the form of tablets (in two strengths), Elavil is a preparation of amitriptyline hydrochloride.

▲/➕ side-effects/warning: *see* AMITRIPTYLINE.

Electrosol (*Macarthys*) is a proprietary non-prescription oral rehydration solution for use in gastroenteritis (diarrhoea and vomiting). Electrosol is produced in the form of oral powder, which should be reconstituted with water, containing SODIUM CHLORIDE, POTASSIUM CHLORIDE and SODIUM BICARBONATE.

Eltroxin (*Glaxo*) is a proprietary preparation of the thyroid hormone thyroxine, used to make up a hormonal deficiency, and to treat associated symptoms (myxoedema). It is produced in the form of tablets (in two strengths) containing thyroxine sodium.

▲/➕ side-effects/warning: *see* THYROXINE SODIUM.

Eludril (*Concept*) is a proprietary non-prescription mouth-wash that has ANTIBACTERIAL and ANTIFUNGAL properties and inhibits the formation of plaque on the teeth. It is also used in the treatment of gum disease and mouth ulcers. Containing the antiseptic chlorhexidine gluconate and chlorbutol, Eludril is not recommended for children aged under six years. An aerosol spray version is also available.

▲/➕ side-effects/warning: *see* CHLORHEXIDINE.

Emeside (*L A B*) is a proprietary preparation of the anti-epileptic drug ethosuximide, available only on prescription, used to treat and suppress petit mal ("absence") seizures. Produced in the form of capsules and as a blackcurrant- or orange-flavoured syrup for dilution (the potency of the syrup once diluted is retained for 14 days), Emeside's blood level may be monitored following the initiation of treatment so that an optimum treatment level can be established.

▲/➕ side-effects/warning: *see* ETHOSUXIMIDE.

*emetics are agents that cause vomiting. Emetics are used mostly to treat poisoning by non-acidic non-corrosive substances, especially drugs in overdose. Some affect the vomiting centre in the brain; others irritate the stomach nerves. Among the best known and most used is IPECACUANHA, but several drugs similarly used as constituents in expectorant preparations can in higher concentrations also cause effective emesis.

Emla (*Astra*) is a proprietary local ANAESTHETIC in the form of a cream for topical application. Available only on prescription, it is used primarily to prevent pain associated with blood tests or the siting of intravenous drips. For it to be effective it needs to be applied approximately half an hour before under an occlusive dressing. It is a combined preparation of the anaesthetics lignocaine and prilocaine, and is presented in a pack that includes dressings.
▲/✚ side-effects/warning: *see* LIGNOCAINE; PRILOCAINE.

Emtexate (*Nordic*) is a proprietary CYTOTOXIC drug, available only on prescription, used in the treatment of leukaemia, lymphomas and some solid tumours. It works by being incorporated into new-forming cells and so preventing normal cell reproduction. Produced in the form of tablets, in vials for injection (in four strengths) and as a powder for reconstitution as a medium for injection, Emtexate is a preparation of methotrexate.
▲/✚ side-effects/warning: *see* METHOTREXATE.

Emulsiderm (*Dermal*) is a proprietary non-prescription skin emollient (softener and soother) in the form of a liquid emulsion that contains benzalkonium chloride and liquid paraffin. It can be rubbed into the skin or added to a bath.
✚ warning: *see* BENZALKONIUM CHLORIDE.

emulsifying ointment is a non-proprietary formulation comprising a combination of wax together with a white soft paraffin and liquid paraffin. It is most commonly used in eczema and should be liberally applied and also added to the bath.

En-De-Kay (*Stafford-Miller*) is a proprietary non-prescription form of fluoride supplement for administration in areas where the water supply is not fluoridated, especially for growing children. Produced in the form of tablets (in three strengths, labelled for children of different ages), as a sugar-free liquid to be used in drops, and as a mouth-wash for dilution, En-De-Kay's active constituent is SODIUM FLUORIDE.

Endoxana (*Degussa*) is a proprietary CYTOTOXIC drug, available only on prescription, used in the treatment of leukaemia, lymphomas and some solid tumours. It works by disrupting the DNA in new-forming cells and so preventing normal cell reproduction. Produced in the form of tablets (in two strengths) and as a powder for reconstitution as a medium for injection, Endoxana is a preparation of cyclophosphamide; it is sometimes prescribed in combination with the drug MESNA.
▲/✚ side-effects/warning: *see* CYCLOPHOSPHAMIDE.

E

Ener-G (*General Designs*) is a proprietary non-prescription gluten-free brown rice bread, for patients whose metabolisms are unable to tolerate the cereal protein gluten (as with coeliac disease). The bread is made without milk, eggs, wheat, soya or refined sugar.

Enrich (*Abbott*) is a proprietary nutritional supplement for patients who are severely undernourished (such as with anorexia nervosa) or who are suffering from some problem with the absorption of food (such as following gastrectomy); it may also be used to feed patients who require a liquid diet through injury or disease. Produced in the form of a lactose- and gluten-free liquid in cans, Enrich contains protein, carbohydrate (including dietary fibre), fats, vitamins and minerals. It is not suitable for children aged under 12 months, or as a sole source of nutrition for children aged under five years.

Ensure (*Abbott*) is a proprietary nutritional supplement for patients who are severely undernourished (such as with anorexia nervosa) or who are suffering from some problem with the absorption of food (such as following gastrectomy); it may also be used to feed patients who require a liquid diet through injury or disease. Produced in the form of a lactose- and gluten-free liquid in cans and bottles (or as a powder for reconstitution in identical form), Ensure contains protein, carbohydrate, fats, vitamins and minerals, and comes in vanilla, coffee and eggnog flavours. It is not suitable for children aged under 12 months. A version with a higher proportion of protein, carbohydrate and fats is also available (under the name Ensure Plus).

Epanutin (*Parke-Davis*) is a proprietary ANTICONVULSANT drug, available only on prescription, used to treat and prevent grand mal (tonic-clonic) and partial (focal) epileptic seizures. Produced in the form of capsules (in three strengths), as chewable tablets (under the name Epanutin Infatabs), and as a suspension for dilution (the potency of the suspension once dilute is retained for 14 days), Epanutin is a preparation of the effective but non-hypnotic drug phenytoin.
▲/✚ side-effects/warning: *see* PHENYTOIN.

Epanutin Ready Mixed Parenteral (*Parke-Davis*) is a form of the proprietary ANTICONVULSANT drug EPANUTIN that is administered to treat the emergency epileptic condition status epilepticus. It may, however, also be used to prevent convulsive seizures during neurosurgical operations and to treat and regularize heartbeat irregularities. Produced in ampoules for injection, it is a solution of phenytoin sodium with propylene glycol.
▲/✚ side-effects/warning: *see* PHENYTOIN.

ephedrine hydrochloride is a SYMPATHOMIMETIC drug used as a VASOCONSTRICTOR. It is used to reduce nasal congestion. However, when it is used in the form of nasal drops there is a danger of rebound swelling in the nose on stopping the medication, if it has been used for too long a period. The medication is of some benefit in asthma, but has been replaced by more specific drugs such as

salbutamol or terbutaline. Administration is oral in the form of
tablets or as an elixir, or topical in the form of nose-drops.

▲ side-effects: there may be changes in heart rate and blood pressure,
anxiety, restlessness, tremor, insomnia, dry mouth and cold
fingertips and toes. Used as a nasal decongestant, there may be
local irritation.

✚ warning: ephedrine hydrochloride should not be administered to
patients who are already taking drugs that affect the action of the
heart; it should be administered with caution to those with
diabetes, reduced blood supply to the heart, high blood pressure
(hypertension) and disorder of the thyroid gland. Prolonged use as a
bronchodilator or as a nasal decongestant may eventually result in
tolerance.

Related articles: AURALGICIN; CAM; EXPULIN; EXPURHIN; HAYMINE;
LOTUSSIN.

Ephynal (*Roche*) is a proprietary non-prescription form of vitamin E
(TOCOPHEROL) supplement, used to make up for vitamin deficiency. It is
produced in the form of tablets (in four strengths) consisting of a
preparation of alpha tocopheryl acetate.

Epilim (*Labaz*) is a proprietary ANTICONVULSANT drug, available only on
prescription, used to treat all forms of epilepsy. Produced in the form
of crushable tablets, as enteric-coated tablets (in two strengths), as a
sugar-free liquid, and as a syrup for dilution (the potency of the syrup
once dilute is retained for 14 days), Epilim is a preparation of the
carboxylic acid derivative sodium valproate.

▲/✚ side-effects/warning: *see* SODIUM VALPROATE.

Epogam (*Scotia*) is a proprietary drug used to treat atopic eczema.
Available only on prescription it is a compound preparation of the
drug gamolenic acid in evening primrose oil together with vitamin E,
produced in the form of capsules.

▲/✚ side-effects/warning: *see* GAMOLENIC ACID.

ergocalciferol is one of the two natural forms of calciferol (vitamin
D), formed in plants by the action of sunlight.

see CALCIFEROL.

ergotamine tartrate is a drug administered to patients who suffer
from migraine that is not relieved by the ordinary forms of pain-
killing drug. A vegetable alkaloid, it is most effectively administered
during the aura – the initial symptoms – of an attack, and probably
works by constricting the cranial arteries. However, although the
pain may be relieved, other symptoms, such as the visual
disturbances and nausea, may not (although other drugs may be
administered to treat those separately). Repeated treatment may in
some patients eventually lead to habituation (addiction); in others it
may cause ergot poisoning, resulting in gangrene of the fingers and
toes, and confusion. Administration is oral in the form of tablets
either for swallowing or to be held under the tongue to dissolve, or as
an aerosol inhalant; one proprietary compound preparation is in the
form of anal suppositories.

E

▲ side-effects: there may be abdominal pain and muscle cramps that may lead to nausea and vomiting. Overdosage or rapid withdrawal of the drug may in turn cause headache.

✚ warning: ergotamine tartrate should not be administered to patients who suffer from vascular disease or any infection. It should not be given to children with hemiplegia migraine (that is, where the migraine is associated with weakness usually of one side of the body). It should be administered with caution to those with kidney, liver or heart disease, or with thyroid gland overactivity. Dosage should be carefully monitored; treatment should not be repeated within four days. It should never be administered on a prophylactic (preventative) basis. Treatment should be withdrawn at once if the patient experiences tingling or numbness at the extremities.

Related articles: CAFERGOT; MEDIHALER-ERGOTAMINE.

Ervevax (*Smith, Kline & French*) is a proprietary VACCINE against German measles (rubella) in the form of a solution containing live but attenuated viruses of the Wistar RA27/3 strain. Available only on prescription, it is administered in the form of injection.

Erymax (*Parke-Davis*) is a proprietary ANTIBIOTIC, available only on prescription. It is a common choice for children as it is generally well tolerated and its spectrum of action is particularly wide (for example, it is used to make children with whooping cough non-infectious, and it may be given to likely contacts to try to prevent the disease). Produced in the form of capsules, Erymax is a preparation of the macrolide erythromycin.

▲/✚ side-effects/warning: *see* ERYTHROMYCIN.

Erymax Sprinkle (*Parke-Davies*) is a proprietary ANTIBIOTIC, available only on prescription used to treat many forms of infection, in particular respiratory or skin infections, and also as an alternative to penicillin antibiotics in patients who are allergic to penicillin. Erymax Sprinkle is a preparation of the antibiotic erythromycin. It is produced in the form of capsules whose contents may be sprinkled on soft food for use with children.

▲/✚ side-effects/warning: *see* ERYTHROMYCIN.

Erythrocin (*Abbott*) is a proprietary ANTIBIOTIC, available only on prescription. It is a common choice for children as it is generally well tolerated and its spectrum of action is particularly wide (for example, it is used to make children with whooping cough non-infectious, and it may be given to likely contacts, in particular the family of a patient with whooping cough, to try to prevent the disease). Produced in the form of tablets (in two strengths), and as a powder for reconstitution as a medium for injection, Erythrocin is a preparation of salts of the macrolide erythromycin. The tablets are not recommended for children.

▲/✚ side-effects/warning: *see* ERYTHROMYCIN.

Erythrolar (*Lagap*) is a proprietary ANTIBIOTIC, available only on prescription. It is a common choice for children as it is generally well tolerated and its spectrum of action is particularly wide (for example, it is used to make children with whooping cough non-infectious, and it may be given to likely contacts to try to prevent the disease). Produced in the form of tablets (in two strengths), and as a suspension for dilution (the potency of the suspension once dilute is retained for five days), Erythrolar is a preparation of salts of the macrolide erythromycin.

▲/✚ side-effects/warning: *see* ERYTHROMYCIN.

erythromycin is a macrolide ANTIBIOTIC with a similar spectrum of action to penicillin, but a different mechanism of action. It inhibits microbial protein synthesis at the ribosome level. It is effective against many gram-positive bacteria including streptococci, mycoplasma, legionella (which causes legionnaire's disease) and chlamydia. It is used in the treatment of soft tissue and respitory tract infections, pneumonia and urethritis, among other infections. It is also used as prophylaxis (preventative therapy) for diphtheria and whooping cough. Erythromycin's principal use is as an alternative to penicillin in individuals who are allergic to penicillin. Bacterial resistance is unfortunately common.

Administration is oral in the form of tablets, as capsules, or as a dilute suspension (mixture), or by injection. Tablets have to be enteric- or film-coated because the drug is inactivated by gastric secretions.

▲ side-effects: large doses may cause nausea and vomiting, and possibly diarrhoea.

✚ warning: one salt of erythromycin (the estolate), a constituent in a proprietary suspension, should not be administered to patients with liver disease; all forms of the drug should be administered with caution to those with impaired liver function.

Related articles: ARPIMYCIN; ERYMAX; ERYTHROCIN; ERYTHROLAR; ERYTHROPED; ILOSONE; RETCIN.

Erythroped (*Abbott*) is a proprietary ANTIBIOTIC, available only on prescription. It is a common choice for children as it is generally well tolerated and its spectrum of action is particularly wide (for example, it is used to make children with whooping cough non-infectious, and it may be given to likely contacts to try to prevent the disease). Produced in the form of a suspension (in three strengths) for dilution (the potency of the suspension once dilute is retained for five days), as sugar-free granules in sachets for solution, and as tablets (under the name Erythroped A), Erythroped is a preparation of salts of the macrolide erythromycin.

▲/✚ side-effects/warning: *see* ERYTHROMYCIN.

Eskamel (*Smith, Kline & French*) is a proprietary non-prescription cream used to treat acne. It contains the KERATOLYTIC agent resorcinol together with SULPHUR.

✚ warning: see RESORCINOL.

Esoderm (*Napp*) is a proprietary non-prescription preparation of the drug lindane, used to treat parasitic infestation by lice (pediculosis)

or by itch-mites (scabies) on the skin surface, particularly under the hair. However, strains of head-lice resistant to lindane have recently emerged, and the drug is not now recommended for use on the scalp. It is produced in the form of a (flammable) alcohol-based lotion, and as a cream shampoo.

▲/✚ side-effects/warning: *see* LINDANE.

ethambutol hydrochloride is an ANTIBIOTIC that is one of the major forms of treatment for tuberculosis. Even so, it is used generally in combination (to cover resistance and for maximum effect) with other antitubercular drugs such as ISONIAZID or rifampicin. Treatment lasts for between 6 and 18 months depending on severity and on the specific drug combination, but the use of ethambutol tends to imply the shorter duration. The drug is also used to prevent the contraction of tuberculosis by relatives. Administration is oral in the form of tablets or as a powder.

▲ side-effects: side-effects are rare, and are mostly in the form of visual disturbances (such as loss of acuity or colour-blindness) which should prove temporary if treatment is withdrawn. A regular ophthalmic check is advised during treatment; because this cannot adequately be performed in young children the drug is not usually prescribed under the age of six.
Related article: MYAMBUTOL.

ethamsylate is a drug that reduces bleeding, although how it does so is not perfectly understood − it may correct abnormal adhesion by the blood platelets on the fibrin matrix (so coagulating the blood). As a haemostatic, it is used particularly to treat haemorrhage from small blood vessels. It is occasionally used to try to prevent brain haemorrhage in very premature babies.

▲ side-effects: there may be nausea with headache; some patients come out in a rash.
✚ warning: ethamsylate should not be administered to patients who are known to have platelet deficiency in the blood.
Related article: DICYNENE.

ethosuximide is an ANTICONVULSANT drug used to treat and suppress petit mal (that is minor epilepsy or absence attacks). Blood level test can be performed and dosage may then be adjusted to the optimum level for each individual patient. Administration is oral in the form of capsules or as a dilute elixir.

▲ side-effects: there may be gastrointestinal disturbances, drowsiness, headache and/or dizziness; some patients experience depression or euphoria. Rarely, there are haematological disorders or psychotic states.
✚ warning: ethosuximide should not be administered to patients with porphyria. Withdrawal of treatment, if undertaken, must be gradual.
Related articles: EMESIDE; ZARONTIN.

etomidate is a general ANAESTHETIC used specifically for the initial induction of anaesthesia. Recovery after treatment is rapid and without any hangover effect, and it causes less of a fall in blood pressure than many other anaesthetics. But there may be pain on injection, when there may also be simultaneous extraneous muscle movements.

▲ side-effects: repeated doses may suppress the secretion of corticosteroid hormones by the adrenal glands.

✚ warning: pain on injection may be overcome by prior administration of suitable premedication (such as a narcotic analgesic). Intravenous injection must be carried out with caution in order to avoid thrombophlebitis.

Related article: HYPNOMIDATE.

Eudemine (*Allen & Hanburys*) is a proprietary preparation of the hyperglycaemic drug diazoxide, available only on prescription, used to treat chronic conditions involving a deficiency of glucose in the bloodstream. Such a condition might occur, for example, if a pancreatic tumour caused excessive secretion of insulin. Also useful in treating an acute hypertensive crisis (apoplexy), Eudemine is produced in the form of tablets and in ampoules for rapid intravenous injection.

▲/✚ side-effects/warning: *see* DIAZOXIDE.

Eumovate (*Glaxo*) is a proprietary CORTICOSTEROID preparation, available only on prescription, used in topical application to treat non-infective inflammation.

Produced in the form of a water-miscible cream and an anhydrous ointment to treat inflammatory skin disorders, such as eczema and some types of dermatitis, and in the form of eye-drops (in two preparations, one additionally containing the ANTIBIOTIC neomycin sulphate under the name Eumovate-N) to treat ophthalmic inflammations, Eumovate is a preparation of the steroid clobetasone butyrate.

▲/✚ side-effects/warning: *see* CLOBETASONE BUTYRATE.

Eumydrin (*Winthrop*) is a proprietary preparation of the ANTICHOLINERGIC antispasmodic drug atropine methonitrate, which was used to relieve muscle spasm in the valve-like sphincter between the stomach and the duodenum (the pylorus) in infants. However, this condition, called pyloric stenosis, is nowadays treated by surgery, which is more effective and safer. Eumydrin is produced in the form of a solution in a dropper bottle (and should be stored in a cool place).

▲/✚ side-effects/warning: *see* ATROPINE METHONITRATE.

Eurax (*Geigy*) is a proprietary non-prescription form of the drug crotamiton, used to treat itching, especially in relation to the effects of infestation by the itch-mite (scabies). It is produced in the form of a lotion and a cream. Another version is available (only on prescription) additionally containing the CORTICOSTEROID hydrocortisone, and used also to treat itching that results from skin inflammation.

▲/✚ side-effects/warning: *see* CROTAMITON; HYDROCORTISONE.

Exelderm (*ICI*) is a proprietary ANTIFUNGAL cream, available only on prescription, used for topical application to skin infections, such as athlete's foot or thrush. The cream should be massaged into the skin;

E

treatment should continue for at least a fortnight after lesions have disappeared. Exelderm is a preparation of the IMIDAZOLE sulconazole nitrate.

▲/✚ side-effects/warning: *see* SULCONAZOLE NITRATE.

Exirel (*Pfizer*) is a proprietary BRONCHODILATOR, available only on prescription, used to treat asthma. Produced in the form of capsules (in two strengths), as an aerosol inhalant, and as a syrup, Exirel is a preparation of the SYMPATHOMIMETIC pirbuterol. It is not recommended for children aged under six years.

▲/✚ side-effects/warning: *see* PIRBUTEROL.

Ex-Lax (*Intercare*) is a proprietary, non-prescription LAXATIVE produced in the form of chocolate and as tablets. It contains phenolphthalein.

▲/✚ side-effects/warning: *see* PHENOLPHTHALEIN.

Exolan (*Dermal*) is a proprietary non-prescription preparation of the drug dithranol triacetate in mild solution, used to treat psoriasis. It is produced in the form of a water-miscible cream for topical application.

▲/✚ side-effects/warning: *see* DITHRANOL.

*expectorants are medicated liquids intended to make it easier to cough up phlegm. They are used particularly in the case of bronchial congestion. (They are not the same as linctuses, which merely comprise liquids thick and soothing enough to relieve sore throats or to loosen a cough. Nor is an expectorant necessarily an elixir, which disguises a potentially horrible taste with a sweetening substance like glycerol or alcohol.) Expectorants may work by irritating the lining of the stomach, so stimulating the reflex secretion of sputum by the glands in the mucous membranes of the upper respiratory tract. However, there is little evidence that expectorants actually work and they are of doubtful benefit. In high dosage, most expectorants can be used as EMETICS (to provoke vomiting).

Expulin (*Galen*) is a proprietary non-prescription cough linctus that is not available from the National Health Service. It is produced as a linctus in two strengths (the weaker labelled as a paediatric version) for dilution (the potency of the linctus once dilute is retained for 14 days), and is a combination of the OPIATE pholcodine, the SYMPATHOMIMETIC ephedrine hydrochloride, the ANTIHISTAMINE chlorpheniramine maleate, and GLYCEROL and menthol. Even the paediatric linctus is not recommended for children aged under three months.

▲/✚ side-effects/warning: *see* CHLORPHENIRAMINE; EPHEDRINE HYDROCHLORIDE; PHOLCODINE.

Expurhin (*Galen*) is a proprietary non-prescription nasal DECONGESTANT for children that is not available from the National Health Service. It is used to relieve all forms of congestion in the upper respiratory tract. Produced in the form of a sugar-free linctus, Expurhin is a combination of the SYMPATHOMIMETIC ephedrine hydrochloride together with the ANTIHISTAMINE chlorpheniramine maleate and MENTHOL. Even as a paediatric linctus, it is not recommended for children aged under three months.

▲/✚ side-effects/warning: *see* CHLORPHENIRAMINE; EPHEDRINE HYDROCHLORIDE.

Exterol (*Dermal*) is a proprietary non-prescription preparation of a urea-hydrogen peroxide complex designed to dissolve and wash out wax in the ears. To be held in the ear with cotton wool for as long as possible, Exterol is produced in the form of ear-drops also containing GLYCEROL.

F

Fabahistin (*Bayer*) is a proprietary ANTIHISTAMINE, available only on prescription, used to treat allergic symptoms in such cases as hay fever and urticaria. Produced in the form of tablets and as a suspension (in either or two diluents), Fabahistin's active constituent is mebhydrolin.
▲/✚ side-effects/warning: *see* MEBHYDROLIN.

Fansidar (*Roche*) is a proprietary ANTIMALARIAL drug, available only on prescription, used to treat patients who are seriously ill with malaria, particularly with strains resistant to the standard drug chloroquine. (A very few strains are resistant also to Fansidar.) It is sometimes alternatively used prophylactically to try to prevent tropical travellers from contracting the disease. Produced in the form of tablets, Fansidar is a compound of the antimalarial pyrimethamine with the ANTIBACTERIAL sulphonamide drug SULFADOXINE. Dosage is critical, and must be carefully monitored.
▲/✚ side-effects/warning: *see* PYRIMETHAMINE.

Fe-Cap (*MCP Pharmaceuticals*) is a proprietary non-prescription preparation of the drug ferrous glycine sulphate, used as an IRON supplement in the treatment of iron deficiency anaemia, and produced in the form of capsules.
▲/✚ side-effects/warning: *see* FERROUS GLYCINE SULPHATE.

Fe-Cap C (*MCP Pharmaceuticals*) is a proprietary non-prescription mineral-and-VITAMIN compound, consisting of capsules containing iron in the form of FERROUS GLYCINE SULPHATE together with ASCORBIC ACID (vitamin C).

Fectrim (*DDSA Pharmaceuticals*) is a proprietary ANTIBIOTIC combination available only on prescription, used especially in infections of the urinary tract, infections such as sinusitis and bronchitis, and infections of the bones and joints. Produced in the form of soluble (dispersible) tablets (in any of three strengths), Fectrim is a preparation of the compound drug co-trimoxazole, made up of the SULPHONAMIDE SULPHAMETHOXAZOLE together with the antibacterial agent TRIMETHOPRIM.
▲/✚ side-effects/warning: *see* CO-TRIMOXAZOLE.

Fenostil Retard (*Zyma*) is a proprietary non-prescription ANTIHISTAMINE used to treat allergic symptoms in such cases as hay fever. Produced in the form of tablets, Fenostil Retard's active constituent is dimethindene maleate.
▲/✚ side-effects/warning: *see* DIMETHINDENE MALEATE.

fenoterol is a SYMPATHOMIMETIC drug used as a BRONCHODILATOR to treat asthmatic attacks. Administration is by aerosol spray or nebulizer; less commonly, injection or infusion is used.
▲ side-effects: there may be tremor of the hands, nervous tension and headache; the heart rate may increase; the potassium level in the bloodstream may drop (hypokalaemia), following an injected dose. *Related article:* BEROTEC.

fentanyl is a narcotic ANALGESIC, used primarily for analgesia during surgery and to supplement other anaesthetics; it may be used also to slow the breathing of an anaesthetized patient. As a narcotic, its proprietary forms are on the controlled drugs list.
▲ side-effects: post-operatively there may be respiratory depression, low blood pressure, slowing of the heart, and nausea (with or without vomiting).
✚ warning: fentanyl should not be administered to patients whose respiration is already impaired by disease or those with myasthenia gravis, hypothyroidism or chronic liver disease. Use on a mother during childbirth may cause respiratory depression in the newborn.
Related article: SUBLIMAZE.

Feospan (*Smith, Kline & French*) is a proprietary non-prescription preparation of the drug ferrous sulphate, used as an IRON supplement in the treatment of iron deficiency anaemia, and produced in the form of spansules (sustained-release capsules). It is not recommended for children aged under 12 months.
▲/✚ side-effects/warning: *see* FERROUS SULPHATE.

Fergon (*Winthrop*) is a proprietary non-prescription preparation of the drug ferrous gluconate, used as an IRON supplement in the treatment of iron deficiency anaemia, and produced in the form of tablets. It is not recommended for children aged under six years.
▲/✚ side-effects/warning: *see* FERROUS GLUCONATE.

Ferrocap (*Consolidated Chemicals*) is a proprietary non-prescription preparation of the drug ferrous fumarate and thiamine hydrochloride, used as an IRON supplement in the treatment of iron deficiency anaemia, and produced in the form of capsules. It is not recommended for children aged under six years.
▲/✚ side-effects/warning: *see* FERROUS FUMARATE.

Ferromyn (*Calmic*) is a proprietary non-prescription preparation of the drug ferrous succinate, used as an IRON supplement in the treatment of iron deficiency anaemia, and produced in the form of tablets and as an elixir.
▲/✚ side-effects/warning: *see* FERROUS SUCCINATE.

Ferromyn S (*Calmic*) is a form of Ferromyn with additional succinic acid.
see FERROMYN.

ferrous fumarate is an IRON-rich drug used to restore iron to the blood in cases of iron deficiency anaemia. Once a patient's blood haemoglobin level has reached normal, treatment should continue for at least three months to replenish fully the stores of iron in the body. Some preparations combine ferrous fumarate with various vitamins, for use particularly as supplements during pregnancy.
▲ side-effects: large doses may cause gastrointestinal upset and diarrhoea; there may be vomiting.

Prolonged treatment may result in constipation.
Related articles: B.C.500 WITH IRON; FERROCAP; FERSAMAL; GALFER; GALFER F.A.; GALFERVIT; GIVITOL.

ferrous gluconate is an IRON-rich drug used to restore iron to the blood in cases if iron deficiency anaemia. Once a patient's blood haemoglobin level has reached normal, treatment should continue for at least three months to replenish fully the stores of iron in the body. Some preparations combine ferrous gluconate with various VITAMINS.
▲ side-effects: large doses may cause gastrointestinal upset and diarrhoea; there may be vomiting. Prolonged treatment may result in constipation.
Related article: FERGON.

ferrous glycine sulphate is a drug used to restore IRON to the blood in cases of iron deficiency anaemia. Once a patient's blood haemoglobin level has reached normal, treatment should continue for at least three months to replenish fully the stores of iron in the body. Some preparations combine ferrous glycine sulphate with various VITAMINS.
▲ side-effects: large doses may cause gastrointestinal upset and diarrhoea; there may be vomiting. Prolonged treatment may result in constipation.
Related articles: FE-CAP; KELFERON; PLESMET.

ferrous succinate is an IRON-rich drug used to restore iron to the blood in cases of iron deficiency anaemia. Once a patient's blood haemoglobin level has reached normal, treatment should continue for at least three months to replenish fully the stores of iron in the body.
▲ side-effects: large doses may cause gastrointestinal upset and diarrhoea; there may be vomiting. Prolonged treatment may result in constipation.
Related articles: FERROMYN; FERROMYN S.

ferrous sulphate is a drug used to restore IRON to the blood in cases of iron deficiency anaemia. Once a patient's blood haemoglobin level has reached normal, treatment should nevertheless continue for at least three months to replenish fully the stores of iron in the body. Some preparations combine dried ferrous sulphate with various vitamins, or with zinc, for use particularly as tonic supplements.
▲ side-effects: large doses may cause gastrointestinal upset and diarrhoea; there may be vomiting. Prolonged treatment may result in constipation.
Related articles: FEOSPAN; FESOVIT; FESOVIT Z; IROFOL C; IRONORM; SLOW-FE.

Fersamal (*Duncan, Flockhart*) is a proprietary non-prescription preparation of the drug FERROUS FUMARATE. It is used as an iron supplement in the treatment of iron deficiency anaemia. In addition to tablets, it is produced in the form of a syrup. Like Fersaday, Fersamal should not be taken simultaneously with tetracycline antibiotics or antacids.

Fesovit (*Smith, Kline & French*) is a proprietary non-prescription compound of the drug ferrous sulphate together with ASCORBIC ACID (vitamin C) and several forms of VITAMIN B. It is not available from the National Health Service. Used as a mineral-and-vitamin supplement in the treatment of iron deficiency anaemia, it is produced in the form of spansules (sustained-release capsules). It is not recommended for children aged under 12 months.
▲/✚ side-effects/warning: *see* FERROUS SULPHATE.

Fersovit Z (*Smith, Kline & French*) is a proprietary non-prescription compound of the drug ferrous sulphate with ZINC SULPHATE, ASCORBIC ACID (vitamin C) and several forms of VITAMIN B. It is not available from the National Health Service. Used as a mineral-and-vitamin supplement in the treatment of iron deficiency anaemia, it is produced in the form of spansules (sustained-release capsules). It is not recommended for children aged under 12 months.
▲/✚ side-effects/warning: *see* FERROUS SULPHATE.

Fisherman's Friend (*Lofthouse of Fleetwood*) is a proprietary non-prescription lozenge for the relief of cold symptoms. It contains liquorice, MENTHOL and aniseed oil.

Flagyl (*May & Baker*) is a proprietary form of the AMOEBICIDAL drug metronidazole, available only on prescription, used to treat bowel infection by such organisms as *Giardia lamblia* (which causes chronic diarrhoea and poor weight gain) and less commonly *Entamoeba histolytica* (which causes amoebic dysentery). It is also used to treat infection by anaerobic bacteria (which thrive in an environment lacking oxygen). It is produced as tablets and a suspension for oral use. Suppositories may be used in patients who have recently had abdominal surgery. An intravenous preparation is also available for infusion.
▲/✚ side-effects/warning: *see* METRONIDAZOLE.

Flamazine (*Smith & Nephew*) is a proprietary ANTIBACTERIAL cream, available only on prescription, used to treat wounds, burns and ulcers, bedsores and skin-graft donor sites. It is a preparation of silver sulphadiazine in a water-soluble base.
▲/✚ side-effects/warning: *see* SILVER SULPHADIAZINE.

Flaxedil (*May & Baker*) is a proprietary SKELETAL MUSCLE RELAXANT, available only on prescription, of the type known as competitive or non-depolarising. It is used during surgical operations, but only after the patient has been rendered unconscious. Produced in ampoules for injection, Flaxedil's active constituent is gallamine triethiodide.
▲/✚ side-effects/warning: *see* GALLAMINE TRIETHIODIDE.

flecainide acetate is a drug used to slow and regularize the heartbeat. Administration is usually first by slow intravenous injection, followed if necessary by infusion, and then orally in the form of tablets.

F

▲ side-effects: there may be dizziness and visual disturbances; rarely, there is nausea and vomiting.
Related article: TAMBOCOR.

Fletcher's Arachis Oil (*Pharmax*) is a proprietary non-prescription form of enema, designed to soften and lubricate impacted faeces within the rectum. It comprises a preparation of ARACHIS OIL that should be warmed before use.

Fletcher's Enemette (*Pharmax*) is a proprietary non-prescription form of enema, designed to soften and lubricate impacted faeces within the rectum. It comprises a preparation of DIOCTYL SODIUM SULPHOSUCCINATE (docusate sodium) with GLYCEROL, MACROGOL OINTMENT and sorbic acid. It is not recommended for children aged under three years.

Flexical (*Bristol-Meyers*) is a proprietary non-prescription gluten-free powder (for reconstitution) that is a complete nutritional diet for patients who are severely undernourished (such as with anorexia nervosa) or who are suffering from some problem with the absorption of food (such as following gastrectomy). Also lactose-free, Flexical contains protein, carbohydrate, fats, vitamins and minerals; it is not suitable for children aged under 12 months, and should not constitute the sole source of nourishment for children of any age.

Florinef (*Squibb*) is a proprietary form of the hormonal substance fludrocortisone acetate, available only on prescription. A mineralocorticoid, it is used to make up a body deficiency in mineralocorticoids (which are essential for the balance of salt and water in the body) resulting from a malfunctioning of the adrenal glands. Florinef is produced in the form of tablets.
▲/✚ side-effects/warning: *see* FLUDROCORTISONE ACETATE.

Floxapen (*Beecham*) is a proprietary ANTIBIOTIC, available only on prescription, used to treat bacterial infections of the skin and of the ear, nose and throat, and especially staphylococcal infections that prove to be resistant to penicillin. Produced in the form of capsules (in two strengths), syrup for dilution (in two strengths; the potency of the dilute syrup is retained for 14 days), and as a powder for reconstitution as injections, Floxapen's active constituent in each case is flucloxacillin or one of its salts.
▲/✚ side-effects/warning: *see* FLUCLOXACILLIN.

Flu-Amp (*Generics*) is a proprietary compound ANTIBIOTIC available only on prescription used to treat bacterial infections. Produced in the form of capsules, Flu-Amp contains the penicillin-like drug ampicillin together with the antibiotic flucloxacillin (which can treat infections that prove to be resistant to penicillin).
▲/✚ side-effects/warning: *see* AMPICILLIN; FLUCLOXACILLIN.

fluclorolone acetonide is a powerful CORTICOSTEROID drug, used in very mild solution to treat severe non-infective inflammations of the skin, particularly eczema that is unresponsive to less powerful drugs, and psoriasis. Administration is as a cream or ointment for topical use. It is not commonly used in children.

▲ side-effects: side-effects depend to some extent on the area of the skin treated. If infection is present, it may spread although the symptoms may not be experienced by the patient. Prolonged treatment may cause thinning of the skin, yet increase hair growth; dermatitis or acne may be present. These side-effects may be worse in children.

✚ warning: like all topical corticosteroids, fluclorolone acetone treats symptoms and does not cure underlying disorders.

flucloxacillin is an ANTIBIOTIC used to treat bacterial infections of the skin and of the ear, nose and throat, and especially staphylococcal infections that prove to be resistant to penicillin. Administration is in the form of capsules, dilute syrup and injection.

✚ warning: flucloxacillin should not be administered to patients who have a history of allergy to penicillin-type antibiotics, or who suffer from impairment of kidney function.

▲ side-effects: there may be sensitivity reactions, including high temperature; the most common side-effect of the drug, however, is diarrhoea.

Related articles: FLOXAPEN; STAFOXIL; STAPHCIL.

flucytosine is a synthesized ANTIFUNGAL drug used to treat systemic infections by yeasts − infections such as candidiasis (or thrush). Administration is oral or by intravenous infusion.

▲ side-effects: there may be diarrhoea, with nausea and vomiting; rashes may occur. Proportions of various blood cells may decrease.

✚ warning: flucytosine should be administered only with caution to patients who suffer from impaired function of the kidneys or liver, or from blood disorders. During treatment there should be regular blood counts and liver-function tests.

Related article: ALCOBON.

fludrocortisone acetate is a hormonal substance, a mineralocorticoid used to make up a body deficiency of mineralocorticoids (which are essential to the balance of salt and water in the body) resulting from a malfunctioning of the adrenal glands.

▲ side-effects: if the dose is excessive there may be high blood pressure, sodium and water retention, and potassium deficiency; there may also be muscular weakness.

Related article: FLORINEF.

flumazanil is a BENZODIAZAPINE antagonist, used to reverse the sedative effects of benzodiazapines used in anaesthetic, intensive care and diagnostic precedures. Administration is by intravenous injection or infusion.

fluocinolone acetonide is a powerful CORTICOSTEROID drug, used in very dilute solution to treat severe non-infective inflammations of the skin. Administration is as a cream, gel, or ointment for topical use. It is not commonly used in children.

▲side-effects: side-effects depend to some extent on the area of the skin treated. If infection is present, it may spread although the symptoms may not be experienced by the patient. Prolonged treatment may cause thinning of the skin, yet increase hair growth; dermatitis or acne may be present. These side-effects may be worse in children.

✚warning: like all topical corticosteroids, fluocinolone acetonide treats symptoms and does not cure underlying disorders.
Related article: SYNALAR.

fluocinonide is a powerful CORTICOSTEROID drug, used in very dilute solution to treat severe non-infective inflammations of the skin, particularly eczema that is unresponsive to less powerful drugs, and some allergic skin conditions. Administration is as a cream or ointment for topical use. It is not commonly used in children.

▲side-effects: side-effects depend to some extent on the area of the skin treated. If infection is present, it may spread although the symptoms may not be experienced by the patient. Prolonged treatment may cause thinning of the skin, yet increase hair growth; dermatitis or acne may occur. These side-effects may be worse in children.

✚warning: like all topical corticosteroids, fluocinonide treats symptoms and does not cure underlying disorders.
Related article: METOSYN.

fluocortolone is a powerful CORTICOSTEROID drug, used in very dilute solution to treat severe non-infective inflammations of the skin, particularly eczema that is unresponsive to less powerful drugs. Administration is as a cream or ointment for topical use. It is not commonly used in children.

▲side-effects: side-effects depend to some extent on the area of the skin treated. If infection is present, it may spread although the symptoms may not be experienced by the patient. Prolonged treatment may cause thinning of the skin, yet increase hair growth; dermatitis or acne may occur. These side-effects may be worse in children.

✚warning: like all topical corticosteroids, fluocortolone treats symptoms and does not cure underlying disorders.
Related article: ULTRADIL PLAIN; ULTRALANUM PLAIN.

Fluor-a-day Lac (*Dental Health Promotion*) is a proprietary non-prescription form of fluoride supplement for administration in areas where the water supply is not fluoridated, especially to growing children. Produced in the form of tablets to be dissolved in the mouth, Fluor-ə-day Lac's active constituent is SODIUM FLUORIDE.

fluorescein sodium is a proprietary diagnostic medium, a water-soluble dye used to distinguish foreign bodies or injured areas in the surface of an eyeball. Alternatively, it may be injected into a retinal vein to check the retinal circulation. When light is shone on the dye, it shows up a brilliant green.
Related articles: MINIMS FLUROESCEIN SODIUM; OPULETS.

Fluorigard (*Hoyt*) is a proprietary non-prescription form of fluoride supplement for administration in areas where the water supply is not fluoridated, especially to growing children. Produced in the form of tablets to be dissolved in the mouth (in two strengths, and in assorted flavours and colours), as drops, and as a mouth wash, Fluorigard's active constituent is SODIUM FLUORIDE.

fluorometholone is a CORTICOSTEROID drug used primarily in the treatment of local eye inflammations in cases where the inflammation is not caused by infection. Administration is as eye-drops.
▲ side-effects: very rarely, and following weeks of treatment, there may be an acute, temporary form of glaucoma in certain patients who are predisposed to it.
✚ warning: as with all corticosteroids, fluorometholone treats only the symptoms and does not treat any underlying disorder. An undetected or misdiagnosed infection may thus get worse although the symptoms may be suppressed.
Related article: FML.

flurandrenolone is a powerful CORTICOSTEROID drug, used in very dilute solution to treat severe non-infective inflammations of the skin, particularly eczema that is unresponsive to less powerful drugs. Administration is as a cream or ointment for topical use. One proprietary form combines it with an antibacterial, antifungal agent. It is not commonly used in children.
▲ side-effects: side-effects depend to some extent on the area of the skin treated. If infection is present, it may spread although the symptoms may not be experienced by the patient. Prolonged treatment may cause thinning of the skin, yet increase hair growth; dermatitis or acne may occur. These side-effects may be worse in children.
✚ warning: like all topical corticosteroids, flurandrenolone by itself treats symptoms and does not cure underlying disorders.
Related article: HAELAN.

Fluvirin (*Evans*) is the name of a series of proprietary flu VACCINES, all comprising inactivated surface antigens of different strains of the influenza virus. None is recommended for children aged under four years.
▲ side-effects: rarely, there is local reaction together with headache and high temperature.
✚ warning: like any flu vaccine, Fluvirin cannot control epidemics and should be used only – in what seems to be the appropriate strain – on people who are at high risk. Fluvirin should not be administered to patients who are markedly allergic to egg or chicken protein (in which vaccine viruses are cultured), or who are pregnant.

FML (*Allergan*) is a proprietary form of ANTI-INFLAMMATORY eye-drops, available only on prescription, used in cases where the inflammation is not caused by injection. The active constituent of FML is the CORTICOSTEROID fluorometholone.
▲/✚ side-effects/warning: *see* FLUOROMETHOLONE.

F

folic acid is a VITAMIN of the B complex, important in the synthesis of nucleic acids (DNA and RNA). Food sources of folic acid include liver and vegetables; consumption is particularly necessary during pregnancy. Deficiency leads to a form of anaemia, which is usually rapidly remedied by oral supplements. Folic acid is prescribed in certain haemolytic anaemias (in which there is an over rapid breakdown of the blood's red cells).
Related articles: FERROGRAD FOLIC; GALFER F.A..

folinic acid is a derivative of FOLIC ACID (a VITAMIN of the B complex), and is used therapeutically to suppress the toxic effects of certain ANTICANCER drugs, especially METHOTREXATE, and to treat some forms of anaemia. Administration is oral in the form of tablets, or by injection or infusion.

Forceval (*Unigreg*) is a proprietary non-prescription mineral-and-VITAMIN compound that is not available from the National Health Service. Used as a supplement to make up body deficiencies, and produced in the form of gelatin capsules in either of two strengths (the weaker one under the trade name Forceval Junior), Forceval contains almost all the vitamins, and calcium, copper, iodine, phosphorus, potassium and zinc.

Forceval Protein (*Unigreg*) is a proprietary, non-prescription, gluten-free powder (for reconstitution) that is a complete nutritional diet for patients who are severely undernourished (such as with anorexia nervosa) or who are suffering from some problem with the absorption of food (such as following gastrectomy). Also lactose- and galactose-free, Forceval Protein contains protein, carbohydrate, vitamins and minerals; it is produced in sachets and tins, and in various flavours.

Not suitable for children aged under 12 months, it should not constitute the sole source of nourishment for children aged under five years.

Formula MCT(1) (*Cow & Gate*) is a proprietary non-prescription powder for reconstitution which is a low-protein high-calorie dietary supplement for patients who suffer from failure of the liver or cystic fibrosis of the pancreas, or following intestinal surgery, when the need is to provide amino acids and protein in a readily available form that does not rely on breakdown by the body. Formula MCT(1) contains triglycerides (fatty acids), protein, carbohydrate, minerals and electrolytes. It does not, however, form a complete diet.

Formula S is a soya-based milk, that is also free of the milk sugar lactose. Therefore it can be used in infants who are either allergic to cows' milk or intolerant to lactose. However, babies can also be allergic to soya milk and should not be changed to this type of milk without good reason.

Fortagesic (*Sterling Research*) is a proprietary narcotic ANALGESIC, a controlled drug that is not available from the National Health

Service. Produced in the form of tablets containing the OPIATE pentazocine together with paracetamol, Fortagesic is not recommended for children under seven years.

▲/✚ side-effects/warning: *see* PARACETAMOL; PENTAZOCINE.

Fortical (*Cow & Gate*) is a proprietary, non-prescription gluten-free liquid that is not available from the National Health Service, and is a carbohydrate-based supplement for patients with kidney failure, liver cirrhosis, or any other condition that needs a high-calorie, low-electrolyte diet requiring minimum absorption. It is available in six flavours.

Fortisip (*Cow & Gate*) is a bland, proprietary, non-prescription, gluten-free liquid that is a complete nutritional diet for patients who are severely undernourished (such as with anorexia nervosa) or who are suffering from some problem with the absorption of food, such as following gastrectomy. Produced in two strengths, Fortisip contains protein, carbohydrate, fats, minerals, and vitamins; as the slightly stronger Fortisip Energy Plus, the liquid is produced in three flavours. Neither form is suitable for children aged under 12 months.

Fortison (*Cow & Gate*) is a bland, proprietary, non-prescription gluten-free liquid that is a complete nutritional diet for patients who are severely undernourished (such as with anorexia nervosa) or who are suffering from some problem with the absorption of food, such as following gastrectomy. Produced in two strengths (Standard and Energy Plus) and with a choice of protein types, Fortison contains protein, carbohydrate, fats, minerals and vitamins. It is not suitable for children aged under 12 months.

Fortral (*Sterling Research*) is a proprietary narcotic ANALGESIC, a controlled drug that is not available from the National Health Service. Produced in the form of tablets, capsules, ampoules for injection and anal suppositories, its active constituent is the OPIATE pentazocine. Fortral suppositories are not recommended for children; as tablets and capsules Fortral is not recommended for children aged under six years; and as injections Fortral is not recommended for children aged under 12 months.

▲/✚ side-effects/warning: *see* PENTAZOCINE.

Fortum (*Glaxo*) is a proprietary broad-spectrum ANTIBIOTIC, available only on prescription, used to treat bacterial infections, particularly infections of the respiratory tract, the ear, nose or throat, the skin, bones and joints, and more serious infections such as septicaemia and meningitis. Produced in the form of powder for reconstitution as a medium for injection or infusion, Fortum is a preparation of the CEPHALOSPORIN ceftazidime.

▲/✚ side-effects/warning: *see* CEFTAZIDIME.

framycetin is a relatively toxic aminoglycoside ANTIBIOTIC, used to treat external bacterial infections. Preparations of framycetin most commonly involve its sulphate form.

▲ side-effects: hypersensitive reactions may occur; there may be temporary kidney malfunction.

✚ warning: application to large areas of the skin may damage the organs of the ears. Framycetin should not be administered to patients who are pregnant, or to those with myasthenia gravis.
Related articles: FRAMYCORT; FRAMYGEN; SOFRADEX; SOFRAMYCIN.

Framycort (*Fisons*) is a proprietary compound, available only on prescription, combining the ANTIBIOTIC framycetin sulphate with the fairly potent steroid hydrocortisone acetate. It is used in the form of an ointment to treat skin infections, particularly on the face or in the urogenital area; as eye-drops to treat bacterial infections such as conjunctivitis; and as ear-drops to treat bacterial infections of the outer ear.

▲/✚ side-effects/warning: *see* FRAMYCETIN; HYDROCORTISONE.

Framygen (*Fisons*) is a proprietary ANTIBIOTIC, available only on prescription, used in the form of eye ointment and eye-drops to treat infections on and around the eyes; as ear-drops to treat infections of the outer ear; and as a cream to treat bacterial skin infections. In all versions, its active constituent is the aminoglycoside framycetin sulphate in very mild solution.

▲/✚ side-effects/warning: *see* FRAMYCETIN.

FreAmine III (*Boots*) is a proprietary form of high-calorie nutritional supplement intended for injection or infusion, available only on prescription. Produced in two strengths, it contains amino acids, nitrogen, phosphate and electrolytes.

Fresubin (*Fresenius Dylade*) is a bland, proprietary, non-prescription, gluten-free liquid that is a complete nutritional diet for patients who are severely undernourished, such as with anorexia nervosa, or who are suffering from some problem with the absorption of food, such as following gastrectomy. Produced in four flavours and three sizes, Fresubin contains protein, carbohydrate, fats, minerals and vitamins. It is not suitable for children aged under 12 months.

Frisium (*Hoechst*) is a proprietary form of the BENZODIAZEPINE clobazam. It is used to treat certain forms of fits, in particular a short-lived variety called myoclonic epilepsy.

▲/✚ side-effects/warning: *see* CLOBAZAM.

frusemide is a powerful DIURETIC which works by inhibiting readsorption in part of the kidney known as the loop of Henle. It is used to treat fluid retention in the tissues (oedema) and to assist a failing kidney. Administration is oral in the form of tablets, or by injection or infusion.

▲ side-effects: the diuretic effect corresponds to dosage; large doses may cause deafness or ringing in the ears (tinnitus). There may be skin rashes.

✚ warning: treatment may cause a deficiency of potassium and sodium in the bloodstream (hypokalaemia, hyponatraemia).
Related article: DIURESAL.

Fucibet (*Leo*) is a proprietary compound, available only on prescription, combining the potent steroid betamethasone with the ANTIBIOTIC fusidic acid. It is used to treat eczema in which bacterial infection is deemed to be present, and is produced in the form of a cream. It is rarely used in children.
▲/✚ side-effects/warning: *see* BETAMETHASONE; FUSIDIC ACID.

Fucidin (*Leo*) is a proprietary narrow-spectrum ANTIBIOTIC, available only on prescription, used mainly against staphylococcal infections – especially skin infections and osteomyletis (bone infection) – that prove to be resistant to penicillin. It is produced in many forms: as tablets, as a suspension, as powder for reconstitution as a medium for infusion, as a gel (with or without a special applicator), as a cream, and as an ointment, all for use as indicated by the location of the infection, and all containing as their active constituent either fusidic acid or one of its salts (particularly sodium fusidate).
▲/✚ side-effects/warning: *see* FUSIDIC ACID.

Fucidin H (*Leo*) is a proprietary compound, available only on prescription, combining the ANTIBIOTIC fusidic acid with the steroid hydrocortisone, and used to treat local skin inflammation deemed to be caused by bacterial infection. It is produced in the form of an ointment, a cream or a gel.
▲/✚ side-effects/warning: *see* FUSIDIC ACID; HYDROCORTISONE.

Fucithalmic (*Leo*) is a proprietary ANTIBIOTIC available only on prescription, used in the form of a gel to treat staphyloccocal infections on and around the eyes. Its active constituent is the antibiotic fusidic acid.
▲/✚ side-effects/warning: *see* FUSIDIC ACID.

Fulcin (*ICI*) is a proprietary ANTIFUNGAL drug, available only on prescription, used to treat fungal infections of the scalp, skin and nails. Produced in the form of tablets (in two strengths) and as a suspension, Fulcin is a preparation of the antibiotic griseofulvin. Treatment may need to continue over several weeks.
▲/✚ side-effects/warning: *see* GRISEOFULVIN.

fungicidal drugs act to destroy fungal infection, and are also known as an antimycotic or antifungal drugs.
see ANTIFUNGAL.

Fungilin (*Squibb*) is a proprietary form of the powerful, but fairly toxic, ANTIFUNGAL drug amphotericin. Available only on prescription, Fungilin is produced in the form of tablets and as a suspension, as lozenges, as an ointment and as a cream, and used in the appropriate form to treat intestinal infection or infections of the urogenital areas (especially candidiasis, or thrush), and infections of the mouth and nose.
▲/✚ side-effects/warning: *see* AMPHOTERICIN.

Fungizone (*Squibb*) is a proprietary form of the ANTIFUNGAL drug amphotericin. Available only on prescription, Fungizone is produced in the form of powder for reconstitution as a medium for intravenous infusion, and used to treat systemic fungal infections.

▲/✚ side-effects/warning: *see* AMPHOTERICIN.

Furadantin (*Norwich Eaton*) is a proprietary ANTIBIOTIC drug, available only on prescription, used to treat infections of the urinary tract. It is produced in the form of tablets (in two strengths) and as a suspension, the active constituent of which is nitrofurantoin.

▲/✚ side-effects/warning: *see* NITROFURANTOIN.

fusidic acid and its salts are narrow-spectrum ANTIBIOTICS used to treat staphylococcal infections − particularly infections of the skin or bone − that prove to be resistant to penicillin.

▲ side-effects: local hypersensitivity reactions may occur; rarely, there may be gastric upset, jaundice, and a reversible change in liver function.

✚ warning: treatment by infusion may require periodic testing of the patient's liver function. Keep fusidic acid ointment, cream and gel away from the eyes.

Related articles: FUCIBET; FUCIDIN; FUCIDIN H.

Fybogel (*Reckitt & Colman*) is a proprietary form of the type of LAXATIVE known as a bulking agent, which works by increasing the overall mass of faeces within the rectum, so stimulating bowel movement. It is used also to soothe the effects of diverticular disease and irritable colon. In the case of Fybogel, the agent involved is ispaghula husk, presented in the form of effervescent grains in sachets for swallowing with water.

▲/✚ side-effects/warning: *see* ISPAGHULA HUSK.

G

Galactomin (*Cow & Gate*) is the name of a proprietary series of powdered milk formulas, which are free from the milk sugar, lactose. Such a diet, free from lactose, is necessary in the rare inborn error of metabolism galactosaemia, or in cases where a baby develops intolerance to lactose and has persistent diarrhoea. Additional vitamins should be given. In the two preparations available (Formulas 17 and 19), Formula 17 has a higher fat content and Formula 19 has fructose as its carbohydrate.

Galcodine (*Galen*) is a proprietary ANTITUSSIVE, available only on prescription, used to encourage the loosening of a dry, painful cough. Produced in the form of an orange-flavoured sugar-free linctus (in two strengths, the weaker under the name Galcodine Paediatric) for dilution (the potency of the dilute linctus is retained for 14 days), galcodine is a preparation of the OPIATE codeine phosphate. It is not recommended for children aged under 12 months.
▲/✚ side-effects/warning: *see* CODEINE PHOSPHATE.

Galenphol (*Galen*) is a proprietary cough suppressant, available only on prescription, used to encourage the loosening of a dry, painful cough. Produced in the form of an aniseed-flavoured sugar-free linctus (in three strengths, the weakest under the name Galenphol Linctus Paediatric, the strongest under the name Galenphol Linctus Strong) for dilution (the potency of the dilute linctus is retained for 14 days), Galenphol is a preparation of the OPIATE pholcodine.
▲/✚ side-effects/warning: *see* PHOLCODINE.

Galfer (*Galen*) is a proprietary non-prescription IRON supplement, used particularly to treat certain forms of anaemia. Produced in the form of capsules, Galfer is a preparation of ferrous fumarate.
▲/✚ side-effects/warning: *see* FERROUS FUMARATE.

Galfer F.A. (*Galen*) is a proprietary non-prescription IRON and VITAMIN supplement, used particularly to prevent iron deficiency or vitamin B deficiency (as sometimes occurs during pregnancy). Produced in the form of capsules, Galfer F.A. is a compound of ferrous fumarate and folic acid.
▲/✚ side-effects/warning: *see* FERROUS FUMARATE; FOLIC ACID.

Galfer-Vit (*Galen*) is a proprietary IRON and VITAMIN supplement that is not available from the National Health Service. It is used to treat certain forms of anaemia in which there is simultaneous vitamin deficiency. Produced in the form of capsules, Galfer-Vit is a compound of various forms of vitamin B (thiamine, riboflavine, PYRIDOXINE and nicotinamide) and ASCORBIC ACID (vitamin C) with ferrous fumarate.
▲/✚ side-effects/warning: *see* FERROUS FUMARATE.

gallamine triethiodide is a SKELETAL MUSCLE RELAXANT of the type known as competitive or non-depolarizing. It is used during surgical operations to achieve long-duration paralysis. Administration is by injection, but only after the patient has been rendered unconscious.
▲ side-effects: there may be a precipitate deceleration in the heart rate.

✚warning: respiration should be assisted throughout treatment.
Related article: FLAXEDIL.

Galpseud (*Galen*) is a proprietary non-prescription form of nasal
DECONGESTANT administered orally. It is produced as tablets and as an
orange-flavoured sugar-free linctus for dilution (the potency of the
linctus once dilute is retained for 14 days), and is a preparation of the
SYMPATHOMIMETIC pseudoephedrine hydrochloride.
▲/✚ side-effects/warning: *see* EPHEDRINE HYDROCHLORIDE.

gamolenic acid is used in the symptomatic relief of atopic ezcema.
▲side-effects: occasionally nausea, indigestion or headaches may
occur.
✚warning: it should be used with caution in patients with epilepsy.

Gantrisin (*Roche*) is a proprietary ANTIBACTERIAL drug, available only
on prescription, used primarily to treat infections of the urinary tract,
but also to relieve lesser infections of the skin and soft tissues and
the respiratory tract, and to treat bacillary dysentery. Produced in
the form of tablets and as a syrup, Gantrisin is a preparation of the
SULPHONAMIDE sulphafurazole.
▲/✚ side-effects/warning: *see* SULPHAFURAZOLE.

Garamycin (*Kirby-Warrick*) is a proprietary ANTIBIOTIC, available only
on prescription, used primarily in the form of drops to treat bacterial
infections of the ear or eye, but also in the form of injections for
children (under the name Garamycin Paediatric) to treat other
bacterial infections, notably those of the urinary tract. In all forms,
Garamycin is a preparation of the aminoglycoside gentamicin.
▲/✚ side-effects/warning: *see* GENTAMICIN.

Gastrovite (*MCP Pharmaceuticals*) is a proprietary non-prescription
mineral-and-VITAMIN compound that is not available from the National
Health Service. The minerals are IRON and CALCIUM, in the form of
ferrous glycine sulphate and calcium gluconate, and the vitamins are
ASCORBIC ACID (vitamin C) and ERGOCALCIFEROL (vitamin D).
▲/✚ side-effects/warning: *see* CALCIUM GLUCONATE; FERROUS GLYCINE
SULPHATE.

Gaviscon (*Reckitt & Colman*) is a proprietary non-prescription ANTACID
(used for the relief of indigestion and flatulence), produced in the form
of tablets containing alginic acid, ALUMINIUM HYDROXIDE, SODIUM
BICARBONATE, magnesium trisilifcate and various sugars. There is also
a liquid version that contains sodium alginate, sodium bicarbonate
and calcium carbonate. Gaviscon is also produced in sachets. This
preparation is often added to feeds in infancy to try and control
troublesome and frequent regurgitation of milk).
✚warning: see MAGNESIUM TRISILICATE.

Gelcotar (*Quinoderm*) is a proprietary preparation of the ANTISEPTIC
COAL TAR, used to treat skin conditions such as dandruff, dermatitis,
eczema and psoriasis. It is produced in the form of a water-micible gel
(with pine tar) and as a liquid shampoo (with cade oil).

*general anaesthetic: *see* ANAESTHETIC

Genisol (*Fisons*) is a proprietary preparation of the ANTISEPTIC coal tar, used to treat skin conditions such as dandruff, dermatitis, eczema and psoriasis. It is produced in the form of a liquid shampoo.

Genotropin 4IU (*Kabi Vitrum*) is a proprietary preparation of human growth hormone (HGH or somatotrophin) in its synthetic form somatropin, available only on prescription. It is used to treat short stature caused by growth hormone deficiency. It is produced in the form of a powder for reconstitution as a medium for injection.
▲/✚ side-effects/warning: *see* SOMATROPIN.

gentamicin is a broad-spectrum ANTIBIOTIC drug, an aminoglycoside used to treat many forms of serious infection, but especially those of the urinary tract, or the blood (septicaemia). It is not capable of being absorbed by the digestive system, so administration is by injection or by topical application in the form of drops, cream or ointment.
▲side-effects: treatment must be discontinued if there are signs of deafness. There may be dysfunction of the kidneys.
✚warning: it should be administered with caution to those with impaired function of the kidneys. Prolonged or high dosage can cause deafness; blood level determinations are performed to make sure an excessive dosage is not given.
Related articles: CIDOMYCIN; GARAMYCIN; GENTICIN; GENTISONE HC; LUGACIN; MINIMS GENTAMICIN.

gentian violet   (or crystal violet) is an ANTISEPTIC dye used to treat certain bacterial and fungal skin infections, or abrasions and minor wounds. Administration is mostly in the form of ointment, paint or lotion, but can, in dilute solution, be oral. The dye is also used to stain specimens for examination under a microscope. A non-proprietary antiseptic paint, used particularly to prepare skin for surgery, combines gentian violet with another dye, brilliant green. Because it is very messy to apply it is little used nowadays
▲side-effects: rarely, there may be nausea and vomiting, with diarrhoea.
✚warning: gentian violet is a dye: it stains clothes as well as skin.

Genticin (*Nicholas*) is a proprietary ANTIBIOTIC, available only on prescription, used to treat any of a number of serious infections, but especially those of the urinary tract and on the skin. Produced in vials or ampoules for injection (in three strengths, the weakest under the name Genticin Paediatric), as a (water-miscible) cream or an (anhydrous greasy) ointment applied topically to treat skin infections, and as eye- or ear-drops, Genticin is a preparation of the aminoglycoside gentamicin.
▲/✚ side-effects/warning: *see* GENTAMICIN.

Genticin HC (*Nicholas*) is a proprietary compound ANTIBIOTIC, available only on prescription, used in the form of a cream and as an ointment to treat skin infections and to soothe the symptoms of

allergic skin conditions. It is a preparation of the aminoglycoside gentamicin sulphate with the CORTICOSTEROID hydrocortisone acetate.
▲/✚ side-effects/warning: *see* GENTAMICIN; HYDROCORTISONE.

Gentisone HC (*Nicholas*) is a proprietary compound ANTIBIOTIC, available only on prescription, used in the form of ear-drops to treat bacterial infections of the outer or middle ear. It is a preparation of the aminoglycoside gentamicin sulphate with the CORTICOSTEROID hydrocortisone acetate.
▲/✚ side-effects/warning: *see* GENTAMICIN; HYDROCORTISONE.

Gentran (*Travenol*) is a proprietary form of the plasma substitute dextran, available only on prescription, used in infusion with either saline (sodium chloride) or glucose to make up a deficiency in the overall volume of blood in a patient, or to prevent thrombosis following surgery. Produced in flasks (bottles) for infusion, there is a choice of two concentrations: Gentran 40 and Gentran 70.
▲/✚ side-effects/warning: *see* DEXTRAN.

Gevral (*Lederle*) is a proprietary non-prescription mineral-and-VITAMIN compound that is not available from the National Health Service. Used to make up mineral and vitamin deficiencies, and produced in the form of capsules, Gevral contains IRON (in the form of FERROUS FUMARATE), CALCIUM, copper, iodine, MAGNESIUM, manganese, phosphorus, POTASSIUM and ZINC; and retinol (vitamin A), vitamin B in the forms of thiamine, riboflavine, PYRIDOXINE, cyanocobalamin, nicotinamide, inositol and pantothenic acid, ASCORBIC ACID (vitamin C), CALCIFEROL (vitamin D) and TOCOPHEROL (vitamin E).

Givitol (*Galen*) is a proprietary non-prescription IRON-and-VITAMIN supplement that is not available from the National Health Service. Produced in the form of capsules, Givitol contains iron in the form of FERROUS FUMARATE, vitamin B in the forms of thiamine, riboflavine, PYRIDOXINE and nicotinamide, and ASCORBIC ACID (vitamin C).

glucagon is a HORMONE produced and secreted by the pancreas to cause an increase in blood sugar levels. It is part of a balancing mechanism complementary to INSULIN, which has the opposite effect. Therapeutically, glucagon is thus administered to patients with low blood sugar levels (hypoglycaemia). Administration is by injection. It may be useful in an emergency to treat hypoglycaemia in children with diabetes. The injection can be given under the skin and is therefore easy to administer.

Glucoplex (*Geistlich*) is a proprietary form of high-energy nutritional supplement intended for infusion into patients who are unable to take food via the alimentary tract. Produced in two strengths (under the names Glucoplex 1000 and Glucoplex 1600) its major constituent is the carbohydrate GLUCOSE.

glucose (or dextrose) is a simple sugar that is an important source of energy for the body − and the sole source of energy for the brain.

Following digestion, it is stored in the liver and muscles in the form of glycogen, and its breakdown into glucose again in the muscles produces energy. The level of glucose in the blood is critical: harmful symptoms occur if the level is too high or too low. Glucose is a common constituent of most fluids used for intravenous infusions. It is also present in oral rehydration solutions.
▲ side-effects: injections of glucose may irritate vascular walls and so tend to promote thrombosis and inflammation.

Glucoven (*MCP Pharmaceuticals*) is a proprietary form of high-energy nutritional supplement intended for infusion into patients who are unable to take food via the alimentary tract. Produced in two strengths (under the names Glucoven 1000 and Glucoven 1600), its major constituent is the natural carbohydrate GLUCOSE, although it also contains ions and trace elements.

glutaraldehyde is a DISINFECTANT much like formaldehyde, but stronger and faster-acting. It is used mostly to sterilize medical and surgical equipment, but may alternatively be used therapeutically (in solution) to treat skin conditions such as warts (particularly verrucas on the soles of the feet) and to remove hard, dead skin.
✚ warning: effects of treatment are not always predictable. Skin treated may become sensitized.
Related articles: GLUTAROL; VERUCASEP.

Glutarol (*Dermal*) is a proprietary non-prescription solution for topical application containing the KERATOLYTIC glutaraldehyde, used to treat warts and to remove hard, dead skin.
✚ warning: see GLUTARALDEHYDE.

Glutenex (*Cow & Gate*) is the name of a proprietary (non-prescription) brand of gluten-free biscuits made without milk, produced for patients with coeliac disease and similar conditions.

glycerol (or glycerin, or glycerine) is a mixture of hydrolized fat and oils. A colourless viscous liquid, it is used therapeutically as a constituent in many emollient skin preparations, as a sweetening agent for medications, and as a LAXATIVE in the form of anal suppositories. Taken orally, glycerol has the short-term effect of reducing pressure within the eyeballs (which may be useful for patients with glaucoma).

Glykola (*Sinclair*) is a proprietary non-prescription IRON supplement that is not available from the National Health Service. Produced in the form of an elixir for dilution (the potency of the elixir once dilute is retained for 14 days), Glykola contains iron (in the form of ferric chloride), caffeine, calcium and kola extract. There is a version for children (produced under the name Glykola Infans) which instead of the caffeine and calcium contains citric acid and the herb gentian.

Glypressin (*Ferring*) is a proprietary preparation of the drug terlipressin, a derivative of the HORMONE VASOPRESSIN. Available only on prescription, Glypressin is used to treat the haemorrhaging of varicose veins in the oesophagus (the tubular channel for food between throat and stomach). It is produced in vials for dilution and injection.

▲/✚ side-effects/warning: *see* TERLIPRESSIN.

gold in the form of its salts (in particular sodium aurothiomalate) is used therapeutically in the treatment of rheumatoid arthritis. Not an anti-inflammatory ANALGESIC like other treatments, however, gold works slowly so that full effects are achieved only after four or five months. Improvement then is significant, not only in the reduction of joint inflammation but also in associated inflammations. Administration is by injection. Gold is increasingly rarely also used in dentistry, occasionally for fillings, but more commonly (as alloys) in crowns, inlays and bridges.

▲/✚ side-effects/warning: *see* SODIUM AUROTHIOMALATE.

Graneodin (*Squibb*) is a proprietary ANTIBIOTIC, available only on prescription, used to treat bacterial infections of the skin and the eye. Produced in the form of an ointment for topical application, Graneodin contains the aminoglycoside neomycin sulphate and gramicidin.

▲/✚ side-effects/warning: *see* NEOMYCIN.

Gregoderm (*Unigreg*) is a proprietary ANTIBIOTIC/ ANTIFUNGAL combination available only on prescription, used to treat inflammation of the skin in which infection is also present. Produced in the form of an ointment for topical application, Gregoderm is a compound of the aminoglycoside antibiotic neomycin sulphate, the antibiotic polymyxin B sulphate and the antifungal nystatin, together with the CORTICOSTEROID hydrocortisone.

▲/✚ side-effects/warning: *see* HYDROCORTISONE; NEOMYCIN; NYSTATIN; POLYMYXIN B SULPHATE.

griseofulvin is a powerful ANTIFUNGAL drug that during treatment – which may be prolonged – is deposited selectively in the skin, hair and nails, and thus prevents further fungal invasion. It is most commonly used for large-scale infections, or to treat infections that prove intractable to other drugs, but can be used equally successfully on ringworm or localized tinea infections (such as athlete's foot). Administration is oral in the form of tablets or as a suspension.

▲ side-effects: there may be headache, with nausea and vomiting; some patients experience a sensitivity to light. Rarely, there may be a rash (which may be mild or serious).

✚ warning: griseofulvin should not be administered to patients who suffer from liver failure or from porphyria.

Related articles: FULCIN; GRISOVIN.

Grisovin (*Glaxo*) is a proprietary ANTIFUNGAL drug, available only on prescription, used to treat infections of the scalp, skin and nails. Produced in the form of tablets (in two strengths), Grisovin is a preparation of the drug griseofulvin. Treatment may need to continue over several weeks.

▲/✚ side-effects/warning: *see* GRISEOFULVIN.

Gypsona (*Smith & Nephew*) is a proprietary form of bandaging impregnated with plaster of Paris, used primarily for the immobilization of a fracture. Soaking the bandage causes the plaster to set hard.

G

Haelan (*Lista*) is a proprietary preparation of the CORTICOSTEROID drug flurandrenolone, available only on prescription, used in the form of a water-miscible cream of an anhydrous ointment as a topical application to treat severe non-infective inflammations of the skin. It is particularly used to treat eczema that is unresponsive to less powerful drugs. In both cream and ointment forms, Haelan is produced in two strengths (the stronger under the name Haelan-X), and in another version that additionally contains the antibacterial, antifungal agent CLIOQUINOL (under the name Haelan-C). There is also an impregnated tape for use as a poultice (marketed under the name Haelan Tape, but not available from the National Health Service). It is rarely used in children.

▲/✚ side-effects/warning: *see* FLURANDRENOLONE.

Haemaccel (*Hoechst*) is a proprietary form of gelatin, a hydrolized animal protein. In a special refined (partly degraded) form available only on prescription, it is used in infusion with saline (sodium chloride) as a means of expanding overall blood volume in patients whose blood volume is dangerously low through shock, particularly in cases of severe burns or septicaemia. It is produced in bottles (flasks) for infusion.

Halciderm (*Squibb*) is a proprietary preparation, in the form of a water-miscible cream for topical application, of the extremely powerful CORTICOSTEROID halcinonide. Available only on prescription, it is used to treat severe non-infective inflammation of the skin, particularly eczema that is unresponsive to less powerful drugs. It is rarely used in children.

▲/✚ side-effects/warning: *see* HALCINONIDE.

halcinonide is a powerful CORTICOSTEROID drug, used in very dilute solution to treat severe non-infective inflammations of the skin, particularly eczema that is unresponsive to less powerful drugs. Administration is in the form of a water-miscible cream for topical application. It is rarely used in children.

▲ side-effects: side-effects depend to some extent on the area of skin treated. Prolonged treatment may cause thinning of the skin, yet increase hair growth; there may be acne or dermatitis. These side-effects may be worse in children.

✚ warning: like all topical corticosteroids, halcinonide by itself treats symptoms and does not cure underlying disorders. If infection is present, it may worsen although the symptoms may be suppressed by the drug.

Related article: HALCIDERM.

halothane is a powerful general ANAESTHETIC that is widely used both for induction and for maintenance of anaesthesia during surgical operations. Used in combination with oxygen or nitrous oxide/oxygen mixtures, halothane vapour is non-irritant and even pleasant to inhale, does not induce coughing, and seldom causes post-operative vomiting. Administration is through a calibrated vaporizer in order to control concentration.

▲ side-effects: there may be liver damage. Repetition of anaesthesia by halothane is inadvisable within three months.

✚ warning: halothane causes a slowing of the heart rate and shallowness of breathing; both must be monitored during anaesthesia to prevent high levels of carbon dioxide or dangerously slow pulse and low blood pressure. The vapour is not good as a muscle relaxant, and muscle relaxants may have to be used in addition during specific types of surgery.

Halycitrol (*L A B*) is a proprietary non-prescription preparation of retinol (vitamin A) and calciferol (vitamin D) that is not available from the National Health Service. Produced in the form of an emulsion, it is used to treat deficiency of either vitamin, or both, but should be taken only under medical supervision, because both vitamins in excess can cause unpleasant side-effects.

▲/✚ side-effects/warning: *see* CALCIFEROL.

Hartmann's solution is another name for sodium lactate in a preparation suitable for intravenous infusion.
see SODIUM LACTATE.

Haymine (*Pharmax*) is a proprietary non-prescription nasal DECONGESTANT that is not available from the National Health Service. Unlike most nasal decongestants, however, it is produced in the form of tablets (for swallowing) and is a compound of the ANTIHISTAMINE chlorpheniramine maleate together with the BRONCHODILATOR ephedrine hydrochloride.

▲/✚ side-effects/warning: *see* CHLORPHENIRAMINE; EPHEDRINE HYDROCHLORIDE.

HBIG (or hepatitis B immunoglobulin) when injected or infused into the body, confers immediate immunity to the potentially dangerous effects of the disease caused by the hepatitis B virus. Prepared from the blood plasma of recent patients, it is used specifically to immunize personnel in medical laboratories and hospitals who may be infected, and to treat babies of mothers infected by the virus during pregnancy. In normal circumstances, however, immunization is with an anti-hepatitis B vaccine.

H-B-Vax (*Merck, Sharp & Dohme*) is a proprietary form of anti-hepatitis B VACCINE, available only on prescription, used on patients with a high risk of infection from the hepatitis B virus mostly through contact with a carrier. Chemically, H-B-Vax consists of an inactivated hepatitis B virus surface antigen derived from the blood plasma of a human carrier and adsorbed on to alum in suspension. It is produced in vials for intramuscular injection; the usual regimen per patient is three doses, at intervals of one month and six months.

✚ warning: *see* HEPATITIS B VACCINE.

Hedex (*Sterling Health*) is a proprietary non-prescription non-narcotic ANALGESIC produced in the form of tablets and as a soluble powder. It contains paracetamol.

▲/✚ side-effects/warning: *see* PARACETAMOL.

Hedex Plus (*Sterling Health*) is a proprietary non-prescription combination ANALGESIC, produced in the form of capsules. It contains paracetamol, caffeine and codeine.

▲/✚ side-effects/warning: *see* CAFFEINE; CODEINE PHOSPHATE; PARACETAMOL.

Heminevrin (*Astra*) is a proprietary SEDATIVE, available only on prescription. Its main use in childhood is to stop fits which have not come under control using other medications, such as intravenous diazepam. It is then used as an intravenous infusion and has no role as a prophylactic agent in epilepsy. It is a preparation of chlormethiazole.

▲/✚ side-effects/warning: *see* CHLORMETHIAZOLE.

Hepanutrin (*Geistlich*) is a proprietary solution intended for intravenous nutrition of patients unable to take food by mouth. Its main constituents are glucose and amino acids.

heparin is a natural ANTICOAGULANT in the body, manufactured by the liver and certain leukocytes (white cells). It can be added to solutions to wash and rinse the interior surfaces of catheters, cannulas and other medical forms of tubing to ensure that blood does not coagulate in them and they remain unobstructed while carrying out their functions.

Heparinised Saline (*Paines & Byrne*) is a proprietary solution (available only on prescription) containing the ANTICOAGULANT heparin sodium, used to wash and rinse the interior surfaces of catheters, cannulas and other medical forms of tubing to ensure that they remain unobstructed while carrying out their functions. The solution has no therapeutic use.

hepatitis B vaccine consists of an inactivated hepatitis B virus surface antigen derived from the blood plasma of a human carrier and adsorbed on to alum in suspension. It is used on patients with a high risk of infection from the hepatitis B virus mostly through contact with a carrier. Administration is by intramuscular injection in the arm or thigh; the usual regimen per patient is three doses, at intervals of one month and six months.

✚ warning: vaccination does not guarantee the avoidance of infection: common sense precautions against infection should still be observed in relation to known carriers.

Hep-Flush (*Burgess*) is a proprietary solution (available only on prescription) containing the ANTICOAGULANT HEPARIN sodium, used to wash and rinse the interior surfaces of catheters, cannulas and other medical forms of tubing to ensure that they remain unobstructed. The solution has no therapeutic use.

Hepsal (*CP Pharmaceuticals*) is a proprietary solution (available only on prescription) containing the ANTICOAGULANT HEPARIN sodium, used to wash and rinse the interior surfaces of catheters, cannulas and other

medical forms of tubing to ensure that they remain unobstructed while carrying out their functions. The solution has no therapeutic use.

heroin is a more familiar term for the narcotic ANALGESIC drug diamorphine.
see DIAMORPHINE.

Herpid (*WB Pharmaceuticals*) is a proprietary form of the ANTIVIRAL drug idoxuridine, prepared in a solution of dimethyl sulphoxide, used to treat skin infections by the viral organisms Herpes simplex (such as cold sores). Available only on prescription, Herpid is produced as a sort of paint for topical application (with a brush).
✚warning: see IDOXURIDINE.

Hewletts Antiseptic Cream (*Astra*) is a proprietary ANTISEPTIC cream for topical application on minor abrasions or burns. Available without prescription, it contains boric acid, hydrous wool fat and ZINC OXIDE.

hexachlorophane is a powerful DISINFECTANT used on the skin. In the form of a cream it is effective against scabies, and is a good substitute for soap in cases of acne or facial infection. It is also produced as a dusting-powder.
▲side-effects: there are occasionally sensitivity reactions, and even more rarely an increased sensitivity to light.
✚warning: hexachlorophane should not be used on areas of raw or abraded skin, and particularly not on raw areas of the skin of infants (in whom neural damage may occur).
Related articles: DERMALEX; STER-ZAC.

hexetidine is a mouthwash or gargle used for routine oral hygiene, to cleanse and freshen the mouth.
Related article: ORALDENE.

HGH is an abbreviation for human growth HORMONE, a hormone produced and secreted by the pituitary gland that promotes growth in the long bones of the limbs and increases protein synthesis. (It is also called somatotrophin.) For therapeutic use, however, HGH extracted from the pituitary gland is not viable; genetic engineering has made possible a form of the hormone using sequences of DNA to create what is known as a growth hormone of human sequence – somatrem – and it is this that can be used in preparations to treat dwarfism and other problems of short stature due to proven growth hormone deficiency. The treatment is given by injection – sometimes daily and continued for many years.
▲/✚ side-effects/warning: *see* SOMATREM.

Hibidil (*ICI*) is a proprietary non-prescription skin DISINFECTANT used to treat wounds and burns, and to provide asepsis during childbirth. Produced in the form of a solution in sachets, for further dilution as required, Hibidil is a preparation of chlorhexidine gluconate.
▲/✚ side-effects/warning: *see* CHLORHEXIDINE.

Hibiscrub *(ICI)* is a proprietary non-prescription DISINFECTANT used instead of soap to wash skin and hands before surgery. Produced in the form of a solution, Hibiscrub is a preparation of chlorhexidine gluconate in a surfactant liquid (a liquid with low surface tension, like a detergent).
▲/✚ side-effects/warning: *see* CHLORHEXIDINE.

Hibisol *(ICI)* is a proprietary non-prescription DISINFECTANT, used to treat minor wounds and burns on the skin and hands. Produced in the form of a solution, Hibisol is a preparation of chlorhexidine gluconate in isopropyl alcohol solvent together with emollients.
▲/✚ side-effects/warning: *see* CHLORHEXIDINE.

Hibitane *(ICI)* is the name of a series of proprietary non-prescription forms of DISINFECTANT, all based on solutions of chlorhexidine gluconate or other chlorhexidine salts. The standard form is that of a powder, used either to prepare solutions of chlorhexidine or to create antiseptic creams or powdered antiseptic compounds. There are two solutions: Hibitane 5% Concentrate (for skin disinfection, following further dilution in water or alcohol) and Hibitane Gluconate 20% (for cavities and the bladder, and to treat urethral infections). Another cream, Hibitane Antiseptic, is used to treat minor wounds and burns by topical application.
▲/✚ side-effects/warning: *see* CHLORHEXIDINE.

Hismanal *(Janssen)* is a proprietary ANTIHISTAMINE drug used primarily to treat allergic symptoms such as hay fever and urticaria. Produced in the form of tablets and as a fruit-flavoured suspension (under the trade name Hismanal Suspension), it is a preparation of astemizole. Hismanal is not recommended for children aged under six years.
▲/✚ side-effects/warning: *see* ASTEMIZOLE.

Histalix *(Wallace)* is a proprietary non-prescription EXPECTORANT and ANTITUSSIVE that is not available from the National Health Service. Produced in the form of a syrup, its active constituents include ammonium chloride, SODIUM CITRATE, DIPHENHYDRAMINE HYDROCHLORIDE and MENTHOL.

Histryl *(Smith, Kline & French)* is a proprietary ANTIHISTAMINE drug used primarily to treat allergic symptoms such as hay fever and urticaria. Produced in the form of spansules (sustained-release capsules) in two strengths (the weaker under the name Histryl Paediatric Spansule), it is a preparation of diphenylpyraline hydrochloride. Histryl, even in its paediatric form, is not recommended for children aged under seven years.
▲/✚ side-effects/warning: *see* DIPHENYLPYRALINE HYDROCHLORIDE.

HNIG is an abbreviation for human normal immunoglobulin, an injection of which − incorporating antibodies in serum − confers immediate immunity to such diseases as infective hepatitis (hepatitis A virus), measles (rubeola), and to some degree at least rubella (German measles). Prepared from more than a thousand pooled donations of blood plasma, it is commonly given to patients at risk. Administration is by intramuscular injection or occasionally by intravenous infusion.

✚ warning: HNIG should not be administered within two weeks following vaccination with live viruses, or within three months before vaccination with live viruses.

*hormones are body substances produced and secreted by glands into the bloodstream, where they are carried to specific organs and areas of tissue on which they have a specific effect. Major types of hormone include CORTICOSTEROIDS (produced mainly in the cortex of the adrenal glands), ADRENALINE from the medulla of the adrenal gland, thyroid hormones (produced by the thyroid gland), the sex hormones (produced mainly by the ovaries or the testes), and the pancreatic hormones (such as INSULIN). Most hormones can be administered therapeutically to make up hormonal deficiency, sometimes in synthetic form.

HTIG is an abbreviation for human tetanus immunoglobulin, a specific form of immunoglobulin (antibodies in serum), used mostly as an added precaution to treat patients with contaminated wounds. (It is generally only a precautionary measure because almost everybody today has established immunity through vaccination from an early age, and vaccination is in any case readily available for those at risk.) Administration is by intramuscular injection. It is available only on prescription.

Human Actraphane (Novo) is a proprietary preparation of mixed human INSULINS, available only on prescription, used to treat and maintain diabetic patients. Produced in vials for injection, Human Actraphane contains both isophane and neutral insulins in a ratio of 70% to 30% respectively.

Human Actrapid (Novo) is a proprietary non-prescription preparation of synthesized neutral human INSULIN, used to treat and maintain diabetic patients. It is produced in vials for injection, and in cartridges for use with a special injector (under the name Human Actrapid Penfill).

Human Initard 50/50 (Nordisk Wellcome) is a proprietary preparation of mixed human INSULINS, available only on prescription, used to treat and maintain diabetic patients. Produced in vials for injection, Human Initard 50/50 contains both hisophane and neutral insulins in equal proportions.

Human Insulatard (Nordisk Wellcome) is a proprietary non-prescription preparation of human isophane INSULIN, used to treat and maintain diabetic patients. It is produced in vials for injection.

Human Mixtard 30/70 (Nordisk Wellcome) is a proprietary non-prescription preparation of mixed human insulins, used to treat and maintain diabetic patients. Produced in vials for injection, Human

Mixtard contains both isophane and neutral insulins in a ratio of 70% and 30% respectively.

Human Monotard (*Novo*) is a proprietary non-prescription preparation of human INSULIN zinc suspension, used to treat and maintain diabetic patients. It is produced in vials for injection.

Human Protaphane (*Novo*) is a proprietary non-prescription preparation of human isophane INSULIN, used to treat and maintain diabetic patients. It is produced in vials for injection.

Human Ultratard (*Novo*) is a proprietary non-prescription preparation of human INSULIN zinc suspension, used to treat and maintain diabetic patients. It is produced in vials for injection.

Human Velosulin (*Nordisk Wellcome*) is a proprietary non-prescription preparation of synthesized neutral human INSULIN, used to treat and maintain diabetic patients. It is produced in vials for injection.

Humotet (*Wellcome*) is a proprietary preparation of anti-tetanus immunoglobulin (HTIG), available only on prescription, used mostly as an added precaution to treat patients with contaminated wounds. (It is generally only a precautionary measure because almost everybody today has established immunity through vaccination from an early age, and vaccination is in any case readily available for those at risk.) It is produced in vials for intramuscular injection.

Humulin I (*Lilly*) is a proprietary non-prescription preparation of human isophane INSULIN, used to treat and maintain diabetic patients. It is produced in vials for injection.

Humulin M1 (*Lilly*) is a proprietary non-prescription preparation of mixed human INSULINS, used to treat and maintain diabetic patients. Produced in vials for injection, Humulin M1 contains both isophane and neutral insulins, in a ratio of 90% to 10% respectively.

Humulin M2 (*Lilly*) is a proprietary non-prescription preparation of mixed human INSULINS, used to treat and maintain diabetic patients. Produced in vials for injection, Humulin M2 contains both isophane and neutral insulins in a ratio of 80% and 20% respectively.

Humulin S (*Lilly*) is a proprietary non-prescription preparation of synthesized neutral human INSULIN, used to treat and maintain diabetic patients. It is produced in vials for injection.

Humulin Zn (*Lilly*) is a proprietary non-prescription preparation of human INSULIN zinc suspension, used to treat and maintain diabetic patients. It is produced in vials for injection.

Hycal (*Beecham*) is a proprietary non-prescription nutritional supplement intended for patients who require a high-energy low-fluid diet low in electrolytes (as with kidney or liver disease). Gluten-free, Hycal contains mostly carbohydrate in the form of corn syrup solids; it is also protein-free and lactose-, fructose- and sucrose-free, and is produced in four flavours.

hydralazine is a vasodilator used to treat heart conditions both acute and chronic; acute in the form of a high blood pressure crisis (apoplexy), and chronic in the form of long-term high blood pressure (in which case simultaneous treatment is administered with a BETA-BLOCKER or a DIURETIC). It is sometimes used to treat congestive heart failure, when it is used in addition to diuretics. Administration is oral in the form of tablets, and by injection or infusion.
▲side-effects: there may be nausea and vomiting. Prolonged high-dosage therapy may cause a vivid red rash.
Related article: APRESOLINE.

hydrochlorothiazide is a THIAZIDE DIURETIC drug used to treat an accumulation of fluid in the tissues (oedema) and high blood pressure (*see* ANTIHYPERTENSIVE). Administration is oral in the form of tablets. It is rarely used in children.
✚warning: hydrochlorothiazide should not be administered to patients who suffer from urinary retention or kidney failure.
▲side-effects: there may be tiredness and a rash. Rarely, there is a sensitivity to light. Potassium supplements may be required.

hydrocortisone is a CORTICOSTEROID hormone, a derivative of cortisone, produced and secreted by the adrenal glands. Sometimes known as cortisol, it is highly important both for the normal metabolism of carbohydrates in the diet and for the neuro-muscular response to stress. Other than to make up hormonal deficiency, hydrocortisone may be administered therapeutically to treat any kind of inflammation (sometimes in combination with ANTIBACTERIAL drugs), including arthritis, and to treat allergic conditions (especially in emergencies). Administration is in many forms.
▲/✚ side-effects/warning: prolonged or high-dosage treatment may lead to peptic ulcers, muscle disorders, bone disorders and (in children) stunting of growth. Another potential result is the onset of adult-type diabetes. In the elderly there may be brittle bones and mental disturbances, particularly depression or euphoria. In addition, treatment with the drug may suppress symptoms of an infection until the infection is far advanced (which may in some cases present its own dangers); treatment should therefore be made as aseptic as possible, and infected areas must not be treated. Withdrawal of treatment must be gradual.
Related articles: ALPHADERM; ALPHOSYL HC; BARQUINOL HC; CANESTEN HC; CHLOROMYCETIN HYDROCORTISONE; COBADEX; CORLAN; CORTACREAM; DAKTACORT; DIODERM; DOME-CORT; ECONACORT; ECZEDERM WITH HYDROCORTISONE; EFCORTELAN; EFCORTELAN SOLUBLE; EFCORTESOL; EURAX-HYDROCORTISONE;

FRAMYCORT; FUCIDIN H; GENTICIN HC; GREGODERM;
HYDROCORTISTAB; HYDROCORTISYL; HYDROCORTONE; NEO-CORTEF;
NYBADEX; NYSTAFORM-HC; QUINOCORT; QUINODERM; SOLU-CORTEF;
TERRA-CORTRIL; TIMODINE; VIOFORM-HYDROCORTISONE.

hydrocortisone acetate is a HYDROCORTISONE salt used as an ANTI-
INFLAMMATORY to treat local inflammation of the joints or of the soft
tissues. Produced in the form of an aqueous suspension, it is
administered by injection. In the treatment of inflamed joints,
injection may be into the joint itself or into the synovial capsule that
acts as a shock-absorber within the joint.
▲/✚ side-effects/warning: see HYDROCORTISONE.
Related articles: CHLOROMYCETIN HYDROCORTISONE;
HYDROCORTISTAB; FRAMYCORT; NEO-CORTEF.

hydrocortisone butyrate is a HYDROCORTISONE salt used as an ANTI-
INFLAMMATORY to treat severe inflammation of the skin that has failed
to respond to treatment with less powerful drugs (as may occur with
some forms of eczema). Administration is topical in the form of cream,
ointment or lotion. It is rarely used in children.
▲/✚ side-effects/warning: see HYDROCORTISONE.
Related article: LOCOID.

hydrocortisone sodium phosphate is a HYDROCORTISONE salt used to
treat deficiency of the HORMONE hydrocortisone. Administration is by
injection, optionally diluted.
▲/✚ side-effects/warning: see HYDROCORTISONE.
Related article: EFCORTESOL.

hydrocortisone sodium succinate is a HYDROCORTISONE SALT USED
PRIMARILY TO TREAT DEFICIENCY OF THE HORMONE hydrocortisone, but also
as an ANTI-INFLAMMATORY to treat inflammation and lesions in and
around the mouth. Administration is by injection, optionally diluted,
or in the form of lozenges.
▲/✚ side-effects/warning: see HYDROCORTISONE.
Related articles: CORLAN; EFCORTELAN SOLUBLE; SOLU-CORTEF.

Hydrocortistab (*Boots*) is a proprietary ANTI-INFLAMMATORY drug,
available only on prescription, in which the active constituent is the
CORTICOSTEROID hormone hydrocortisone. Produced in the form of
tablets and in vials for injection, Hydrocortistab is used to treat
inflammation in allergic conditions. Produced in the form of a cream
and an ointment, Hydrocortistab is used to treat severe skin
inflammations, such as eczema and various forms of dermatitis.
▲/✚ side-effects/warning: see HYDROCORTISONE.

Hydrocortisyl (*Roussel*) is a proprietary ANTI-INFLAMMATORY drug,
available only on prescription, in which the active constituent is the
CORTICOSTEROID hormone hydrocortisone. Produced in the form of a
cream and an ointment, Hydrocortisyl is used to treat severe skin
inflammations, such as eczema and various forms of dermatitis.
▲/✚ side-effects/warning: see HYDROCORTISONE.

Hydrocortone (*Merck, Sharp & Dohme*) is a proprietary form of the CORTICOSTEROID hormone hydrocortisone, used to make up hormonal deficiency and to treat inflammation, shock, and certain allergic conditions. Available only on prescription, Hydrocortisone is produced in the form of tablets (in two strengths).
▲/✚ side-effects/warning: *see* HYDROCORTISONE.

hydrogen peroxide is a general DISINFECTANT used in solution and as a cream to cleanse and deodorize wounds and ulcers, to clean ears in the form of ear-drops, and as a mouth wash and gargle for oral hygiene. Some preparations available require further dilution: a 6% solution is the maximum concentration recommended for use on the skin. Solutions stronger will bleach fabric.

hydrotalcite is an ANTACID complex that is readily dissociated internally for rapid relief of dyspepsia, and has deflatulent properties. Administration is oral in the form of tablets that can be chewed, or in suspension. It is not recommended for children aged under six years. *Related article:* ALTACITE.

hyoscine (also known as scopolamine, particularly in the USA) is a powerful alkaloid drug derived from plants of the belladonna family. By itself it is an effective SEDATIVE and HYPNOTIC — it is often used together with the OPIATE PAPAVERETUM as a premedication prior to surgery — and an ANTI-EMETIC (in which capacity it is found in travel-sickness medications). In the form of its bromide salts, hyoscine has additional antispasmodic properties without the side-effects usually associated with other antispasmodic drugs that directly affect the central nervous system (and is thus particularly useful in treating disorders of the muscular walls of the stomach and intestines, such as the symptoms of colic). It is also used (in solution) in ophthalmic treatments to paralyze the muscles of the pupil of the eye either for surgery or to rest the eye following surgery. Administration is oral in the form of tablets, by injection, or as eye-drops.
▲ side-effects: there may be drowsiness, dizziness and dry mouth; sometimes there is also blurred vision and difficulty in urinating.
✚ warning: hyoscine (or its bromide salts) should not be administered to patients with glaucoma; it should be administered with caution to those with heart or intestinal disease, or urinary retention.
Related articles: BUSCOPAN; OMNOPON-SCOPOLAMINE.

Hypnomidate (*Janssen*) is a proprietary general ANAESTHETIC used primarily for initial induction of anaesthesia. Available only on prescription, it is produced in ampoules for injection (in two strengths, the stronger for dilution), and is a preparation of etomidate. It should not be allowed to come into contact with plastic equipment.
▲/✚ side-effects/warning: *see* ETOMIDATE.

*hypnotics are a type of drug that induces sleep by direct action on various centres of the brain. They are used mainly to treat insomnia, and to calm patients who are mentally ill. Best known and most used hypnotics are the BENZODIAZEPINES (such as diazepam and nitrazepam), other medications useful in children include CHLORAL HYDRATE and some of the ANTIHISTAMINES.

Hypnovel is a proprietary preparation of the powerful BENZODIAZEPINE midazolam, available only on prescription, used mainly for sedation, particularly as a premedication prior to surgery, for the initial induction of anaesthesia, or for the short-term anaesthesia required for endoscopy or minor surgical examinations. Its effect is often accompanied by a form of amnesia. It is produced in ampoules for infusion (in two strengths).

Hypotears (*Cooper Vision*) is a proprietary non-prescription compound of polyethylene glycol with POLYVINYL ALCOHOL, used to supplement the film of tears over the eye when the mucus that normally constitutes that film is intermittent or missing through disease or disorder. It is produced in the form of drops to be used every three to four hours (or as required).

Hypurin Isophane (*CP Pharmaceuticals*) is a proprietary non-prescription preparation of highly purified beef isophane INSULIN, used to treat and maintain diabetic patients. It is produced in vials, for injection.

Hypurin Lente (*CP Pharmaceuticals*) is a proprietary non-prescription preparation of highly purified beef INSULIN zinc suspension, used to treat and maintain diabetic patients. It is produced in vials, for injection.

Hypurin Neutral (*CP Pharmaceuticals*) is a proprietary non-prescription preparation of highly purified beef neutral INSULIN, used to treat and maintain diabetic patients. It is produced in vials, for injection.

Hypurin Protamine Zinc (*CP Pharmaceuticals*) is a proprietary non-prescription preparation of highly purified beef protamine zinc INSULIN, used to treat and maintain diabetic patients. It is produced in vials, for injection.
▲/✚ side-effects/warning: *see* INSULIN.

Ibular (*Lagap*) is a proprietary ANTI-INFLAMMATORY non-narcotic ANALGESIC, available only on prescription, used to treat the pain of rheumatic and other musculo-skeletal disorders. Produced in the form of tablets, Ibular is a preparation of ibuprofen.
▲/✚ side-effects/warning: *see* IBUPROFEN.

ibuprofen is a non-steroid ANTI-INFLAMMATORY non-narcotic ANALGESIC drug used primarily to treat the pain of rheumatism and other musculo-skeletal disorders, but also sometimes to treat other forms of pain, including menstrual pain (dysmenorrhoea). Administration is oral in the form of tablets or sustained-release capsules, or as a syrup.
▲ side-effects: administration with or following meals reduces the risk of gastrointestinal disturbance and nausea. But there may be headache, dizziness and ringing in the ears (tinnitus), and some patients experience sensitivity reactions or blood disorders. Occasionally there is fluid retention.
Related articles: APSIFEN; BRUFEN; EBUFAC; IBULAR; MOTRIN; PAXOFEN.

Ichthaband (*Seton*) is a proprietary form of bandaging impregnated with ZINC PASTE (15%) and ichthammol (2%), used to treat and dress chronic forms of eczema.
▲/✚ side-effects/warning: *see* ICHTHAMMOL.

ichthammol is a thick, dark brown liquid derived from bituminous oils, used for its mildly ANTISEPTIC properties in ointments or in glycerol solution for the topical treatment of ulcers and inflammation on the skin. Milder than COAL TAR, ichthammol is useful in treating the less severe forms of eczema. A popular mode of administration is in an impregnated bandage with ZINC PASTE.
▲ side-effects: some patients experience skin irritation; the skin may become sensitized.
✚ warning: ichthammol must not be placed in contact with broken skin surfaces.
Related articles: ICHTHABAND; ICHTHOPASTE.

Ichthopaste (*Smith & Nephew*) is a proprietary form of bandaging impregnated with ZINC PASTE (6%) and ichthammol (2%), used to treat and dress chronic forms of eczema.
▲/✚ side-effects/warning: *see* ICHTHAMMOL.

Idoxene (*Spodefell*) is a proprietary ANTIBIOTIC eye ointment, available only on prescription, used to treat local viral infections, particularly of *Herpes simplex*. It is a solute preparation of idoxuridine.
▲/✚ side-effects/warning: *see* IDOXURIDINE.

idoxuridine is an ANTIVIRAL drug used primarily in very mild solution to treat viral infections (such as herpes simplex) in and around the mouth or eye. It works by inhibiting the growth of the viruses. Administration is as a paint for topical application, as eye-drops or as eye ointment.
✚ warning: because idoxuridine contains iodine, treatment may cause initial irritation and/or stinging.

Related articles: HERPID; IDOXENE; IDURIDIN; KERECID; OPHTHALMADINE.

Iduridin (*Ferring*) is a proprietary ANTIVIRAL drug, available only on prescription, used to treat infections of the skin by herpes simplex (cold sores). Produced in the form of a lotion or paint, for topical application either with a dropper or its own applicator, Iduridin is a solution of idoxuridine in the organic solvent dimethyl sulphoxide (DMSO).
✚warning: see IDOXURIDINE.

Ilosone (*Dista*) is a proprietary broad-spectrum ANTIBIOTIC, one of the macrolides, used to treat many forms of infection. It is a common choice for children as it is generally well tolerated and its spectrum of action is particularly wide (for example, it is used to make children with whooping cough non-infectious, and it may be given to likely contacts to try to prevent the disease). Administration is oral in the form of tablets, as capsules, or a dilute suspension (mixture) or by injection. However, patients often complain that injection is uncomfortable. Tablets have to be enteric- or film-coated because the drug is inactivated by gastric secretions. Ilsone is a preparation of erythromycin estolate.
▲/✚ side-effects/warning: *see* ERYTHROMYCIN.

Imferon (*CP Pharmaceuticals*) is a proprietary preparation of IRON and DEXTRAN, administered in infusion or by injection to patients who are in need of substantial replacement of iron and who, perhaps because of malabsorption, cannot be given iron orally. Administration by infusion is slow – over six to eight hours. It is rarely, if ever, necessary to use this in childhood. Oral iron therapy is much preferred.
✚warning: stringent tests must first be carried out to ensure that the patient will not suffer any allergic reaction: if hypersensitivity reactions do occur, they are usually violent. For this reason, treatment by infusion must be supervised throughout and for a time afterwards; there must also be full facilities for emergency cardio-respiratory resuscitation immediately available. Imferon should not be administered to patients with severe disease of the kidneys or liver, and should not be administered by infusion to asthmatic patients.

*imidazoles are a group of ANTIFUNGAL drugs active against most fungi and yeasts. The most common condition that they are used to treat is thrush. Best known and most used imidazoles include clotrimazole, miconazole, ketoconazole and econazole.
see CLOTRIMAZOLE; ECONAZOLE NITRATE; KETOCONAZOLE; MICONAZOLE.

imipramine is an ANTIDEPRESSANT drug of a type that has fewer sedative properties than many others. As is the case with many such drugs, imipramine can also be used to treat bed wetting at night by children (aged over seven years). However, there is a tendency for patients to relapse on stopping medication. It may be particularly useful when a child is away from home to save embarrassment.

Administration is oral in the form of tablets or as a syrup, or by injection.

▲ side-effects: there are few when taken for bedwetting, as the dosage is low.

✚ warning: these tablets are dangerous if taken in overdose and should be kept in a safe place.

Related article: TOFRANIL.

*immunization against specific diseases is effected by either of two means. Active immunity is conferred by vaccination, in which live antigens that have been rendered harmless (attenuated) or dead ones (inactivated) are administered by injection or by mouth so that the body's own defence mechanisms are required to deal with them (by manufacturing antibodies) and with anything like them that they encounter again. This method gives long-lasting but protection. Passive immunity is conferred by the injection of a quantity of blood serum already containing antibodies (immunoglobulins); this method gives immediate protection which eventually wears off.

see IMMUNOGLOBULINS; VACCINES.

*immunoglobulins are proteins of a specific structure, which act as antibodies in the bloodstream. Created in response to the presence of a specific antigen, immunoglobulins circulate with the blood to give systemic defence and protection as part of the immune system. Classified according to a differentiation of class and function, immunoglobulins may be administered therapeutically by injection or infusion to confer immediate (passive) immunity.

see IMMUNIZATION.

Related article: HNIG.

*immunosuppressants are drugs used to inhibit the body's resistance to the presence of infection or foreign bodies. In this capacity, such drugs may be used to suppress tissue rejection following donor grafting or transplant surgery (although there is then the risk of unopposed infection). Commonly used medications include CYCLOSPORIN and AZATHIOPRINE.

Imodium (*Janssen*) is a proprietary ANTIDIARRHOEAL drug, available only on prescription, which works by reducing the speed at which material travels along the intestines. Produced in the form of capsules, and as a syrup, Imodium is a preparation of the OPIATE loperamide hydrochloride. It is not usually recommended for children aged under four years.

▲/✚ side-effects/warning: *see* LOPERAMIDE HYDROCHLORIDE.

Imperacin (*ICI*) is a proprietary broad-spectrum ANTIBIOTIC, available only on prescription, used to treat serious infections by bacteria and other micro-organisms (such as chlamydia and rickettsia), and to relieve severe acne. Produced in the form of tablets, Imperacin is a preparation of the TETRACYCLINE oxytetracycline dihydrate. It is not recommended for children aged under 12 years.

▲/✚ side-effects/warning: *see* OXYTETRACYCLINE.

Imuran (*Wellcome*) is a proprietary preparation of the CYTOTOXIC drug azathioprine, used to suppress tissue rejection following donor grafting or transplant surgery, particularly in cases where corticosteroids have already been used excessively and/or failed to be fully effective. Available only on prescription, Imuran is produced in the form of tablets (in two strengths), and as a powder for reconstitution as a medium for injection.

indomethacin is a non-steroidal ANTI-INFLAMMATORY non-narcotic ANALGESIC drug used to treat rheumatic and muscular pain caused by inflammation and/or bone degeneration, particularly at the joints. It is not usually used in children for this purpose. Administration is mostly oral in the form of tablets, capsules, sustained-release capsules or as a liquid, but its use in anal suppositories is especially effective for the relief of pain overnight and stiffness in the morning. Indomethacin is given to some premature babies to help close a structure called a Patent Ductus Arteriosus, which is a vascular connection between the systemic and pulmonary blood circulations.
▲ side-effects: gastrointestinal disturbance and fluid retention are quite common.

*influenza vaccines are recommended only for persons at high risk of catching known strains of influenza. This is because the influenza viruses A and B are constantly changing in physical form, and antibodies manufactured in the body to deal with one strain at one time will have no effect at all on the same strain at another time. Consequently, it is only possible to provide vaccine for any single strain once it has already shown itself to be endemic. Moreover, during times when no influenza strain is endemic, vaccination against influenza is positively discouraged. The World Health Organisation makes an annual recommendation on the strains of virus for which stocks of vaccine should be prepared. Administration is by injection of surface-antigen vaccine: a single dose for adults (unless the specific strain is in the process of changing again and two slightly different doses are required), two doses over five weeks or so for children.
Related articles: FLUVIRIN; INFLUVAC SUB-UNIT.

Influvac Sub-unit (*Duphar*) is the name of a series of proprietary influenza vaccines consisting of inactivated surface antigens of the influenza virus. None is recommended for children aged under four years.
▲ side-effects: rarely, there is local reaction together with headache and high temperature.
✚ warning: like any influenza vaccine, Influvac Sub-unit cannot control epidemics and should be used only − in what seems to be the appropriate strain − to treat people who are at high risk: the elderly, patients with cardiovascular problems, and medical staff. Influvac Sub-unit should not be administered to patients who are markedly allergic to egg or chicken protein (in which vaccine viruses are cultured), or who are pregnant.

Initard 50/50 (*Nordisk Wellcome*) is a proprietary non-prescription preparation of mixed pork INSULINS used to treat and maintain diabetic patients. Produced in vials for injection, Initard 50/50 contains both neutral and isophane insulins in equal proportions.

Initard 50/50 Human
see HUMAN INITARD 50/50.

Instant Carobel (*Cow & Gate*) is a proprietary non-prescription powder, used to thicken milk and therefore may be helpful in infants with troublesome regurgitation. Carobel is a preparation of carob seed flour.

Insulatard (*Nordisk Wellcome*) is a proprietary non-prescription preparation of pork isophane INSULIN, used to treat and maintain diabetic patients. It is produced in vials for injection.

Insulatard, Human
see HUMAN INSULATARD.

insulin is a protein hormone produced and secreted by the islets of Langerhans within the pancreas. It has the effect of reducing the level of glucose (sugar) in the bloodstream, and is meant as one half of a balancing mechanism with opposing hormones which increase the blood sugar level. Its absence (in the disorder called diabetes mellitus) therefore results in high levels of blood sugar that can rapidly lead to severe symptoms, and potentially coma and death. Most diabetics therefore take some form of insulin on a regular (daily) basis, generally by injection. All children with diabetes need to take insulin. Modern genetic engineering has permitted the production of quantities of the human form of insulin that are now replacing the former insulins extracted from oxen (beef insulin) or pigs (pork insulin). There is also a difference in absorption time between insulin with an acid pH (acid insulin injection) and neutral insulin. Other insulin preparations are intermediate-acting (and require administration twice daily, on a "biphasic" basis) or long-acting (and require only once-daily administration). These include insulin zinc suspension (long-acting) and isophane insulin (suitable for the initiation of biphasic regimes). Many diabetic patients use more than one type of insulin in proportions directly related to their own specific needs.

Intal (*Fisons*) is a proprietary preparation of sodium cromoglycate, available only on prescription, used in the form of an inhalant to prevent asthma attacks. The drug is thought to work by effectively inhibiting the release of histamine and other mediators in the membranes of the bronchial passages. Intal is produced in several modes both in liquid form and as a powder: in an aerosol (in two strengths, the stronger under the trade name Intal 5), in an automatic insufflator (under the trade name Halermatic) and in solution for a power-operated nebuliser. It is produced in the form of dry powder inhalation cartridges (Spincaps) for use with an inhaler

called a spinhaler. Under the trade name Intal Compound, sodium cromoglycate is combined with the BETA-RECEPTOR STIMULANT isoprenaline sulphate.
▲/✚ side-effects/warning: *see* ISOPRENALINE; SODIUM CROMOGLYCATE.

Intralipid (*KabiVitrum*) is a proprietary form of high-energy nutritional supplement intended for infusion into patients who are unable to take food via the alimentary canal. Produced in two strengths (under the trade names Intralipid 10% and Intralipid 20%), its major constituent is fat emulsion derived from soya bean oils and from eggs.

Intraval Sodium (*May & Baker*) is a proprietary GENERAL ANAESTHETIC, available only on prescription, used mainly for the induction of anaesthesia or for short-duration effect during minor surgical procedures. Produced in the form of a powder for reconstitution as a medium for injections (in two strengths), and in ampoules and bottles (flasks), Intraval Sodium is a preparation of thiopentone sodium.
▲/✚ side-effects/warning: *see* THIOPENTONE SODIUM.

Intropin (*American Hospital Supply*) is a proprietary preparation of the powerful SYMPATHOMIMETIC drug dopamine hydrochloride, used to treat cardiogenic shock. Dosage is critical − too much OR too little may have harmful effects. It is produced in the form of a liquid (in two strengths) for dilution and infusion.
▲/✚ side-effects/warning: *see* DOPAMINE.

iodine is an element required in small quantities in the diet for healthy growth and development. Good dietary sources are sea food and iodized salt. Internally, iodine is concentrated in the thyroid gland in the neck, because the gland utilizes iodine in the production of the thyroid hormones. The element is thus administered therapeutically to make up for dietary deficiency leading to hypothyroidism, and radioactive isotopes of iodine are used in the diagnosis and treatment of thyroid gland disorders. More mundanely, iodine is still commonly used as an ANTISEPTIC (either as AQUEOUS IODINE SOLUTION or as POVIDINE-IODINE).
▲ side-effects: there may be sensitivity reactions, resulting in symptoms like those of a heavy cold; a rash may also occur. Prolonged treatment with iodine may lead to insomnia and depression.

Ionax Scrub (*Alcon*) is a proprietary non-prescription gel and is a preparation of the ANTISEPTIC BENZALKONIUM CHLORIDE together with abrasive polyethylene granules within a foaming aqueous-alcohol base. It is used to treat acne, or to cleanse the skin before the application of further acne treatments.

Ionil T (*Alcon*) is a proprietary preparation of the ANTISEPTICS BENZALKONIUM CHLORIDE and COAL TAR together with the astringent ANTIFUNGAL drug SALICYLIC ACID, all within an alcohol base. It is used to treat seborrhoeic dermatitis of the scalp, and is accordingly produced as a shampoo. If required for strictly medical reasons it is available on prescription.

ipecacuanha (or ipecac) is an extract from the roots of a Brazilian shrub that is an irritant to the digestive system. It is a powerful emetic (used to make a child vomit in some instances of non-corrosive poisoning), but in smaller doses it is also used in non-proprietary mixtures and in proprietary tinctures and syrups as an expectorant. ✚ warning: high dosage can cause severe gastric upset.

Ipral (*Squibb*) is a proprietary ANTIBIOTIC, available only on prescription, used to treat infections of the urinary tract. Produced in the form of tablets (in two strengths) and as a sugar-free suspension for children (under the trade name Ipral Paediatric) for dilution (the potency of the suspension once dilute is retained for 14 days), Ipral is a preparation of the drug trimethoprim.
▲/✚ side-effects/warning: *see* TRIMETHOPRIM.

ipratropium is an ANTICHOLINERGIC drug that has the properties of a BRONCHODILATOR, and is (in the form of ipratropium bromide) accordingly used to treat asthma. Administration is by inhalation, from an aerosol or from a nebuliser.
Related article: ATROVENT.

Irofol C (*Abbott*) is a proprietary non-prescription IRON-and-VITAMIN compound that is not available from the National Health Service. As an iron and a vitamin supplement, it is used particularly during pregnancy. It contains iron (in the form of ferrous sulphate), FOLIC ACID (a B vitamin) and ASCORBIC ACID (vitamin C), and is produced in the form of sustained-release tablets.

iron is a metallic element essential to the body in several ways, and especially important in its role as transporter of oxygen around the body (in the form of the red blood cell constituent oxyhaemoglobin); it is also retained in the muscles. Dietary deficiency of iron leads to anaemia; good food sources include meats, particularly liver. Iron is administered therapeutically mostly to make up a dietary deficiency (and so treat anaemia). Supplements may be administered orally (in the form of FERROUS FUMARATE, FERROUS GLUCONATE, FERROUS GLYCINE SULPHATE, FERROUS SUCCINATE, FERROUS SULPHATE and other salts). There are also many iron-and-vitamin supplements available to prevent deficiencies of either (particularly during pregnancy).

Ironorm (*Wallace*) is three preparations of a mineral-and-VITAMIN compound. It is available without prescription as a tonic (or elixir) containing IRON (in the form of ferric ammonium citrate), calcium, phosphorus, most forms of vitamin B, and liver extract. Available only on prescription are capsules containing iron (in the form of FERROUS SULPHATE), several forms of vitamin B, ascorbic acid (vitamin C) and fractionated liver. Also available only on prescription are ampoules of the plasma-and-iron infusion fluid, iron dextran complex.

Iso-Autohaler (*Lewis*) is a proprietary BETA-RECEPTOR STIMULANT, available only on prescription, used in the form of an inhalant to treat bronchial asthma. Produced in an aerosol, Iso-Autohaler is a preparation of isoprenaline sulphate. This has generally been replaced in therapy by more selective drugs such as salbutamol and terbutaline.

▲/✚ side-effects/warning: *see* ISOPRENALINE.

Isocal (*Mead Johnson*) is a proprietary non-prescription gluten-free liquid that is a complete nutritional diet for patients who are severely undernourished (such as with anorexia nervosa) or who have some problem of absorption of food (such as following gastrectomy). Also lactose-free, Isocal contains protein, carbohydrate and fats, with vitamins and minerals, but is unsuitable as the sole source of nutrition for children, and unsuitable altogether for children aged under 12 months.

Isogel (*Allen & Hanburys*) is a proprietary form of the type of laxative known as a bulking agent, which works by increasing the overall mass of faeces within the rectum, so stimulating bowel movement. It is thus used both to relieve constipation and to relieve diarrhoea, and also in the control of faecal consistency for patients with a colostomy. Produced in the form of granules for solution in water, Isogel is a preparation of ispaghula husk.

▲/✚ side-effects/warning: *see* ISPAGHULA HUSK.

Isomil (*Abbott*) is a proprietary non-prescription gluten-free powder that when reconstituted is a complete nutritional diet for patients – especially infants – who are unable to tolerate milk or milk sugars. Also therefore milk protein-free and lactose-free, Isomil contains protein, carbohydrate and fats, with vitamins and minerals.

isoniazid is an ANTITUBERCULAR drug used, as is normal in the treatment of tuberculosis, in combination with other antibacterial drugs to defeat bacterial resistance. It is also administered to prevent the contraction of tuberculosis by close associates of an infected patient. Administration is oral in the form of tablets or as a non-proprietary elixir, or by injection.

▲ side-effects: there may be nausea with vomiting. Jaundice may result. High dosage may lead to sensitivity reactions, including a rash.

Related article: RIMIFON.

isoprenaline is a compound substance closely related to the hormone ADRENALINE. In the form of isoprenaline sulphate it is a BETA-RECEPTOR STIMULANT and BRONCHODILATOR produced as an inhalant or in the form of tablets to be held under the tongue, and was used primarily to treat the bronchospasm of asthma. However, it is rarely used for this purpose nowadays. In the form of isoprenaline hydrochloride, however, it is a SYMPATHOMIMETIC administered by injection, and is used to treat extremely slow heart rate and some heart diseases.

▲ side-effects: there may be headache, nervous tension, tremor of the hands, sweating, increased heart rate and heartbeat irregularities, and a decrease in blood potassium levels. Administration as an inhalant results in few of these side-effects.

✚warning: isoprenaline should be administered with caution to patients with heart disease or excessive secretion of thyroid hormones (hyperthyroidism), or who are diabetic (in which case regular blood sugar counts are essential during treatment).
Related article: DUO-AUTOHALER; ISO-AUTOHALER; MEDIHALER-ISO.

Isopto (*Alcon*) is a series of proprietary preparations of various drugs, all available only on prescription, each used in the form of eye-drops to treat infections and glaucoma, and to facilitate inspection of the eye. The range comprises Isopto Alkaline (comprising simply the synthetic tear medium hypromellose); Isopto Atropine (comprising ATROPINE SULPHATE); Isopto Carbachol (comprising carbachol and the synthetic tear medium hypromellose); Isopto Carpine (comprising PILOCARPINE hydrochloride, in any of five strengths, and the synthetic tear medium hypromellose); Isopto Cetamide (comprising SULPHACETAMIDE sodium and the synthetic tear medium hypromellose); Isopto Epinal (comprising the hormone ADRENALINE and the synthetic tear medium hypromellose); Isopto Frin (comprising PHENYLEPHRINE hydrochloride and the synthetic tear medium hypromellose); and Isopto Plain (comprising simply the synthetic tear medium hypromellose, at half the strength of Isopto Alkaline).

isotretinoin is a powerful drug, derived from retinol (vitamin A), and used for the systemic treatment of severe acne that has failed to respond to more usual therapies. Full medical supervision is required during treatment, which may last for three or four months – during which (from about the second to the fourth week) there may actually be an exacerbation of the acne; if treatment fails, repeat courses should not be given. Administration is oral in the form of capsules (generally from hospitals only).

▲side-effects: dry lips and mucous membranes, sore eyes, and joint and muscle pains are not uncommon; there may also be nose-bleeds and temporary hair loss.

✚warning: blood fat levels and liver function should be regularly checked.

ispaghula husk is a high-fibre substance used as a LAXATIVE because it is an effective bulking agent – it increases the overall mass of faeces within the rectum, so stimulating bowel movement. It is also particularly useful in soothing the symptoms of diverticular disease and irritable colon. Administration is oral, generally in the form of granules or a powder for solution in water.

▲side-effects: there may be flatulence, so much as to distend the abdomen.

✚warning: preparations of ispaghula husk should not be administered to patients with obstruction of the intestines, or failure of the muscles of the intestinal wall; it should be administered with caution to those with ulcerative colitis. Fluid intake during treatment should be higher than usual.
Related articles: AGIOLAX; FYBOGEL; ISOGEL; METAMUCIL.

itraconazole is a broad-spectrum ANTIFUNGAL agent of the triazole
family, used to treat fungal infections on the skin. In particular,
itraconazole is used to treat resistant candidiasis (thrush or
moniliasis) and infections of the skin or finger-nails by *tinea*
organisms (such as athlete's foot).

▲ side-effects: there may be nausea, abdominal pains and dyspepsia.

✚ warning: itraconazole should not be administered to patients who
have impaired liver function or who are pregnant.

Jacksons (*Ernest Jackson*) are proprietary non-prescription throat lozenges. They contain acetic acid, camphor, benzoic acid and menthol.

Jectofer (*Astra*) is a proprietary compound of iron sorbitol and citric acid, available only on prescription, used to replace IRON in patients with iron-deficiency anaemia. It is produced as a dark brown liquid for intramuscular injection. It is rarely used in children, as oral preparations of iron are preferred.
▲side-effects: rarely, there are heartbeat irregularities.
✚warning: Jectofer should not be administered to patients with liver or kidney disease.

Jexin (*Duncan, Flockhart*) is a proprietary SKELETAL MUSCLE RELAXANT, available only on prescription, of the type known as competitive or non-depolarizing. It is used during surgical operations, but only after the patient has been rendered unconscious. Produced in ampoules for injection, Jexin's active constituent is tubocurarine chloride.
▲/✚ side-effects/warning: *see* TUBOCURARINE.

Joy-Rides (*Stafford-Miller*) is a proprietary non-prescription ANTICHOLINERGIC formulation for the treatment of motion sickness. It contains the atropine-like drug hyoscine.
▲/✚ side-effects/warning: *see* HYOSCINE.

Juvela (*G F Dietary Supplies*) is a proprietary non-prescription brand of gluten-free bread- and cake-mix, produced for patients with coeliac disease and other forms of gluten sensitivity. There is also a low-protein milk-free version for patients suffering from defects of protein metabolism such as phenylketonuria (PKU).

Kabiglobulin (*KabiVitrum*) is a proprietary preparation of human normal immunoglobulin (HNIG), part of the plasma of the blood that is directly concerned with immunity. Administered by intramuscular injection, Kabiglobulin is used to protect patients at risk from contact with hepatitis A virus or measles (rubeola), to give at least some protection against rubella (German measles), or to enhance immunity in patients who have suffered serious shock (as for example from crush injuries or large-scale burns).
➕warning: *see* HNIG.

Kamillosan (*Norgine*) is a proprietary, non-prescription, water-based OINTMENT, used to treat and soothe nappy rash, cracked nipples and chapping on the hands. Its active constituents are various essences of chamomile.

kanamycin is a broad-spectrum ANTIBIOTIC of the aminoglycoside family, with activity against gram-positive bacteria but used primarily against serious infections caused by gram-negative bacteria. It is not orally absorbed and is therefore given by injection or infusion for the treatment of, for example, septicaemia. Because of its toxicity to the ear (ototoxicity) potentially resulting in deafness, and its toxicity to the kidney (nephrotoxicity), treatment should be limited in duration. Because of the relatively frequent occurrence of bacterial resistance in some coliform bacteria, kanamycin has largely been replaced by gentamicin. It is not frequently used in children because of this toxicity.
▲side-effects: prolonged or high dosage may be damaging to the ear causing deafness and balance disorders; treatment must be discontinued if this occurs; there may also be reversible kidney damage.
➕warning: because the drug is excreted by the kidney great care must be taken in patients with impaired kidney function. In such cases, and/or where dosage is high or prolonged, regular checks on kanamycin concentrations in the blood must be carried out.
Related article: KANNASYN.

Kannasyn (*Winthrop*) is a proprietary form of the aminoglycoside ANTIBIOTIC kanamycin sulphate, available only on prescription, used to treat serious bacterial infections. It is produced in the form of a solution and as powder for reconstitution, in both cases for injection.
▲/➕ side-effects/warning: *see* KANAMYCIN.

Kaodene (*Boots*) is a proprietary, non-prescription liquid preparation used to treat diarrhoea, containing the adsorbent kaolin with the opiate codeine phosphate. It is not recommended for children aged under five years or patients with chronic liver disease (because it may cause sedation). In particular, fluid intake should be increased to more than normal. Prolonged use should be avoided.
▲/➕ side-effects/warning: *see* CODEINE PHOSPHATE.

kaolin is a white clay (china clay) which, when purified (and sometimes powdered), is used as an adsorbent, particularly in

ANTIDIARRHOEAL preparations (with or without opiates such as CODEINE PHOSPHATE or MORPHINE) but also to treat food poisoning and some digestive disorders. Occasionally used in poultices, it is additionally found in some dusting powders.
Related articles: KAODENE; KAOPECTATE.

Kaopectate (*Upjohn*) is a proprietary non-prescription suspension of the ANTIDIARRHOEAL adsorbent kaolin, in a form suitable for dilution (the potency of the dilute mixture is retained for 14 days) before being taken orally. During treatment, fluid intake should be increased to more than normal.

Kay-Cee-L (*Geistlich*) is a proprietary non-prescription form of potassium supplement, used to treat patients with deficiencies and to replace potassium in patients taking potassium-depleting drugs such as diuretics. It is produced in the form of a red syrup (not for dilution) containing potassium chloride.

Kefadol (*Dista*) is a proprietary ANTIBIOTIC, available only on prescription, used to treat bacterial infections, but also to provide freedom from infection during surgery. Produced in the form of a powder for reconstitution as injections, Kefadol is a compound of the cephalosporin cephamandole with sodium carbonate.
▲/✚ side-effects/warning: *see* CEPHAMANDOLE.

Keflex (*Lilly*) is a proprietary ANTIBIOTIC, available only on prescription, used to treat bacterial infections. Produced in the form of capsules (in two strengths), tablets (in two strengths) and as a suspension (for dilution, in two strengths). Keflex is a preparation of the cephalosporin cephalexin.
▲/✚ side-effects/warning: *see* CEPHALEXIN.

Keflin (*Lilly*) is a proprietary ANTIBIOTIC, available only on prescription, used to treat bacterial infections, but also to provide freedom from infection during surgery. Produced in the form of powder for reconstitution as injections, Keflin is a preparation of the cephalosporin cephalothin.
▲/✚ side-effects/warning: *see* CEPHALOTHIN.

Kefzol (*Lilly*) is a proprietary ANTIBIOTIC, available only on prescription, used to treat bacterial infections, but also to provide freedom from infection during surgery. Produced in the form of powder for reconstitution as injections, Kefzol is a preparation of the cephalosporin cephazolin.
▲/✚ side-effects/warning: *see* CEPHAZOLIN.

Kelferon (*MCP Pharmaceuticals*) is a proprietary non-prescription preparation of the drug ferrous glycine sulphate, used as an IRON supplement in the treatment of iron-deficiency anaemia, and produced in the form of tablets.
▲/✚ side-effects/warning: *see* FERROUS GLYCINE SULPHATE.

Kelocyanor (*Lipha*) is a proprietary CHELATING AGENT, available only on prescription, that is an emergency antidote to cyanide poisoning. It is produced in the form of ampoules for injection, containing dicobalt edetate in glucose solution.

Kemicetine (*Farmitalia Carlo Erba*) is a proprietary broad-spectrum ANTIBIOTIC, available only on prescription. Produced in the form of powder for reconstitution as injections, Kemicetine is a preparation of the powerful drug chloramphenicol which, because of its potential toxicity, is generally only used to treat life-threatening infections.
▲/✚ side-effects/warning: *see* CHLORAMPHENICOL.

Kenalog (*Squibb*) is a proprietary form of the anti-inflammatory glucocorticoid (corticosteroid) drug triamcinolone acetonide, available only on prescription. Produced in the form of pre-filled hypodermics, Kenalog is used in two different ways in order to achieve either of two distinct purposes: intramuscular injection relieves allergic states (such as hay fever or pollen induced asthma) and some collagen disorders, and can reduce severe dermatitis; injection directly into a joint relieves pain, swelling and stiffness (such as with rheumatoid arthritis, bursitis and tenosynovitis). It is not recommended for children aged under six years.
▲/✚ side-effects/warning: *see* TRIAMCINOLONE ACETONIDE.

Keralyt (*Westwood*) is a proprietary non-prescription gel containing salicylic acid, used to treat thickened patches of skin (hyperkeratoses), as occur in some forms of eczema, in ichthyosis and in psoriasis. Each evening the gel is smoothed on to cleansed skin and held by bandaging overnight; it is washed off each morning.
▲/✚ side-effects/warning: *see* SALICYLIC ACID.

*keratolytics are drugs and preparations intended to clear the skin of thickened, horny patches (hyperkeratoses) and scaly areas, as occur in some forms of eczema, ichthyosis and psoriasis, and in the treatment of acne. The standard, classic keratolytic is salicylic acid, generally used in very mild solution. Others include ichthammol, coal tar, etretinate and dithranol (which is the most powerful), several of which can usefully be applied in the form of paste inside an impregnated bandage.
Related articles: COAL TAR; DITHRANOL; ICHTHAMMOL; SALICYLIC ACID; ZINC PASTE.

Kerecid (*Smith, Kline & French*) is a proprietary preparation, available only on prescription, used to treat *Herpes simplex* infections of the eye. Containing a mild solution of the antiviral agent idoxuridine, it is produced in the form of eye-drops (with polyvinyl alcohol) for use during the day, and eye ointment for use overnight.

Keri (*Westwood*) is a proprietary non-prescription lotion used to soften dry skin and to relieve itching. Active constituents include liquid paraffin and lanolin oil. It is produced in a pump pack, and is intended to be massaged into the skin.

Ketalar (*Parke-Davis*) is a proprietary preparation of the general ANAESTHETIC ketamine, in the form of ketamine chloride. Available only on prescription, Ketalar is produced as vials for injection (in three strengths).
▲/✚ side-effects/warning: *see* KETAMINE.

ketamine is a general ANAESTHETIC that is used mainly for minor surgery on children, in whom hallucinogenic side-effects seem to appear less often than in adults. Ketamine increases muscle tone, maintains good air passages, and has good analgesic qualities at doses too low for actual anaesthesia. Administration is either by intramuscular injection or by intravenous infusion.
▲ side-effects: Transient hallucinations may occur.
✚ warning: ketamine should not be administered to patients who suffer from high blood pressure (hypertension) or who are mentally ill.
Related article: KETALAR.

ketoconazole is a broad-spectrum ANTIFUNGAL agent, an IMIDAZOLE that is surprisingly effective when taken orally, used to treat deep-seated fungal infections (mycoses) or superficial ones that have not responded to other treatment. In particular, ketoconazole is used to treat resistant candidiasis (thrush, or moniliasis) and dermatophytic infections of the skin or fingernails.
▲ side-effects: liver damage may occur − and to a serious extent; rarely there may be an itching skin rash, or nausea.
✚ warning: ketoconazole should not be administered to patients who have impaired function of the liver.
Related article: NIZORAL.

ketotifen is an ANTIHISTAMINE that may be prescribed in an effort to prevent asthmatic attacks. However, experimental evidence suggests that it is of little benefit. It may be used to treat other allergic disorders. Administration should be simultaneous with a meal.
▲/✚ side-effects/warning: ketotifen may cause drowsiness and dryness in the mouth.
Related article: ZADITEN.

Ketovite (*Paines & Byrne*) is a proprietary MULTIVITAMIN supplement, available only on prescription, used as an adjunct in synthetic diets. Produced in the form of tablets and a liquid, both forms are intended to be taken daily following a specified regimen. The tablets contain thiamine (vitamin B_1), riboflavine (vitamin B_2), PYRIDOXINE (vitamin B_3), cyanocobalamin (vitamin B_{12}), nicotinamide (of the vitamin B complex), FOLIC ACID (of the B complex), ASCORBIC ACID (vitamin C) and other useful factgors; the sugar-free liquid contains retinol (vitamin A), CYANOCOBALAMIN (vitamin B_{12}), and a form of CALCIFEROL (vitamin D) in a purified water base.

Kloref (*Cox Pharmaceuticals*) is a proprietary non-prescription form of POTASSIUM supplement, used to treat patients with deficiencies and to replace potassium in patients taking potassium-depleting drugs such as diuretics. It is produced in the form of effervescent tablets and (under the name Kloref-S) sachets of granules containing potassium chloride, potassium bicarbonate and betaine hydrochloride.

Konakion (*Roche*) is a proprietary form of VITAMIN K — or phytomenadione — used in newborn infants to prevent haemorrhage which may result from deficiency of this vitamin, and to treat patients deficient in the vitamin because of fat malabsorption. It is produced in the form of (non-prescription) tablets, and ampoules for injection (available in two strengths, only on prescription).

Kwells (*Nicholas-Kiwi*) is a proprietary ANTICHOLINERGIC non-prescription anti-motion sickness preparation containing hyoscine.
▲/✚ side-effects/warning: *see* HYOSCINE.

labetalol hydrochloride is a mixed BETA-BLOCKER and alpha-blocker used to treat high blood pressure (hypertension) and to control blood pressure during surgery. Administration is oral in the form of tablets, and by injection. It is not commonly recommended for children.
▲ side-effects: there may be lethargy and debility, headache and/or tingling of the scalp; rashes may break out. Higher dosages may lead to low blood pressure (hypotension).
✚ warning: labetalol hydrochloride should be administered with caution to patients who have heart failure, who are already taking drugs to control the heart rate, or who have a history of bronchospasm.
Related article: LABROCOL.

Labrocol (*Lagap*) is a proprietary form of the mixed BETA-BLOCKER and alpha-blocker labetalol hydrochloride, available only on prescription, used to treat high blood pressure (*see* ANTIHYPERTENSIVE) and to control the heart rate during surgery. Produced in the form of tablets (in three strengths), Labrocol is not commonly recommended for children.
▲/✚ side-effects/warning: *see* LABETALOL HYDROCHLORIDE.

Lacticare (*Stiefel*) is a proprietary non-prescription skin emollient (softener and soother), used to treat chronic conditions of dry skin. Produced in the form of a lotion for topical application, Lacticare contains the simple sugar lactic acid and a moisturizer.

lactulose is a LAXATIVE that works by causing a volume of fluid to be retained in the colon through osmosis. Its action also discourages the increase of ammonia-producing microbes – although it may take up to 48 hours to have full effect (this property may be useful in liver failure).
▲ side-effects: rarely, there is nausea and vomiting.
✚ warning: lactulose should not be administered to patients with any form of intestinal obstruction.
Related article: DUPHALAC.

lanolin (or hydrous wool fat) is a non-proprietary skin emollient (softener and soother) commonly used also as a base for other medications. It has some antibacterial properties, but in some patients can cause a sensitivity reaction (in the form usually of an eczematous rash).

Lanoxin (*Wellcome*) is a proprietary form of the powerful heart stimulant digoxin (a CARDIAC GLYCOSIDE), available only on prescription, used to treat heart failure and severe heartbeat irregularity. It is produced in the form of tablets (in several strengths, under the names Lanoxin, Lanoxin 125 and Lanoxin PG), as an elixir (under the name Lanoxin PG Elixir) and in ampoules for injection (under the name Lanoxin Injection).
▲/✚ side-effects/warning: *see* DIGOXIN.

Laractone (*Lagap*) is a proprietary DIURETIC drug, available only on prescription, used to treat accumulation of fluids within the tissues

(oedema), particularly when due to cirrhosis of the liver. Produced in the form of tablets (in two strengths), Laractone is a preparation of the weak potassium-sparing diuretic spironolactone.
▲/✚ side-effects/warning: *see* SPIRONOLACTONE.

Laratrim (*Lagap*) is a proprietary broad-spectrum ANTIBACTERIAL, available only on prescription, used to treat infections of the urinary tract, the sinuses or the middle ear. It is produced in the form of tablets (in two strengths, the stronger under the name Laratrim Forte) and as a suspension (in two strengths, Laratrim Paediatric Suspension and Laratrim Adult Suspension), Laratrim is a compound combination of the drug trimethoprim and the sulphonamide, sulphamethoxazole – a compound itself known as co-trimoxazole.
▲/✚ side-effects/warning: *see* CO-TRIMOXAZOLE.

Largactil (*May & Baker*) is a proprietary preparation of the powerful PHENOTHIAZINE drug chlorpromazine hydrochloride, used primarily to treat patients who are undergoing behavioural disturbances (as a major TRANQUILLIZER), or who are psychotic (as an ANTIPSYCHOTIC), particularly schizophrenic. It is also used to treat severe anxiety, or as an anti-emetic sedative prior to surgery. Available only on prescription, Largactil is produced in the form of tablets (in three strengths), as a syrup (under the name Largactil Syrup), as a suspension (under the name Largactil Forte Suspension), as anal suppositories (under the name Largactil Suppositories), and in ampoules for injection (under the name Largactil Injection). In the form of suppositories Largactil is not recommended for the treatment of children.
▲/✚ side-effects/warning: *see* CHLORPROMAZINE.

Lasix (*Hoechst*) is a proprietary DIURETIC drug, available only on prescription, used to treat accumulation of fluids within the tissues (oedema), particularly when due to heart, kidney or liver disease, or associated with high blood pressure (hypertension). Produced in the form of tablets (in three strengths, the third under the name Lasix 500 for use in hospitals only), as a syrup for children (under the name Lasix Paediatric Liquid), and in ampoules for injection (under the name Lasix Injection).
▲/✚ side-effects/warning: *see* FRUSEMIDE.

Lassar's paste is a non-proprietary formulation of ZINC OXIDE, salicylic acid and starch in white soft paraffin. Applied topically, it is used to treat hard, layered, dead skin. The compound must not be put on broken or inflamed skin.

latamoxef disodium is a broad-spectrum cephalosporin ANTIBIOTIC used to treat many bacterial infections. Administration is by injection.
▲ side-effects: there may be hypersensitivity reactions, including effects on the composition of the blood (on which it may have an anticoagulating influence). Rarely there is diarrhoea.

✚warning: it should be administered with caution to those known to have penicillin sensitivity. Dosage should be reduced in patients with impaired kidney function.
Related article: MOXALACTAM.

*laxatives are preparations that promote defecation and so relieve constipation. There are several types. One major type is faecal softeners (which soften the faeces for easier evacuation); they include LIQUID PARAFFIN. Another type is the bulking agent (which increases the overall volume of the faeces in the rectum and thus stimulates bowel movement); bulking agents are mostly what is also called fibre, and include BRAN, ISPAGHULA HUSK, METHYLCELLULOSE and sterculia. A third type is the stimulant laxative, which acts on the intestinal muscles to increase motility; many old-fashioned remedies are stimulants of this kind, including CASCARA, CASTOR OIL, figs, and SENNA – but there are modern variants too, such as BISACODYL, DIOCTYL SODIUM SULPHOSUCCINATE (docusate sodium) and SODIUM PICOSULPHATE. Some laxatives work by bringing in water from surrounding tissues, so increasing overall liquidity: such osmotic laxatives include MAGNESIUM HYDROXIDE, MAGNESIUM SULPHATE and LACTULOSE.

Laxoberal (*Windsor*) is a proprietary non-prescription LAXATIVE that is not available from the National
Health Service. A stimulant laxative, Laxoberal is produced in the form of a liquid containing sodium picosulphate.
▲/✚ side-effects/warning: *see* SODIUM PICOSULPHATE.

Ledclair (*Sinclair*) is a proprietary CHELATING AGENT, an antidote to poisoning by heavy metals, especially by lead, available only on prescription. Produced in liquid form in ampoules for injection, and as a cream for topical use on areas of skin that have become broken or sensitive through contact with the metals, Ledclair's active constituent is sodium calciumedetate.
▲/✚ side-effects/warning: *see* SODIUM CALCIUMEDETATE.

Ledercort (*Lederle*) is a proprietary form of the anti-inflammatory glucocorticoid (CORTICOSTEROID) drug triamcinolone, available only on prescription. Produced in the form of tablets (in two strengths) and, as triamcinolone acetonide, as a water-based cream and an anhydrous ointment, Ledercort treats inflammations of the skin (such as severe eczema), and particularly inflammations arising as a result of allergy.
▲/✚ side-effects/warning: *see* TRIAMCINOLONE; TRIAMCINOLONE ACETONIDE.

Ledermycin (*Lederle*) is a proprietary ANTIBIOTIC, available only on prescription, used to treat infections of soft tissues, particularly of the upper respiratory tract. Produced in the form of tablets (in two strengths, the stronger under the name Ledermycin Tablets), Ledermycin is a preparation of the TETRACYCLINE demeclocycline hydrochloride. It is not used in children aged under 12 years.
▲/✚ side-effects/warning: *see* DEMECLOCYCLINE HYDROCHLORIDE.

Lederspan (*Lederle*) is a proprietary CORTICOSTEROID drug, available only on prescription, used to treat INFLAMMATION of the joints and the soft tissues. Produced in the form of a suspension in vials for injection (in two concentrations), Lederspan's active constituent is the corticosteroid triamcinolone hexacetonide.

▲/✚ side-effects/warning: *see* TRIAMCINOLONE HEXACETONIDE.

Lem-sip (*Nicholas-Kiwi*) is a proprietary non-prescription cold relief preparation containing the non-narcotic ANALGESIC paracetamol, the SYMPATHOMIMETIC phenylephrine, sodium citrate and ascorbic acid.

▲/✚ side-effects/warning: *see* ASCORBIC ACID; PARACETAMOL; PHENYLEPHRINE; SODIUM CITRATE.

Lenium (*Winthrop*) is a proprietary non-prescription cream shampoo containing SELENIUM SULPHIDE, a salt thought to act as an antidandruff agent. Lenium should not be used within 48 hours of a hair colorant or a permanent wave.

Lentard MC is a proprietary non-prescription preparation of the protein hormone INSULIN, in the form of insulin zinc suspension, used to treat diabetic patients. Containing highly purified beef and pork insulins, Lentard MC's effect is of intermediate duration, intended to maintain background residual levels of the hormone. It is produced in vials for injection.

Leo K (*Leo*) is a proprietary non-prescription form of POTASSIUM supplement, used to treat patients with deficiencies and to replace potassium in patients taking potassium-depleting drugs such as diuretics. It is produced in the form of tablets containing potassium chloride.

▲/✚ side-effects/warning: *see* POTASSIUM CHLORIDE.

levamisole is an ANTHELMINTIC drug used specifically to treat infestation by roundworms. Effective, it is also well tolerated and side-effects are rare. Occasionally there may be mild nausea.

Lidocaton is a proprietary preparation of the local ANAESTHETIC lignocaine, used in cartridges for dental surgery.

▲/✚ side-effects/warning: *see* LIGNOCAINE.

lignocaine is primarily a local ANAESTHETIC, the drug of choice for very many topical or minor surgical procedures, especially in dentistry (because it is absorbed directly through mucous membranes). It is, for example, used on the throat to prepare a patient for bronchoscopy. For a greater duration of action it may be combined with adrenaline. It also has an anti-arrythmic action and may be used to treat heartbeat irregularities. Administration is (in the form of lignocaine hydrochloride) by infiltration, injection or infusion, or topically as a gel, an ointment, a spray, a lotion, or as eye-drops.

✚ warning: lignocaine should not be administered to patients with the neuromuscular disease myasthenia gravis; it should be administered with caution to those with heart or liver failure (in order not to cause depression of the central nervous system and convulsions), or from epilepsy.

▲ side-effects: when used to treat heartbeat irregularities there is generally a slowing of the heart rate and a fall in blood pressure. *Related articles:* LIDOCATON; LIGNOSTAB; MINIMS; LIGNOCAINE AND FLUOROSCEIN; NEO-LIDOCATON; XYLOCAINE; XYLOTOX.

Lignostab is a proprietary preparation of the local ANAESTHETIC lignocaine, used in cartridges for dental surgery.
▲/✚ side-effects/warning: *see* LIGNOCAINE.

Lincocin (*Upjohn*) is a proprietary ANTIBIOTIC, available only on prescription, used to treat serious infections of the tissues and bones (particularly infections that prove to be resistant to penicillin). Produced in the form of capsules, as a syrup for dilution (the potency of the syrup once dilute is retained for 14 days) and in ampoules for injection, Lincocin is a preparation of lincomycin.
▲/✚ side-effects/warning: *see* LINCOMYCIN.

lincomycin is an ANTIBIOTIC that is now used less commonly than it once was (because of side-effects) to treat infections of bones and joints, and peritonitis (inflammation of the peritoneal lining of the abdominal cavity). Administration is oral in the form of capsules and as a dilute syrup, or by injection or infusion.
▲ side-effects: diarrhoea or other symptoms of colitis may appear during treatment. There may be nausea and vomiting.
✚ warning: lincomycin should not be administered to patients suffering from diarrhoea; if diarrhoea or other symptoms of colitis appear during treatment, administration must be halted at once. This is because lincomycin is especially disposed towards promoting colitis (particularly in mature or elderly women), causing potentially severe symptoms. It should be administered with caution to patients with impaired liver or kidney function.
Related article: LINCOCIN.

*linctuses are medicated syrups, thick and soothing enough to relieve sore throats or loosen a cough. (A linctus is not the same as an expectorant, however, which is intended to make it easier to cough sputum up. Nor is it necessarily an elixir, which disguises a potentially horrible taste with a sweetening substance like glycerol or alcohol).

lindane (or gamma benzene hexachloride) is a drug used to treat parasitic infestation by lice (pediculosis) or by itch-mites (scabies) on the skin surface, particularly under the hair. However, strains of head-lice resistant to lindane have recently emerged, and the drug is now not recommended for use on the scalp. Administration is topical in the form of a lotion or a shampoo, to be left wet as long as possible.
▲ side-effects: side-effects are rare, but a few patients suffer minor skin irritation.
✚ warning: keep lindane away from the eyes.
Related articles: ESODERM; LOREXANE; QUELLADA.

liniments are medicated lotions for rubbing into the skin; many contain alcohol and/or camphor, and are intended to relieve minor muscle indispositions. Some liniments are alternatively produced for application on a surgical dressing.

Lioresal (*Ciba*) is a proprietary SKELETAL MUSCLE RELAXANT, available only on prescription, used to treat muscle spasm caused by injury or disease in the central nervous system, for example, spasticity associated with cerebral palsy. Produced in the form of tablets and as a sugar-free liquid for dilution (the potency of the diluted liquid is retained for 14 days), Lioresal is a preparation of baclofen.
▲/✚ side-effects/warning: *see* BACLOFEN.

liothyronine sodium is a form of the natural thyroid HORMONE triiodothyronine, used to make up a hormonal deficiency (hypothyroidism) and to treat the associated symptoms (myxoedema). It may also be used in the treatment of goitre. Administration is oral in the form of tablets, or by injection.
Related article: TERTROXIN.

Lipobase (*Brocades*) is a proprietary non-prescription skin emollient (softener and soother), used to treat dry conditions of the skin (especially in alternation with corticosteroid preparations). Produced in the form of a cream, Lipobase contains stearyl alcohol in a paraffin base, and is a base in which other medications can be applied topically.

liquid paraffin is an old-fashioned but effective LAXATIVE. It is a constituent of a number of proprietary laxatives and some non-proprietary formulations. But it can also be used as a tear-substitute, administered as an eye ointment for patients in whom tear production is dysfunctioning.
▲ side-effects: little is absorbed in the intestines; seepage of the paraffin may thus occur from the anus, causing local irritation. Prolonged use may interfere with the internal absorption of fat-soluble vitamins.
✚ warning: prolonged or continuous use of liquid paraffin as a laxative is to be avoided.
Related articles: AGAROL; PETROLAGAR.

Liquifilm Tears (*Allergan*) is a proprietary non-prescription tear-substitute, used to lubricate the eyes of patients whose tear producing apparatus is not working properly. Produced in the form of eye drops, Liquifilm Tears is a solution of POLYVINYL ALCOHOL.

Liquigen (*Scientific Hospital Supplies*) is a proprietary non-prescription gluten-free milk substitute, produced for patients recovering from intestinal surgery or with chronic disease of the liver or of the pancreas; it may also be used for patients on the special diet associated with epilepsy. Produced in the form of an emulsion, Liquigen is a preparation of neutral lipids.

Locasol New Formula (*Cow & Gate*) is a milk substitute for people who suffer from high calcium levels. Produced in the form of powder,

Locasol New Formula is a preparation of protein, carbohydrate, fat, lactose, vitamins and minerals.

Lockets (*Mars*) are a proprietary non-prescription cold relief preparation containing honey, GLYCEROL, citric acid, menthol and eucalyptus.
▲/✚ side-effects/warning: *see* MENTHOL.

Locobase (*Brocades*) is a proprietary non-prescription skin emollient (softener and soother), used to treat dry conditions of the skin (especially in alternation with corticosteroid preparations). Produced in the form of a water-miscible cream and an anhydrous ointment, Locobase is a base in which other medications can be applied topically to the skin.

Locoid (*Brocades*) is a proprietary CORTICOSTEROID, available only on prescription, used to treat serious non-infective inflammatory skin conditions, such as eczema. Produced in the form of a water-miscible cream, in a fatty cream base (under the name Lipocream), ointment and a scalp lotion, Locoid is a preparation of the steroid hydrocortisone butyrate. Another version of Locoid additionally containing the broad-spectrum ANTIBIOTIC chlorquinaldol is also available (under the trade name Locoid C), produced in the form of a cream and an ointment.
▲/✚ side-effects/warning: *see* HYDROCORTISONE BUTYRATE.

Locorten-Vioform (*Zyma*) is a proprietary ANTIBACTERIAL AND ANTIFUNGAL, available only on prescription, used to treat infections in the ear. Produced in the form of ear-drops, Locorten-Vioform is a compound of CLIOQUINOL and the minor CORTICOSTEROID flumethasone pivalate.
▲/✚ side-effects/warning: *see* CLIOQUINOL.

Lofenalac (*Bristol-Myers*) is a proprietary non-prescription nutritional supplement, used to nourish patients with amino-acid abnormalities (such as phenylketonuria). Produced in the form of a powder, Lofenalac contains protein, carbohydrate, fats, vitamins and minerals. It is gluten-, sucrose- and lactose-free.

Lomotil (*Gold Cross*) is a proprietary ANTIDIARRHOEAL drug available only on prescription, which works by reducing the speed at which material travels along the intestines. Produced in the form of tablets and as a sugar-free liquid for dilution (with glycerol: the potency of the diluted liquid is retained for 14 days), Lomotil is a preparation of the OPIATE diphenoxylate hydrochloride and the ANTI-CHOLINERGIC belladonna alkaloid, atropine sulphate. It is not recommended for children aged under two years.
▲/✚ side-effects/warning: *see* ATROPINE SULPHATE; DIPHENOXYLATE HYDROCHLORIDE.

loperamide hydrochloride is an ANTIDIARRHOEAL drug which acts on the sympathetic nervous system to inhibit peristalsis — the waves of muscular activity that force along the intestinal contents — so reducing motility. Although loperamide is an OPIATE, even prolonged treatment is unlikely to cause dependence; it also has fewer sedative effects on patients than other opiates used to treat chronic diarrhoea. Administration is oral in the form of capsules or as a dilute syrup.

▲ side-effects: there may be a rash.

Related articles: ARRET; IMODIUM.

lorazepam is an ANXIOLYTIC and ANTIDEPRESSANT drug, one of the BENZODIAZEPINES. In children it may be used as a premedication before surgery or as a sedative.

Administration is oral in the form of tablets.

▲ side-effects: concentration and speed of reaction are affected. Drowsiness, dizziness, headache, dry mouth and shallow breathing are all fairly common.

Related article: ATIVAN.

Lorexane (*Care*) is a proprietary non-prescription preparation of the parasiticidal drug lindane, used to treat infestation of the skin of the trunk and limbs by itch-mites (scabies) or by lice (pediculosis). It is produced in the form of a water-miscible cream and (under the name Lorexane No. 3) as a shampoo.

▲/✚ side-effects/warning: *see* LINDANE.

*lotions are medicated liquids used to bathe or wash skin conditions, the hair or the eyes. In many cases lotions should be left wet after application for as long as possible.

Lotussin (*Searle*) is a proprietary non-prescription ANTIHISTAMINE EXPECTORANT and cough mixture that is not available from the National Health Service. Produced in the form of a syrup for dilution (the potency of the mixture once dilute is retained for 14 days), Lotussin is a compound of the cough suppressant dextromethorphan hydrobromine, the antihistamine diphenhydramine hydrochloride, the SYMPATHOMIMETIC ephedrine hydrochloride and the EXPECTORANT guaiphenesin. It is not recommended for children aged under 12 months.

▲/✚ side-effects/warning: *see* DEXTROMETHORPHAN; DIPHENHYDRAMINE HYDROCHLORIDE; EPHEDRINE HYDROCHLORIDE.

Lugacin (*Lagap*) is a proprietary ANTIBIOTIC, available only on prescription, used to treat serious infections in various parts of the body. Produced in ampoules for injection, Lugacin is a preparation of the aminoglycoside gentamicin.

▲/✚ side-effects/warning: *see* GENTAMICIN.

Lugol's solution is a non-proprietary solution of iodine and potassium iodide in water (and is also known as aqueous iodine solution). It is used as an iodine supplement for patients suffering from an excess of thyroid hormones in the bloodstream (thyrotoxicosis), especially prior to thyroid surgery.

▲/✚ side-effects/warning: *see* IODINE.

lymecycline is a broad-spectrum ANTIBIOTIC, one of the tetracyclines, used to treat infections of many kinds. Administration is oral in the form of capsules.

▲ side-effects: there may be nausea and vomiting, with diarrhoea. Some patients experience a sensitivity to light. Rarely, there are allergic reactions.

✚ warning: lymecycline should not be administered to patients with kidney failure or who are aged under 12 years. It should be administered with caution to those with impaired liver function. *Related article:* TETRALYSAL.

lypressin (or 8-lysine vasopressin) is one of two major forms of the antidiuretic HORMONE vasopressin, used to treat pituitary-originated diabetes insipidus. Administration of lypressin is topical in the form of a nasal spray.

▲/✚ side-effects/warning: *see* VASOPRESSIN. *Related article:* SYNTOPRESSIN.

8-lysine vasopressin is a chemical name for lypressin. *see* LYPRESSIN.

Mac (*Beecham Health Care*) are proprietary non-prescription throat sweets containing sucrose and glucose syrups, menthol and amylmetacresol.

Macrodantin (*Norwich Eaton*) is a proprietary ANTIBIOTIC drug, available only on prescription, used to treat infections of the urinary tract. It works by interfering with the DNA of specific bacteria. Produced in the form of capsules (in two strengths), Macrodantin is a preparation of the antibacterial nitrofurantoin. It is not normally recommended for children aged under 30 months.
▲/✚ side-effects/warning: *see* NITROFURANTOIN.

Macrodex (*Pharmacia*) is a proprietary form of Dextran 70 intravenous infusion, available only on prescription, used to make up a deficiency in the overall volume of blood in a patient, or to prevent thrombosis following surgery. It is produced in flasks, and prepared in a glucose or a saline matrix.
▲/✚ side-effects/warning: *see* DEXTRAN.

macrogol ointment is a skin emollient (softener and soother) consisting of a compound of two water-soluble constituent macrogols (polyethelene glycols); unlike most emollient ointments, therefore, it is readily washed off − a property that is sometimes useful.

Magnapen (*Beecham*) is a proprietary compound ANTIBIOTIC, available only on prescription, used to treat bacterial infection where the causative organism has not been identified or where penicillin-resistant bacterial infection is probable. Produced in the form of capsules, as a syrup (under the name Magnapen Syrup), as a powder for reconstitution as a syrup, and in vials for injections (under the name Magnapen Injection), Magnapen is a preparation of the broad-spectrum penicillin-like antibiotic ampicillin together with the anti-staphylococcal antibiotic flucloxacillin. It should not be used for blind treatment of infections because many organisms are now resistant.
▲/✚ side-effects/warning: *see* AMPICILLIN; FLUCLOXACILLIN.

magnesium is a metallic element necessary to the body; ingested as a trace element in the diet, it is important to the functioning of the nerves and muscles. Good dietary sources include green vegetables. Therapeutically, magnesium is used in the form of its salts. Magnesium carbonate, hydroxide, oxide ("magnesia") and trisilicate are ANTACIDS; MAGNESIUM SULPHATE (Epsom salt/salts) is a saline LAXATIVE; magnesium deficiency is usually treated with supplements of MAGNESIUM CHLORIDE.
▲/✚ side-effects/warning: *see* MAGNESIUM CARBONATE; MAGNESIUM HYDROXIDE; MAGNESIUM TRISILICATE.

magnesium carbonate is a natural ANTACID that also has LAXATIVE properties. As an antacid it is actually comparatively weak, but fairly long-acting. Used to relieve indigestion and to soothe duodenal ulcer pain, it is commonly combined with other antacids. Administration is oral, most commonly in the form of a non-proprietary water-based mixture that also includes sodium bicarbonate.

▲ side-effects: there may be belching – due to the internal liberation of carbon dioxide – and diarrhoea.

✚ warning: magnesium carbonate should be administered with caution to patients with impaired function of the kidney, or who are taking any other form of drug.
Related articles: ALUDROX; DIOVOL.

magnesium chloride is the form of MAGNESIUM most commonly used to make up a deficiency of the metallic element in the body (as may occur through prolonged diarrhoea or vomiting.

magnesium hydroxide (or hydrated magnesium oxide – "magnesia") is a natural ANTACID that also has LAXATIVE properties. As an antacid it is actually comparatively weak, but fairly long-acting. Used to relieve indigestion and to soothe duodenal ulcer pain, it is sometimes combined with other antacids. Administration is oral in the form of tablets or as an aqueous suspension.

▲ side-effects: there may be diarrhoea.

✚ warning: magnesium hydroxide should be administered with caution to patients with impaired function of the kidney, or who are taking any other form of drug.
Related article: DIOVOL.

magnesium sulphate (or Epsom salt/salts) is a LAXATIVE that works by preventing the resorption of water within the intestines. It is sometimes also used as a MAGNESIUM supplement, administered to patients whose bodies are deficient in the mineral. And as a paste with glycerol, it is used topically to treat boils and carbuncles.

magnesium trisilicate is a natural ANTACID that also has absorbent properties. As an antacid it is long-acting. Used to relieve indigestion and to soothe peptic ulcer pain, it is sometimes combined with other antacids. Administration is oral in the form of tablets or as an aqueous suspension.

✚ warning: magnesium trisilicate should be administered with caution to patients with impaired function of the kidney, or who are taking any other form of drug.
Related article: GAVISCON.

Malarivon (*Wallace*) is a proprietary ANTIMALARIAL drug, available only on prescription, used both to prevent and to treat malaria. Produced in the form of an elixir, Malarivon is a preparation of the powerful drug chloroquine.

▲/✚ side-effects/warning: *see* CHLOROQUINE.

malathion is a powerful drug used to treat infestations by lice (pediculosis) or by itch-mites (scabies). Administration is topical in the form of a lotion or a shampoo, but treatment should not take place more than once a week for more than three weeks in succession. Some of the proprietary forms are highly inflammable.

✚ warning: avoid contact with the eyes.
Related articles: DERBAC-M; PRIODERM; SULFO-M.

Maloprim (*Wellcome*) is a proprietary ANTIMALARIAL drug, available only on prescription, used to prevent travellers to tropical areas from contracting the disease. Produced in the form of tablets, Maloprim is a compound of the SULPHONE dapsone together with the catalytic enzyme-inhibitor pyrimethamine (which is particularly useful in relation to malarial strains resistant to chloroquine). Treatment is weekly, not daily, but must be continued for at least four weeks after the patient leaves the tropical area.

▲/✚ side-effects/warning: *see* DAPSONE; PYRIMETHAMINE.

mannitol is a form of sugar that cannot be metabolized. Therapeutically, it is used primarily to lower pressure within the head when there is brain swelling.

▲ side-effects: there may be high body temperature with chills.

✚ warning: treatment may in the short term expand the overall blood volume, and should not be administered to patients with heart complaints or fluid on the lungs (pulmonary oedema). An escape of mannitol into the tissues from the site of infusion or from a blood vessel causes inflammation.

Marcain (*Astra*) is a proprietary form of the local ANAESTHETIC drug bupivacaine, used particularly when duration of treatment is to be prolonged. Administration is thus most commonly as a nerve block injection, or as a lumbar puncture or epidural. Available only on prescription, Marcain is produced in ampoules by itself (in four strengths, the strongest under the name Marcain Heavy), and with additional adrenaline (in two strengths, under the name Marcain with Adrenaline).

▲/✚ side-effects/warning: *see* ADRENALINE; BUPIVACAINE HYDROCHLORIDE.

Maxamaid XP (*Scientific Hospital Supplies*) is a proprietary, non-prescription, orange-flavoured powder consisting of a virtually complete nutritional supplement for patients with amino-acid abnormalities (such as phenylketonuria). It thus contains amino acids (except phenylalanine), carbohydrate, vitamins and trace elements; it is also gluten-free. Maxamaid XP is not recommended for children aged under two years.

Maxidex (*Alcon*) is a proprietary compound, available only on prescription, used to treat inflammation of the surface of the eye. Produced in the form of eye-drops, Maxidex is a combination of the CORTICOSTEROID dexamethasone with the water-soluble cellulose derivative hypromellose (the basis of "artificial tears", a spreading agent).

▲/✚ side-effects/warning: *see* DEXAMETHASONE.

Maxijul (*Scientific Hospital Supplies*) is the name of a proprietary non-prescription series of preparations consisting of nutritional supplements for patients who require a high-energy low-fluid diet. Consisting mostly of polyglucose polymer, sodium and potassium, the standard form of Maxijul is produced as a gluten-, sucrose-, lactose-, galactose- and fructose-free powder. There is also a liquid form (in three flavours, under the name Maxijul Liquid) and a form with less sodium and potassium (under the name Maxijul LE).

Maxitrol (*Alcon*) is a proprietary compound, available only on prescription, used to treat inflammation of the surface of the eye. Produced in the form of eye-drops for daytime use, and as an ointment for use overnight, Maxitrol is a combination of the CORTICOSTEROID dexamethasone and the ANTIBIOTICS neomycin and polymyxin B sulphate; the eye-drops also contain the water-soluble cellulose derivative hypromellose (the basis of "artificial tears", a spreading agent).
    ▲/✚ side-effects/warning: *see* DEXAMETHASONE; NEOMYCIN; POLYMYXIN B SULPHATE.

Maxolon (*Beecham*) is an effective ANTI-EMETIC drug used to prevent vomiting caused by gastrointestinal disorders or by chemotherapy or radiotherapy in the treatment of cancer. Available only on prescription, Maxolon's primary constituent − metoclopramide hydrochloride − works by action on the vomiting centre in the brain and by encouraging the flow of stomach contents into the intestine. It is produced in the form of tablets, in liquid form (under the name Maxolon Paediatric Liquid), as a syrup (under the name Maxolon Syrup) and in ampoules for injection (under the name Maxolon Injection and Maxolon High Dose).
    ▲/✚ side-effects/warning: *see* METOCLOPRAMIDE.

Maxtrex (*Farmitalia Carlo Erba*) is a proprietary preparation of the ANTICANCER drug methotrexate, available only on prescription, used to treat some forms of leukaemia, certain solid tumours, and other conditions in which abnormal cell replication is occurring. For this reason it may also be used to treat severe psoriasis. It is produced in the form of a solution (in two strengths) in vials, and as tablets (in two strengths, under the name Maxtrex Tablets).
    ▲/✚ side-effects/warning: *see* METHOTREXATE.

MCT Oil (*Bristol-Myers*) is a proprietary non-prescription form of fats (lipids) used as a nutritional supplement for patients whose metabolism finds fat absorption difficult or impossible (for instance following intestinal surgery, with cirrhosis of the liver, or with cystic fibrosis of the pancreas).

MCT(1) (*Cow & Gate*) is a proprietary non-prescription nutritional supplement for patients whose capacity for food absorption has been reduced (for instance following intestinal surgery, with chronic liver disease, or with cystic fibrosis of the pancreas). In the form of a powder for reconstitution, MCT(1) contains protein, carbohydrate, and fats (triglycerides); it is also low in lactose and sucrose-free.

measles vaccine is a VACCINE against measles (rubeola), available only on prescription. It is a powdered preparation of live but attenuated measles viruses for administration by injection. It is not usually recommended for children aged under 12 months.

▲side-effects: there may be inflammation at the site of injection. Occasionally a mild measles-like illness may develop about a week after the vaccination.

✚warning: it should not be administered to patients who suffer from any infection, particularly tuberculosis; who have known immune-system abnormalities; or who are already taking corticosteroid drugs (except for replacement therapy), cytotoxic drugs or undergoing radiation treatment.

mebendazole is an ANTHELMINTIC drug used in the treatment of infections by roundworm, threadworm, whipworm and hookworm. A powerful drug generally well tolerated, it is the treatment of choice for patients of all ages over two years.

▲side-effects: side-effects are uncommon, but there may be diarrhoea and abdominal pain.

✚warning: mebendazole should not be administered to patients who are aged under two years.
Related article: VERMOX.

mebhydrolin is an ANTIHISTAMINE used to treat allergic conditions such as hay fever and urticaria, some forms of dermatitis, and some sensitivity reactions to drugs. Its additional sedative properties are useful in the treatment of some allergic conditions. Administration is oral in the form of tablets or a dilute suspension (mixture).

▲side-effects: sedation may affect capacity for speed of thought and movement; there may be nausea, headache and/or weight gain, dry mouth, gastrointestinal disturbances and visual problems.
Related article: FABAHISTIN.

mecillinam is a penicillin-type ANTIBIOTIC, it may be used to treat urinary infections. Administration is in the form of injection.

▲side-effects: there may be sensitivity reactions ranging from a minor rash to urticaria and joint pains, and (occasionally) to high temperature or anaphylactic shock. High doses may in any case cause convulsions.

✚warning: mecillinam should not be administered to patients known to be allergic to penicillins; it should be administered with caution to those with impaired kidney function.
Related article: SELEXIDIN.

meclozine is an ANTIHISTAMINE used primarily as an ANTI-EMETIC in the treatment or prevention of motion sickness and vomiting. Administration (as meclozine hydrochloride, generally with a form of vitamin B) is oral in the form of tablets.

▲side-effects: concentration and speed of thought may be affected. There is commonly dry mouth and drowsiness; there may also be headache, blurred vision and gastrointestinal disturbances.

✚warning: meclozine should be administered with caution to patients with epilepsy or liver disease.

Medicoal (*Lundbeck*) is a proprietary non-prescription adsorbent preparation for oral administration, used to treat patients suffering from poisoning or a drug overdose. It works by binding the toxic material to itself before being excreted in the normal way. Produced in the form of granules for effervescent solution in water, Medicoal is a preparation of charcoal.

Medihaler-Duo (*Riker*) is a proprietary BRONCHODILATOR available only on prescription, used in the form of an inhalant to treat bronchial asthma. It is produced in a metered-dosage aerosol, Medihaler-Duo is a compound preparation of the SYMPATHOMIMETICS isoprenaline hydrochloride and phenylephrine bitartrate. It is no longer used in children as drugs such as salbutamol and terbutaline are more specific and safer.
▲/✚ side-effects/warning: *see* ISOPRENALINE; PHENYLEPHRINE.

Medihaler-Epi (*Riker*) is a proprietary BRONCHODILATOR, available only on prescription, used in the form of an inhalant to treat bronchial asthma and chronic bronchitis. Produced in a metered-dosage aerosol, Medihaler-Epi is a preparation of the SYMPATHOMIMETIC adrenaline acid tartrate. It is no longer used in children as drugs such as salbutamol and terbutaline are more specific and safer.
▲/✚ side-effects/warning: *see* ADRENALINE.

Medihaler-Ergotamine (*Riker*) is a proprietary anti-migraine treatment, available only on prescription, used in the form of an inhalant to treat migraine and recurrent vascular headache. Produced in a metered-dosage aerosol, Medihaler-Ergotamine is a preparation of the vegetable alkaloid, ergotamine tartrate. It is not recommended in children aged under ten years.
▲/✚ side-effects/warning: *see* ERGOTAMINE TARTRATE.

Medihaler-Iso (*Riker*) is a proprietary BRONCHODILATOR, available only on prescription, used in the form of an inhalant to treat bronchial asthma and chronic bronchitis. Produced in a metered-dosage aerosol (in two strengths, the stronger under the trade name Medihaler-Iso Forte), it is a preparation of the SYMPATHOMIMETIC isoprenaline sulphate. It is no longer used in children as drugs such as salbutamol and terbutaline are more specific and safer.
▲/✚ side-effects/warning: *see* ISOPRENALINE.

Medilave (*Martindale*) is a proprietary non-prescription preparation for topical application, used to relieve pain in sores and ulcers in the mouth. Produced in the form of a gel, Medilave is a preparation of the local ANAESTHETIC benzocaine and the ANTISEPTIC cetylpyridinium chloride, and is not recommended for children aged under six months.
▲/✚ side-effects/warning: *see* BENZOCAINE.

Medised (*Martindale/Panpharma*) is a proprietary non-prescription compound non-narcotic ANALGESIC that is not available from the National Health Service. Used to treat pain, Medised is produced in the form of tablets (which are not recommended for children aged under three months). Medised is a combination of the analgesic paracetamol and the ANTIHISTAMINE promethazine hydrochloride.

▲/✚ side-effects/warning: *see* PARACETAMOL; PROMETHAZINE HYDROCHLORIDE.

Meditar (*Brocades*) is a proprietary non-prescription preparation used to treat eczema and psoriasis. Produced in the form of a wax stick for topical application, Meditar is a specialized form of COAL TAR.

Medocodene (*Medo*) is a proprietary non-prescription compound ANALGESIC that is not available from the National Health Service. Used to treat pain anywhere in the body, and produced in the form of tablets, Medocodene is a combination of the analgesic paracetamol and the OPIATE codeine phosphate (a combination itself known as co-codamol). Medocodene is not recommended for children aged under six years.
▲/✚ side-effects/warning: *see* CODEINE PHOSPHATE; PARACETAMOL.

Medrone (*Upjohn*) is a proprietary preparation of the anti-inflammatory CORTICOSTEROID drug methylprednisolone, available only on prescription, used to treat allergies. It is produced in the form of tablets (in three strengths) and as a lotion (which additionally contains the KERATOLYTIC aluminium chlorhydroxide).
▲/✚ side-effects/warning: *see* METHYLPREDNISOLONE.

mefenamic acid is a non-steroidal ANTI-INFLAMMATORY non-narcotic ANALGESIC. It is primarily used to treat mild to moderate pain in rheumatic disease and other musculo-skeletal disorders, although it may also be used either to reduce high body temperature (especially in children) or to lessen the pain of menstrual problems.
▲ side-effects: there may be drowsiness and dizziness; some patients experience nausea; gastrointestinal disturbances may eventually result in peptic ulceration.
✚ warning: mefenamic acid should not be administered to patients with inflammations in the intestines, peptic ulcers, or impaired liver or kidney function.
Related article: PONSTAN.

Mefoxin (*Merck, Sharp & Dohme*) is a proprietary broad-spectrum ANTIBIOTIC, available only on prescription, used to treat bacterial infections and to ensure asepsis during surgery. Produced in the form of a powder for reconstitution as a medium for injection, Mefoxin is a preparation of the CEPHALOSPORIN cefoxitin.
▲/✚ side-effects/warning: *see* CEFOXITIN.

Mengivax (A&C) (*Merieux*) is a VACCINE designed to give protection against the organism meningococcus, which can cause serious infection including meningitis. It may be indicated for travellers intending to go to parts of the world where the risk of meningococcal infection is much higher than in the United Kingdom, such as parts of Africa. It may be given to adults and children aged over 18 months.

Megozzones (*Kirby-Warrick Pharmaceuticals*) are proprietary non-prescription throat pastilles containing MENTHOL, benzoin and liquorice.

menadiol sodium phosphate is an analogue of VITAMIN K
(phytomenadione) which because it is water-soluble − whereas other
forms are only fat-soluble − is primarily used in oral application to
treat vitamin deficiency caused by the malabsorption of fats in the
diet (perhaps through obstruction of the bile ducts or liver disease).
The vitamin is necessary on a regular basis to maintain the presence
in the blood of clotting factors.
Administration is both oral in the form of tablets, and by injection.
Related article: SYNKAVIT.

menthol is a white, crystalline substance derived from peppermint oil
(an essential oil in turn derived from a plant of the mint family). It is
used, with or without the volatile substance eucalyptus oil, mostly in
inhalations meant to clear nasal or catarrhal congestion in conditions
such as rhinitis or sinusitis. It is also included in many proprietary
cold lozenges and preparations.
Related articles: BENYLIN DECONGESTANT; EXPULIN; EXPURHIN; HISTALIX;
PHYTOCIL; TERCODA.

Mentholatum (*Mentholatum*) is a proprietary non-prescription
preparation for the relief of cold symptoms produced in the form of
ANTISEPTIC lozenges, balm, deep heat lotion, and spray. These
preparations contain MENTHOL, camphor, eucalyptus oil, methyl
salicilate and amylmetacersol.

mepacrine hydrochloride is a synthetic drug used primarily to treat
infection by the intestinal protozoan *Giardia lamblia*: giardiasis
occurs throughout the world, particularly in children, and is
contracted by eating contaminated food. The drug more commonly
used to treat it, however, is METRONIDAZOLE. Mepacrine can also be
used to assist in the treatment of most forms of malaria.

mepyramine is an ANTIHISTAMINE used to treat the symptoms of
allergic conditions such as hay fever and urticaria, and − as an anti-
emetic − to treat or prevent nausea and vomiting, especially in
connection with motion sickness or the vertigo caused by infection of
the middle or inner ear. Administration (as mepyramine maleate) is
oral in the form of tablets.
▲ side-effects: sedation may affect capacity for speed of thought and
movement; there may be headache, and/or weight gain, dry mouth,
gastrointestinal disturbances and visual problems.

mequitazine is an ANTIHISTAMINE, used to treat the symptoms of
allergic conditions such as hay fever and urticaria. Administration is
oral in the form of tablets.
▲ side-effects: concentration and speed of thought and movement
may be affected. There may be nausea, headache, and/or weight
gain, dry mouth, gastrointestinal disturbances and visual
problems.

Merbentyl (*Merrell*) is a proprietary ANTICHOLINERGIC drug, available
only on prescription, used to treat gastrointestinal disorders that

result from muscle spasm in the stomach or intestinal walls. Produced in the form of tablets (in two strengths, the stronger under the name Merbentyl 20) and as a syrup for dilution (the potency of the syrup once dilute is retained for 14 days), Merbentyl is a preparation of dicyclomine hydrochloride and is not recommended for children aged under six months.

▲/✚ side-effects/warning: *see* DICYCLOMINE HYDROCHLORIDE.

Merieux Inactivated Rabies Vaccine is a proprietary preparation of rabies vaccine for administration to medical personnel and relatives who may come into contact with patients who have been bitten by an animal that might or might not have been rabid. Available only on prescription, the vaccine is of a type known as human diploid cell vaccine and has no known contra-indications. It is freeze-dried and produced in vials with a diluent for injection.

see RABIES VACCINE.

Merieux Tetavax (*Merieux*) is a proprietary preparation of tetanus vaccine, adsorbed on to a mineral carrier (in the form of aluminium hydroxide) and produced in syringes and in vials for injection.

see TETANUS VACCINE.

Merocaine (*Merrell*) is a proprietary non-prescription local anaesthetic, used to treat painful mouth and throat infections. Produced in the form of lozenges, Merocaine is a preparation of the local anaesthetic benzocaine together with the minor ANTISEPTIC cetylpyridinium chloride. It is not recommended for children.

▲/✚ side-effects/warning: *see* BENZOCAINE.

Merocet (*Merrell*) is a proprietary non-prescription mouth-wash which is a preparation of the ANTISEPTIC cetylpyridinium chloride. Although it can (but need not) be used in dilute form, it is not recommended for children aged under six years.

Merocets (*Merrell*) are proprietary non-prescription lozenges that are a preparation of the ANTISEPTIC CETYLPYRIDINIUM CHLORIDE, used in general oral hygiene.

Meruvax II (*Morson*) is a proprietary VACCINE against German measles (rubella) in the form of a solution containing live but attenuated viruses of the Wistar RA27/3 strain. Available only on prescription, it is administered in the form of an injection.

see RUBELLA VACCINE.

mesna is a synthetic drug that has the remarkable property of reducing the incidence of the serious form of cystitis (inflammation of the bladder) that is a toxic complication of the use of the CYTOTOXIC drugs cyclophosphamide and ifosfamide, without inhibiting the cytotoxic effects of the drugs. Used therefore as an adjunct in the treatment of certain forms of cancer, mesna is administered by injection.

▲ side-effects: overdosage may cause gastrointestinal disturbances and headache, with tiredness.

Mestinon (*Roche*) is a proprietary form of the drug pyridostigmine bromide, which has the effect of increasing the activity of the neurotransmitter acetylcholine that transmits the neural instructions of the brain to the muscles. It is thus used primarily to treat the neuromuscular disease myasthenia gravis, but may also be used to stimulate intestinal motility and so promote defecation. Available only on prescription, Mestinon is produced in the form of tablets and in ampoules for injection.
▲/✚ side-effects/warning: *see* PYRIDOSTIGMINE.

Metabolic Mineral Mixture (*Scientific Hospital Supplies*) is a proprietary non-prescription mineral supplement, used to supplement special diets. Produced in the form of a powder, it contains various mineral salts.

Metamucil (*Searle*) is a proprietary non-prescription LAXATIVE of the type known as a bulking agent, which works by increasing the overall mass of faeces within the rectum, so stimulating bowel movement. It is also used to soothe the effects of diverticular disease and irritable colon, and to control the consistency of faecal material in patients who have had a colostomy. Produced in the form of a gluten-free powder, Metamucil is a preparation of ispaghula husk.
▲/✚ side-effects/warning: *see* ISPAGHULA HUSK.

Metanium (*Bengué*) is a proprietary non-prescription astringent, used to relieve nappy rash and other macerated skin conditions. Produced in the form of an ointment, Metanium is a preparation of titanium salts in a silicone base.

methadone is a powerful and long-acting narcotic ANALGESIC used both to relieve severe pain and – like several narcotic analgesics – to suppress coughs. Administration (in the form of methadone hydrochloride) is oral in the form of tablets, as a linctus, or by injection.
▲ side-effects: there is commonly constipation, drowsiness and dizziness. High dosage may result in respiratory depression.
✚ warning: methadone should not be administered to patients with liver disease, raised intracranial pressure, or head injury. It should be administered with caution to those with asthma, low blood pressure (hypotension), underactivity of the thyroid gland (hypothyroidism) or impaired liver or kidney function.
Related article: PHYSEPTONE.

methicillin is a PENICILLIN derivative used primarily to treat staphylocci resistant to penicillin. This is because methicillin is not inactivated by the enzymes produced, for example, by certain Staphylococci. However, because administration is only by injection or infusion, other similar penicillin derivatives that can be administered orally have rather superseded methicillin. It has largely been replaced by such antibiotics as flucloxacillin. Methicillin remains important in the laboratory as organisms are still tested for sensitivity to it. The term methicillin resistant staphylococcus aureus (MRSA) describes an organism highly resistant to most antibiotics.

M

▲ side-effects: there may be sensitivity reactions ranging from a minor rash to urticaria and joint pains, and (occasionally) to high body temperature or anaphylactic shock. High dosage may in any case cause convulsions.

✚ warning: methicillin should not be administered to patients known to the allergic to penicillins; it should be administered with caution to those with impaired kidney function.

methionine is an antidote to poisoning by the analgesic paracetamol (which has the greatest toxic effect on the liver). Administration is oral in the form of tablets; dosage depends on the results of blood level tests every four hours.

methohexitone sodium is a general ANAESTHETIC used for both the induction and the maintenance of general anaesthesia in surgical operations; administration is intravenous (generally in 1% solution). It is less irritant to tissues than some other anaesthetics, and recovery afterwards is quick, but the induction of anaesthesia is not particularly smooth.

▲ side-effects: induction may cause hiccups and involuntary movements. The patient may feel pain on the initial injection.

✚ warning: maintenance of anaesthesia is usually in combination with other anaesthetics. Induction may take up to 60 seconds.
Related article: BRIETAL SODIUM.

methotrexate is a CYTOTOXIC drug used primarily in the treatment of lymphoblastic leukaemia, but also to treat other lymphomas and the lymphatic cancer Hodgkin's disease, as well as some solid tumours. It works by inhibiting the activity of an enzyme essential to the DNA metabolism in cells, and is administered orally or by injection.

▲ side-effects: there is commonly nausea and vomiting; there may also be hair loss. The capacity of the bone-marrow to produce blood cells is reduced. The drug may also cause inflammation in various body tissues.

✚ warning: methotrexate should not be administered to patients with severely impaired kidney function, or who have fluid within the pleural cavity. Leakage of the drug into the tissues at the site of injection may cause tissue damage. Regular blood counts are essential during treatment.
Related articles: EMTEXATE; MAXTREX.

methylcellulose is a high-fibre substance used as a LAXATIVE because it is an effective bulking agent – it increases the overall mass of faeces within the rectum, so stimulating bowel movement. It is also particularly useful in soothing the symptoms of diverticular disease and irritable colon. Administration is oral, generally in the form of tablets, granules for solution, or a mixture.

▲ side-effects: there may be flatulence, so much as to distend the abdomen.

✚ warning: preparations of methylcellulose should not be administered to patients with obstruction of the intestines, or failure of the muscles of the intestinal wall; it should be

administered with caution to those with ulcerative colitis. Fluid
intake during treatment should be higher than usual.
Related articles: CELEVAC; COLOGEL.

methylprednisolone is a CORTICOSTEROID used primarily to treat the
symptoms of inflammation or allergic reaction, but useful also in the
treatment of fluid retention in the brain or of shock. Administration
(as methylprednisolone, methylprednisolone acetate or
methylprednisolone sodium succinate) is oral in the form of tablets, or
by injection or infusion.
▲ side-effects: treatment of susceptible patients may engender a
euphoria, or a state of confusion or depression. Rarely, the patient
suffers from a peptic ulcer.
✛ warning: in children, prolonged administration of
methylprednisolone may lead to stunting of growth. The effects of
potentially serious infections may be masked by the drug during
treatment. Withdrawal after a prolonged course of treatment must
be gradual.
Related articles: DEPO-MEDRONE; MEDRONE; MIN-I-MIX
METHYLPREDNISOLONE; SOLU-MEDRONE.

methysergide is a potentially dangerous drug used, generally under
strict medical supervision in a hospital, to prevent severe recurrent
migraine and similar headaches in patients for whom other forms of
treatment have failed. It is rarely used in childhood.
▲ side-effects: there is initial nausea, drowsiness and dizziness; there
may also be fluid retention and consequent weight gain, spasm of
the arteries, numbness of the fingers and toes, increased heart rate
and even psychological changes. the most worrying side-effect is an
occasional tendency to a fibrotic (scarring) reaction in certain parts
of the body.
✛ warning: methysergide should not be administered to patients with
heart, lung, liver or kidney disease, or who suffer from collagen
disorders. It should be administered with caution to those with
peptic ulcer. Withdrawal of treatment should be gradual, although
no course of treatment should last for more than six months at a
time.
Related article: DESERIL.

metoclopramide is an effective ANTI-EMETIC drug used to prevent
vomiting caused by gastrointestinal disorders or by chemotherapy or
radiotherapy in the treatment of cancer. It works both by action on
the vomiting centre of the brain and by encouraging the flow of
stomach contents into the intestine, and has fewer side-effects than
many other anti-emetics (such as the phenothiazine derivatives).
Administration (as metoclopramide hydrochloride) is oral in the form
of tablets and syrups, or by injection. Some children and adolescents
are very sensitive to metoclopramide and bizarre and alarming
muscular spasms can result.
▲ side-effects: side-effects are relatively uncommon, especially in male
patients. There may, however, be mild neuromuscular symptoms,
drowsiness and constipation.

✚warning: It should be used with caution on children; and it should not be administered to patients who have had gastrointestinal surgery within the previous four days; it should be administered with caution to those with impaired kidney function, or who are children or elderly. Dosage should begin low and gradually increase. The effects of the drug may mask underlying disorders.
Related articles: MAXOLON; METOX; MIGRAVESS; MYGDALON; PRIMPERAN.

Metosyn (*Stuart*) is a proprietary CORTICOSTEROID preparation, available only on prescription, used to treat inflammations of the skin (such as severe eczema) in patients not responding to less potent corticosteroids. Produced in the form of a water-miscible cream, as a paraffin-based ointment, and as a scalp lotion, Metosyn is a preparation of the potent steroid fluocinonide. It is rarely used in children.

▲/✚ side-effects/warning: *see* FLUOCINONIDE.

Metox (*Steinhard*) is a proprietary preparation of the ANTI-EMETIC drug metoclopramide hydrochloride, available only on prescription, used to relieve symptoms of nausea and vomiting caused by gastrointestinal disorders, or by chemotherapy or radiotherapy in the treatment of cancer. It is produced in the form of tablets. In some children, the drug causes muscular spasms.
▲/✚ side-effects/warning: *see* METOCLOPRAMIDE.

Metrolyl (*Lagap*) is a proprietary ANTIBIOTIC and ANTIPROTOZOAL, available only on prescription, used to treat many forms of infection including those caused by anaerobic bacteria, by protozoa, or by amoebae. Produced in the form of tablets (in two strengths), as anal suppositories (in two strengths), and in solution for intravenous infusion, Metrolyl is a preparation of metronidazole.
▲/✚ side-effects/warning: *see* METRONIDAZOLE.

metronidazole is an ANTIMICROBIAL with ANTIBIOTIC and ANTIPROTOZOAL properties. Its antibiotic spectrum is narrow, being limited to activity against strictly anaerobic bacteria. It acts by interfering with DNA replication. The other group of microbes it is active against are the protozoa, specifically, *Entamoebe histolytica* (causes amoebic dysentery), *Giardia lamblia* (causes giardiasis, an infection of the small intestine) and *Trichomonas vaginalis* (causes vaginitis). Resistance is rare and this drug has radically improved the success of treating anaerobic infections such as may be found in peritonitis, pelvic abscess, brain abscess and wound infections. One reason for its activity in such situations is its ability to penetrate and remain effective in the presence of pus. Administration is oral in the form of tablets or a suspension, topical in the form of anal suppositories, or by injection or infusion.
▲ side-effects: these are uncommon — but there may be nausea and vomiting, with drowsiness, headache and gastrointestinal disturbances; gastrointestinal effects may be reduced by taking the drug during or after food. Some patients experience a discoloration of the urine. Prolonged treatment may eventually give rise to

neuromuscular disorders or even seizures reminiscent of epilepsy
with high doses.

➕warning: metronidazole should not be taken regularly on a high-
dosage basis. It should be administered with caution to patients
with impaired liver function. During treatment patients must avoid
alcohol consumption (the presence of alcohol in the body during
treatment gives rise to most unpleasant side-effects), including
gripe water which contains alcohol.
Related articles: FLAGYL; METROLYL; NIDAZOL; ZADSTAT.

metronidazole benzoate is the form in which the broad-spectrum
ANTIBIOTIC metronidazole is administered in a suspension.
see METRONIDAZOLE.

Mevillin-L (*Evans*) is a proprietary VACCINE against measles (rubeola),
available only on prescription. It is a powdered preparation of live but
attenuated measles viruses for administration within a diluent by
injection.

▲side-effects: there may be inflammation at the site of injection.
Rarely, there may be high temperature, cough and sore throat, a
rash, swelling of the lymph glands and/or pain in the joints.

➕warning: mevillin-L should not be administered to patients with
any infection, particularly tuberculosis; who are markedly allergic
to eggs, that is, when they are thought to have had a life-
threatening reaction to eggs in the past (the viruses are cultured in
chick embryo tissue); who have known immune-system
abnormalities; who are pregnant; hypersensitive to neomycin or
polymyxin; or who are already taking corticosteroid drugs,
cytotoxic drugs or are undergoing radiation treatment. It should be
administered with caution to those with epilepsy or any other
condition potentially involving convulsive fits.

mezlocillin is a derivative of the broad-spectrum penicillin-type
ANTIBIOTIC ampicillin that is additionally effective in treating some
infections by bacteria resistant to ampicillin. Administration is by
injection or infusion.

▲side-effects: there may be sensitivity reactions ranging from a
minor rash to urticaria and joint pains, and (occasionally) to high
temperature and anaphylactic shock. High doses may in any case
cause convulsions.

➕warning: mezlocillin should not be administered to patients known
to be allergic to penicillins; it should be administered with caution
to those with impaired kidney function.
Related article: BAYPEN.

Micolette (*Ayerst*) is a proprietary non-prescription form of small
enema administered rectally to promote defecation, especially pre- or
post-operatively or before rectal examination by endoscope. Produced

in single-dose disposable packs with a nozzle, Micolette is a preparation that includes sodium citrate, sodium laurysulphoacetate and GLYCEROL in a viscous solution. It is not recommended for children aged under three years.

miconazole is an ANTIFUNGAL drug used in the treatment of many forms of fungal infection, most commonly thrush, generally by topical application (for instance, as an oral gel, as a spray powder, or as a water-miscible cream), although tablets are also available for use in recurrent or resistant infection and as an injection for systemic infections. In solution, the drug may be used for irrigation of the bladder.

▲side-effects: rarely, there is irritation of the skin or minor sensitivity reaction. Miconazole may cause nausea and vomiting. *Related articles:* DAKTARIN; DERMONISTAT.

Micralax (*Smith, Kline & French*) is a proprietary non-prescription form of small enema administered rectally to promote defecation, especially before labour or rectal examination by endoscope. Produced in single-dose disposable packs with a nozzle, Micralax is a preparation that includes sodium citrate, sodium alkylsulphoacetate and sorbic acid in a viscous solution. It is not recommended for children aged under three years.

Micro-K (*Merck*) is a proprietary non-prescription form of potassium supplement, used to treat patients with deficiencies and to replace potassium in patients taking potassium-depleting drugs such as diuretics or the THIAZIDE diuretics. Produced in the form of sustained-release capsules, Micro-K is a preparation of potassium chloride.

✚warning: Micro-K should not be used in patients with advanced renal failure. It should be discontinued if it produces ulceration or obstruction of the small bowel.

Mictral (*Winthrop*) is a proprietary ANTIBIOTIC, available only on prescription, used primarily to treat infections of the urinary tract, including cystitis. Produced in the form of granules in a sachet for solution in water, Mictral's major active constituents are the ANTIBACTERIAL drug nalidixic acid and sodium citrate. It is not recommended for infants aged under three months, and is best avoided altogether in children aged under one year as it may raise the pressure inside the head (raised intracranial pressure).

▲/✚ side-effects/warning: *see* NALIDIXIC ACID.

midazolam is an ANXIOLYTIC drug, one of the BENZODIAZEPINES, used primarily to provide sedation for minor surgery such as dental operations or as a premedication prior to surgical procedures and, because it also has some SKELETAL MUSCLE RELAXANT properties, to treat some forms of spasm. Prolonged use results in tolerance. Administration is by injection.

▲side-effects: there may be drowsiness, dizziness, headache, dry mouth and shallow breathing; hypersensitivity reactions may occur.

✚ warning: concentration and speed of thought and movement are often affected. Midazolam should be administered with caution to patients with respiratory difficulties (it sometimes causes a sharp fall in blood pressure). Abrupt withdrawal of treatment should be avoided.
Related article: HYPNOVEL DIAZEPAM.

Migraleve (*International Labs*) is a proprietary non-prescription compound ANALGESIC and ANTIHISTAMINE, used to treat migraine. Produced in the form of tablets, Migraleve is a preparation of the antihistamine buclizine hydrochloride, the analgesic paracetamol and the OPIATE codeine phosphate; tablets without buclizine hydrochloride are also available separately or in a duo-pack. These preparations are not recommended for children aged under ten years. They should never be prescribed prophylactically.
▲/✚ side-effects/warning: *see* CODEINE PHOSPHATE; PARACETAMOL.

Migravess (*Bayer*) is a proprietary compound non-narcotic ANALGESIC, available only on prescription, used to treat migraine. Produced in the form of tablets (in two strengths, the stronger under the name Migravess Forte), Migravess is a preparation of the analgesic aspirin together with the ANTI-EMETIC metoclopramide hydrochloride. It is not recommended for children aged under ten years.
▲/✚ side-effects/warning: *see* ASPIRIN; METOCLOPRAMIDE.

Mildison (*Brocades*) is a proprietary ANTI-INFLAMMATORY drug, available only on prescription; its active constituent is the CORTICOSTEROID hydrocortisone. It is produced in the form of a lipocream in a fatty cream basis. Mildison is used to treat severe skin inflammations such as eczema and various forms of dermatitis.
▲/✚ side-effects/warning: *see* HYDROCORTISONE.

Milupa LPD (*Milupa*) is a proprietary non-prescription nutritional supplement for patients who suffer from disorders of amino acid metabolism. Produced in the form of a powder for reconstitution as a low protein drink, it contains low-protein and low-mineral whey, starch, sucrose and vegetable oil.

Minafen (*Cow & Gate*) is a proprietary non-prescription nutritional preparation, used to feed infants and young children who have the amino acid metabolic abnormality phenylketonuria (PKU). Produced in the form of a powder, Minafen is a preparation of protein, fat, carbohydrate, vitamins and minerals, and is low in the amino acid phenylalanine. It is not, however, usable as a complete diet.

Min-i-Jet Adrenaline (*International Medication Systems*) is a proprietary form of the natural catecholamine adrenaline, available only on prescription, used as a SYMPATHOMIMETIC drug to treat bronchial asthma and in the emergency treatment of acute allergic reactions. However, it is rarely used to treat asthma nowadays. Produced in disposable syringes for injection (straight into the heart muscle if necessary), Min-i-Jet Adrenaline is a preparation of adrenaline hydrochloride.

▲/✚ side-effects/warning: *see* ADRENALINE.

Min-i-Mix Methylprednisolone (*International Medication Systems*) is a proprietary CORTICOSTEROID, available only on prescription, used to suppress inflammation or allergic symptoms, to relieve fluid retention around the brain, or to treat shock. Produced in the form of powder for reconstitution as a solution for injection, it is a preparation of methylprednisolone sodium succinate.

▲/✚ side-effects/warning: see METHYLPREDNISOLONE.

Minims Amethocaine (*Smith & Nephew*) is a proprietary local ANAESTHETIC for topical application and ophthalmic procedures available only on prescription. Produced in the form of single-dose eye-drops, Minims Amethocaine is a preparation of amethocaine hydrochloride.

▲/✚ side-effects/warning: *see* AMETHOCAINE HYDROCHLORIDE.

Minims Atropine Sulphate (*Smith & Nephew*) is a proprietary ANTICHOLINERGIC mydriatic drug, available only on prescription, used to dilate the pupils and paralyse certain eye muscles for the purpose of ophthalmic examination, especially in young children, or occasionally to assist in antibiotic treatment. It is produced in the form of single-dose eye-drops (and is a preparation of the anticholinergic drug atropine sulphate).

▲/✚ side-effects/warning: *see* ATROPINE SULPHATE.

Minims Benoxinate (*Smith & Nephew*) is a proprietary local ANAESTHETIC, available only on prescription, used to relieve pain in the eyes especially during minor surgery or ophthalmic examination. Produced in the form of single-dose eye-drops, Minims Benoxinate is a preparation of oxybuprocaine hydrochloride.

▲/✚ side-effects/warning: *see* OXYBUPROCAINE.

Minims Castor Oil (*Smith & Nephew*) is a proprietary non-prescription form of eye-drops consisting of castor oil, for use as a lubricant in removing foreign bodies from the eye.

Minims Chloramphenicol (*Smith & Nephew*) is a proprietary ANTIBIOTIC for topical application, available only on prescription, used to treat bacterial infections in the eye. Produced in the form of single-dose eye-drops, Minims Chloramphenicol is a preparation of chloramphenicol.

▲/✚ side-effects/warning: *see* CHLORAMPHENICOL.

Minims Cyclopentolate (*Smith & Nephew*) is a proprietary ANTI-CHOLINERGIC mydriatic drug, available only on prescription, used to dilate the pupils and paralyse certain eye muscles for the purpose of ophthalmic examination (or occasionally to assist in antibiotic treatment). Produced in the form of single-dose eye-drops, it is a preparation of the drug cyclopentolate hydrochloride.

▲/✚ side-effects/warning: *see* CYCLOPENTOLATE HYDROCHLORIDE.

Minims Fluorescein Sodium (*Smith & Nephew*) is a proprietary non-prescription dye used in the diagnosis of certain disorders of the eye – for instance, to locate abrasions and foreign bodies. Produced in the form of single-dose eye-drops, it is a preparation of FLUORESCEIN SODIUM.

Minims Gentamicin (*Smith & Nephew*) is a proprietary ANTIBIOTIC, available only on prescription, used to treat bacterial infections in the eye. Produced in the form of single-dose eye-drops, Minims Gentamicin is a preparation of the aminoglycoside gentamicin sulphate.
▲/✚ side-effects/warning: *see* GENTAMICIN.

Minims Homatropine (*Smith & Nephew*) is a proprietary ANTI-CHOLINERGIC, mydriatic drug, available only on prescription, used to dilate the pupils and paralyse certain eye muscles for the purpose of ophthalmic examination (or occasionally to assist in antibiotic treatment). Produced in the form of single-dose eye-drops, it is a preparation of the ATROPINE derivative homatropine hydrobromide.

Minims Lignocaine and Fluorescein (*Smith & Nephew*) is a proprietary local ANAESTHETIC, available only on prescription. Produced in the form of single-dose eye-drops, Minims Lignocaine and Fluorescein is a preparation of lignocaine hydrochloride together with the diagnostic dye FLUORESCEIN SODIUM.
▲/✚ side-effects/warning: *see* LIGNOCAINE.

Minims Neomycin (*Smith & Nephew*) is a proprietary ANTIBIOTIC, available only on prescription, used to treat bacterial infections in the eye. It is produced in the form of single-dose eye-drops.
▲/✚ side-effects/warning: *see* NEOMYCIN.

Minims Phenylephrine (*Smith & Nephew*) is a proprietary non-prescription SYMPATHOMIMETIC, used to dilate the pupils and paralyse certain eye muscles for the purpose of ophthalmic examination (or occasionally to assist in antibiotic treatment). Produced in the form of single-dose eye-drops, it is a preparation of the SYMPATHOMIMETIC phenylephrine hydrochloride.
▲/✚ side-effects/warning: *see* PHENYLEPHRINE.

Minims Pilocarpine (*Smith & Nephew*) is a proprietary parasympathomimetic miotic drug, available only on prescription, used in the treatment of glaucoma. It works by improving drainage in the trabecular meshwork of the eyeball. Produced in the form of eye-drops (in three strengths), it is a preparation of pilocarpine nitrate.
▲/✚ side-effects/warning: *see* PILOCARPINE.

Minims Prednisolone (*Smith & Nephew*) is a proprietary CORTICOSTEROID, available only on prescription, used to treat non-infective inflammatory conditions in and around the eye. Produced in the form of eye-drops, it contains prednisolone sodium phosphate.
▲/✚ side-effects/warning: *see* PREDNISOLONE.

Minims Sodium Chloride (*Smith & Nephew*) is a proprietary non-prescription preparation of saline solution used for the irrigation of the eyes, and to facilitate the first-aid removal of harmful substances. It is produced in the form of single-dose eye-drops.
▲/✚ side-effects/warning: *see* SODIUM CHLORIDE.

Minims Sulphacetamide Sodium (*Smith & Nephew*) is a proprietary ANTIBACTERIAL, available only on prescription, used to treat local infections in the eye. Produced in the form of single-dose eye-drops, it is a preparation of the SULPHONAMIDE sulphacetamide sodium.
▲/✚ side-effects/warning: *see* SULPHACETAMIDE.

Minims Thymoxamine (*Smith & Nephew*) is a proprietary miotic drug, available only on prescription, used to constrict the pupil after dilation caused by the administration of a SYMPATHOMIMETIC drug (for the purpose usually of ophthalmic examination). Produced in the form of single-dose eye-drops, it is a preparation of thymoxamine hydrochloride.

Minims Tropicamide (*Smith & Nephew*) is a proprietary mydriatic drug, available only on prescription, used to dilate the pupils and paralyse certain eye muscles for the purpose of ophthalmic examination (or occasionally to assist in antibiotic treatment). Produced in the form of single-dose eye-drops, it is a preparation of the short-acting ANTICHOLINERGIC drug tropicamide.
▲/✚ side-effects/warning: *see* TROPICAMIDE.

Minocin (*Lederle*) is a proprietary broad-spectrum ANTIBIOTIC, available only on prescription, used to treat many forms of infection but particularly those of the respiratory tract, skin and soft tissue (including acne). Produced in the form of tablets (in two strengths), Minocin is a preparation of the TETRACYCLINE minocycline hydrochloride. It should not be given to children aged under 12 years.
▲/✚ side-effects/warning: *see* MINOCYCLINE.

minocycline is a broad-spectrum ANTIBIOTIC, a TETRACYCLINE with a wide range of action. Administration is oral in the form of tablets.
▲ side-effects: there may be nausea and vomiting, with diarrhoea; dizziness and vertigo are quite common, especially in female patients. Rarely, there are sensitivity reactions.
✚ warning: minocycline should not be administered to patients who are aged under 12 years. It should be administered with caution to those who are lactating or who have impaired liver or kidney function.
Related article: MINOCIN.

Mintezol (*Merck Sharp & Dohme*) is a proprietary non-prescription ANTHELMINTIC drug, used to treat intestinal infestations by threadworm and guinea worm, and to assist in the treatment of resistant infections by hookworm, whipworm and roundworm. Produced in the form of tablets, Mintezol is a preparation of thiabendazole.
▲/✚ side-effects/warning: *see* THIABENDAZOLE.

Miochol (*CooperVision*) is a proprietary preparation of the parasympathomimetic drug acetylcholine chloride, available only on prescription, used mainly to contract the pupil of the eye for the purpose of surgery on the iris, the cornea, or other sections of the exterior of the eye. It is produced in the form of a solution for intra-ocular irrigation.

Miraxid (*Leo*) is a proprietary compound ANTIBIOTIC preparation, available only on prescription, used to treat infections in the respiratory tract, the ear and the urinary tract. Produced in the form of tablets (in two strengths, the stronger under the name Miraxid 450, which is not recommended for children) and as a suspension for children, Miraxid is a compound preparation of the penicillins pivampicillin and pivmecillinam hydrochloride.

▲/✚ side-effects/warning: *see* PIVAMPICILLIN; PIVMECILLINAM.

Mixtard 30/70 (*Nordisk Wellcome*) is a proprietary non-prescription preparation of mixed pork INSULINS used to treat and maintain diabetic patients. Produced in vials for injection, Mixtard 30/70 is a preparation of both neutral (30%) and isoplhane (70%) insulins. HUMAN MIXTARD 30/70 is also available.

MMR vaccine is a combined measles, mumps and rubella vaccine using live but weakened strains of the viruses (prepared in chick embryos). Rarely the mumps component has been thought to cause a mild viral meningitis, but this is less common than the incidence of viral meningitis complicating natural mumps, and such a complication settles on its own. Less commonly convulsions and encephalitis (inflammation of the brain) have been associated with the vaccine. This may be related to either the measles or the mumps component. Such complications are again more common after infection with either natural measles or mumps.

▲ side-effects: as with single measles vaccine there may be fever (it is a good idea to have paracetamol available if fever occurs, especially if the child has a tendency to develop febrile convulsions) and/or a rash about a week after (a rash does not mean that a child is infectious); there may also be parotid gland swelling about two to three weeks after vaccination.

✚ warning: it should not be given to immunocompromised children; to children allergic to neomycin or kanamycin; who have had an anaphylactic reaction to egg; with acute febrile illness. It should not be given within three months of an immunoglobulin injection.

MMR II (*Wellcome*) is a proprietary VACCINE preparation for measles, mumps and rubella.

Modrasone (*Kirby-Warrick*) is a proprietary ANTI-INFLAMMATORY CORTICOSTEROID drug, available only on prescription, used in topical application to treat severe skin inflammation, such as eczema and various forms of dermatitis. Produced in the form of a cream and as an ointment, Modrasone is a preparation of the corticosteroid alclometasone dipropionate. It is not commonly recommended for use in childhood.

▲/✚ side-effects/warning: *see* ALCLOMETASONE DIPROPIONATE.

Molcer (*Wallace*) is a proprietary non-prescription form of ear-drops designed to soften and dissolve ear-wax (cerumen), and commonly prescribed for use at home two nights consecutively before syringing of the ears in a doctor's surgery. Its solvent constituent is dioctyl sodium sylphosuccinate (also called docusate sodium).

✚ warning: Molcer should not be used if there is inflammation in the ear, or where there is any chance that an eardrum has been perforated.

Monaspor (*Ciba*) is a proprietary ANTIBIOTIC, available only on prescription, used to treat many forms of infection, especially those of the respiratory tract, certain bone and soft tissue infections, and those caused by the organism *Pseudomonas aeruginosa*. It is also sometimes used to ensure asepsis during surgery. Produced in the form of a powder for reconstitution as a medium for injection, Monaspor is a preparation of the cephalosporin cefsulodin sodium.

▲/✚ side-effects/warning: *see* CEFSULODIN.

monosulfiram is a parasitocidal drug used mainly in topical application to treat skin surface infestation by the itch-mite (scabies). In this it is particularly valuable in treating children. Administration is in the form of a dilute spiritous solution (generally applied topically after a hot bath).

▲ side-effects: rarely, there are sensitivity reactions.

✚ warning: keep the solution away from the eyes. During treatment, patients should avoid alcohol consumption (if absorbed, the drug may give rise to a severe reaction – as does the closely-related drug disulfiram – in the presence of alcohol).

Monotard MC (*Nova*) is a proprietary non-prescription highly purified pork INSULIN zinc suspension, used to treat and maintain diabetic patients. It is produced in vials for injection.

Monotrim (*Duphar*) is a proprietary ANTIBIOTIC, available only on prescription, commonly used to treat various bacterial infections, and infections of the urinary tract. Produced in the form of tablets (in two strengths), as a sugar-free suspension for dilution (the potency of the suspension once dilute is retained for 14 days), and in ampoules for injection, Monotrim is a preparation of the antibacterial drug trimethoprim. This antibiotic is not recommended for children aged under six weeks.

▲/✚ side-effects/warning: *see* TRIMETHOPRIM.

Monovent (*Lagap*) is a proprietary BETA-RECEPTOR STIMULANT BRONCHODILATOR, available only on prescription, used to relieve the bronchial spasm associated with asthma. Produced in the form of tablets, as sustained-release tablets (under the name Monovent SA), and as a syrup for dilution (the potency of the syrup once dilute is retained for 14 days), Monovent is a preparation of terbutaline sulphate.

▲/✚ side-effects/warning: *see* TERBUTALINE.

Morhulin (*Napp*) is a proprietary non-prescription skin emollient (softener and soother), used to treat nappy rash and bedsores. Produced in the form of an ointment, Morhulin is a preparation of cod-liver oil and ZINC OXIDE in a wool fat and paraffin base.

✚warning: wool fat causes sensitivity reactions in some patients.

morphine is a powerful narcotic ANALGESIC that is the principal alkaloid of opium. It is widely used to treat severe pain and to soothe the associated stress and anxiety; it may be used in treating shock (with care since it lowers blood pressure), in suppressing coughs (although it may cause nausea and vomiting), and in reducing peristalsis (the muscular waves that urge material along the intestines) as a constituent in some antidiarrhoeal mixtures. It is also sometimes used as a premedication prior to surgery, or to supplement anaesthesia during an operation. Tolerance occurs extremely readily; dependence (addiction) may follow. Administration is oral and by injection; given by injection, morphine is more active. Proprietary preparations that contain morphine (in the form of morphine, morphine tartrate, morphine hydrochloride or morphine sulphate) are all on the controlled drugs list.

▲side-effects: there may be nausea and vomiting, loss of appetite, urinary retention and constipation. There is generally a degree of sedation, and euphoria which may lead to a state of mental - detachment or confusion.

✚warning: morphine should not be administered to patients with depressed breathing (the drug may itself cause a degree of respiratory depression), or who have raised intracranial pressure or head injury. It should be administered with caution to those with low blood pressure (hypotension), impaired liver or kidney function, or underactivity of the thyroid gland (hypothyroidism). Prolonged treatment should be avoided.

Related articles: CYCLIMORPH; NEPENTHE.

Morsep (*Napp*) is a proprietary non-prescription skin emollient (softener and soother), used to treat urinary dermatitis and nappy rash. Produced in the form of a cream, Morsep is a preparation of the ANTISEPTIC CETRIMIDE, retinol (vitamin A), and CALCIFEROL (vitamin D).

Motilium (*Janssen*) is a proprietary preparation of the ANTINAUSEANT and ANTI-EMETIC drug domperidone, available only on prescription. It works by inhibiting the action of the natural substance dopamine on the vomiting centre of the brain, and may be used to treat nausea and vomiting in gastrointestinal disorders, or during treatment with cytotoxic drugs or radiotherapy. It is produced in the form of tablets, as a sugar-free suspension and as anal suppositories.

▲/✚ side-effects/warning: *see* DOMPERIDONE.

Motrin (*Upjohn*) is a proprietary ANTI-INFLAMMATORY non-narcotic ANALGESIC, available only on prescription, used to treat the pain of rheumatic and other musculo-skeletal disorders. Produced in the form of tablets (in four strengths), Motrin is a preparation of ibuprofen.
▲/✚ side-effects/warning: *see* IBUPROFEN.

Moxalactam (*Lilly*) is a proprietary broad-spectrum ANTIBIOTIC, available only on prescription, used to treat many forms of bacterial infection. Produced in the form of a powder for reconstitution as a medium for injection, Moxalactam is a preparation of the CEPHALOSPORIN latamoxef disodium.
▲/✚ side-effects/warning: *see* LATAMOXEF SODIUM.

MSUD Aid (*Scientific Hospital Supplies*) is a proprietary essential and non-essential amino acid mixture, used as a nutritional supplement for patients with the congenital abnormality maple syrup urine disease. Produced in the form of a powder containing vitamins, minerals and trace elements, it is isoleucine-, leucine- and valine-free, but does not consist of a complete diet.

Multibionta (*Merck*) is a proprietary MULTIVITAMIN solution, available only on prescription, for addition to infusion solutions to feed patients who for one reason or another cannot be fed via the alimentary canal. Produced in ampoules, Multibionta is a preparation of retinol (vitamin A), thiamine (vitamin B₁), riboflavine (vitamin B₂), PYRIDOXINE (vitamin B₅), nicotinamide (of the B complex), dexpanthenol (of the B complex), ASCORBIC ACID (vitamin C) and TOCOPHERYL ACETATE (vitamin E).

Multilind (*Squibb*) is a proprietary ANTIFUNGAL preparation, available only on prescription, used in topical application to treat fungal infections, especially forms of candidiasis (such as thrush), and to relieve the symptoms of nappy rash. Produced in the form of an ointment, Multilind is a preparation of the ANTIFUNGAL agent nystatin together with ZINC OXIDE.
▲/✚ side-effects/warning: *see* NYSTATIN.

*multivitamin preparations contain selections of various VITAMINS. There are a large number of such preparations available, and are mostly used as dietary supplements and for making up vitamin deficiencies. Choice of a particular multivitamin depends on its content; they are not usually available on the National Health.

Multivitamins (*Evans*) is a proprietary non-prescription MULTIVITAMIN preparation that is not available from the National Health Service. Produced in the form of tablets, Multivitamins is a preparation of retinol (vitamin A), thiamine (vitamin B₁), riboflavine (vitamin B₂), nicotinamide (of the B complex), ASCORBIC ACID (vitamin C) and CALCIFEROL (vitamin D).

Multivite (*Duncan, Flockhart*) is a proprietary non-prescription MULTIVITAMIN preparation for use in vitamin deficiency states that is not available from the National Health Service. Produced in the form of pellets, Multivite is a preparation of retinol (vitamin A), thiamine (vitamin B₁), ASCORBIC ACID (vitamin C) and CALCIFEROL (vitamin D).

Mumpsvax (*Morson*) is a proprietary mumps vaccine, available only on prescription. Produced in the form of powder in a single-dose vial with diluent, Mumpsvax is a preparation of live but attenuated viruses that when injected cause the body to provide itself with antibodies against the virus. It is not recommended for children aged under one year.

mupirocin (or pseudomonic acid) is an ANTIBIOTIC drug, unrelated to any other antibiotic, used in topical application to treat bacterial skin infection. Administration is in the form of a water-miscible cream. It is used to eradicate the highly resistant organism methicillin resistant *Staphylococcus aureus* (MRSA) from the nose. Some people carry this organism in their noses and this may be important in the spread of infection within a hospital.
▲ side-effects: topical application may sting.
✚ warning: mupirocin should be administered with caution to patients with impaired kidney function.
Related article: BACTROBAN.

*muscle relaxants are agents that reduce tension in or paralyse muscles. They include antispasmodic drugs or SMOOTH MUSCLE RELAXANTS, which relieve spasm (rigidity) in smooth muscles that are not under voluntary control (such as the muscles of the respiratory tract or of the intestinal walls − or of blood vessels). They also include those drugs that are used in surgical operations to paralyse skeletal muscles that are normally under voluntary control (neuromuscular blocking drugs); such drugs work either by competing with the neurotransmitter acetylcholine at receptor sites between nerve and muscle (non-depolarizing) or by imitating the action of acetylcholine and so blocking the receptor sites (depolarizing). Non-depolarizing muscle relaxants include TUBOCURARINE CHLORIDE, GALLAMINE TRIETHIODIDE, ALCURONIUM CHLORIDE and VECURONIUM BROMIDE; depolarizing muscle relaxants include SUXAMETHONIUM CHLORIDE. Antagonists used to reverse the effects of one of these two drug types once surgery has finished prolong the effect of the other drug type. Patients receiving a muscle relaxant during surgery must have their respiration assisted or controlled. Other drugs relax skeletal muscle spasm by an action on the spinal cord, and these SKELETAL MUSCLE RELAXANTS include baclophen and certain of the benzodiazepines.

Myambutol (*Lederle*) is a proprietary ANTITUBERCULAR drug, available only on prescription, used for the prevention and treatment of tuberculosis in conjunction with other drugs. Produced in the form of tablets (in two strengths) and as an oral powder, Myambutol is a preparation of ethambutol hydrochloride.
▲/✚ side-effects/warning: *see* ETHAMBUTOL HYDROCHLORIDE.

Myciguent (*Upjohn*) is a proprietary ANTIBIOTIC, available only on prescription, used to treat infections of the skin and the eye. Produced

in the form of an ointment and an eye ointment, Myciguent is a preparation of the aminoglycoside neomycin sulphate.
▲/✚ side-effects/warning: *see* NEOMYCIN.

Mycota (*Crookes Products*) is a proprietary non-prescription ANTIFUNGAL preparation, used in topical application to treat skin infections caused by Tinea organisms (such as athlete's foot). Produced in the form of a cream, as a dusting powder, and as an aerosol spray, Mycota is a preparation of undecenoic acid and its salts.

Mydriacyl (*Alcon*) is a proprietary ANTICHOLINERGIC mydriatic drug, available only on prescription, used to dilate the pupils and paralyse certain eye muscles, generally for the purpose of ophthalmic examination (but occasionally to assist in antibiotic treatment). Produced in the form of eye-drops (in two strengths), Mydriacyl is a preparation of tropicamide.
▲/✚ side-effects/warning: *see* TROPICAMIDE.

Mydrilate (*Boehringer Ingelheim*) is a proprietary ANTICHOLINERGIC mydriatic drug, available only on prescription, used to dilate the pupils and paralyse certain eye muscles, generally for the purpose of ophthalmic examination (but occasionally to assist in antibiotic treatment). Produced in the form of eye-drops (in two strengths), Mydrilate is a preparation of cyclopentolate hydrochloride.
▲/✚ side-effects/warning: *see* CYCLOPENTOLATE HYDROCHLORIDE.

Mygdalon (*DDSA Pharmaceuticals*) is a proprietary ANTI-EMETIC, available only on prescription, used to treat nausea and vomiting, especially when associated with gastrointestinal disorders, during radiotherapy, or accompanying treatment with CYTOTOXIC drugs. Produced in the form of tablets, Mygdalon is a preparation of metoclopramide hydrochloride.
▲/✚ side-effects/warning: *see* METOCLOPRAMIDE.

Myocrisin (*May & Baker*) is a proprietary preparation of one of the salts of gold, available only on prescription, used to treat rheumatoid arthritis. Produced in ampoules (in five strengths) for injection, Myocrisin is a preparation of sodium aurothiomalate.
▲/✚ side-effects/warning: *see* SODIUM AUROTHIOMALATE.

Mysoline (*ICI*) is a proprietary ANTICONVULSANT, available only on prescription, used to treat and prevent epileptic attacks, especially grand mal (tonic-clonic) and partial (focal) seizures (but not petit mal epilepsy). Produced in the form of tablets and an oral suspension, Mysoline is a preparation of primidone. It is not commonly used nowadays.
▲/✚ side-effects/warning: *see* PRIMIDONE.

nabilone is a synthetic cannabinoid (a drug derived from cannabis) used to relieve some of the toxic side-effects, particularly the nausea and vomiting, associated with chemotherapy in the treatment of cancer. However, it too has significant side-effects. Administration is oral in the form of capsules.

▲ side-effects: drowsiness, dry mouth and decreased appetite are common; there may also be an increase in the heart rate, dizziness on rising from a sitting or lying position (indicating low blood pressure), and abdominal cramps. Some patients experience psychological effects such as euphoria, confusion, depression, hallucinations and general disorientation. There may be headache, blurred vision and tremors.

✚ warning: nabilone should be administered with caution to patients with severely impaired liver function or unstable personality. The patient's concentration and speed of reaction are affected.
Related article: CESAMET.

nalbuphine hydrochloride is a narcotic ANALGESIC that is very similar to morphine (although it has fewer side-effects and possibly less addictive potential). Like morphine, it is used primarily to relieve moderate to severe pain, especially during or after surgery. Administration is by injection.

▲ side-effects: shallow breathing, urinary retention, constipation, and nausea are all common; tolerance and dependence (addiction) are possible. There may also be drowsiness and pain at the site of injection (where there may also be tissue damage).

✚ warning: nalbuphine should not be administered to patients who suffer from head injury or intracranial pressure; it should be administered with caution to those with impaired kidney or liver function, asthma, depressed respiration, insufficient secretion of thyroid hormones (hypothyroidism) or low blood pressure (hypotension).

Nalcrom (*Fisons*) is a proprietary compound mast cell stabilizer available only on prescription, used to assist in the treatment of allergy to specific foods. Produced in the form of capsules, Nalcrom is a preparation of sodium cromoglycate, a drug that prevents some cellular allergic response. It is not recommended for children aged under two years.

▲/✚ side-effects/warning: *see* SODIUM CROMOGLYCATE.

nalidixic acid is an ANTIBIOTIC used primarily to treat infection of the urinary tract. Administration is oral in the form of tablets, as a dilute suspension, and as an effervescent solution.

▲ side-effects: nausea, vomiting, diarrhoea and gastrointestinal disturbance are fairly common, but there may also be sensitivity reactions (such as urticaria or a rash). A very few patients experience visual disturbances and convulsions.

✚ warning: nalidixic acid should not be administered to patients who suffer from epilepsy, or who are aged under three months – preferably it should be avoided in infancy as it may raise the pressure within the head (intracranial pressure). It should be

administered with caution to those with kidney or liver
dysfunction. During treatment it is advisable for patients to avoid
strong sunlight.
Related articles: MICTRAL; NEGRAM; URIBEN.

naloxone is a powerful OPIATE antagonist drug used primarily (in the
form of naloxone hydrochloride) as an antidote to an overdose of
narcotic ANALGESICS. Quick but short-acting, it effectively reverses the
respiratory depression, coma and convulsions that follow overdosage
of opiates. It is most commonly used to treat respiratory depression in
newborn infants whose mothers were given Pethidine or some other
narcotic analgesic during labour. Administration is by intramuscular
or intravenous injection. Naloxone is also used to treat patients at the
end of operations to reverse respiratory depression caused by narcotic
analgesics.
✚ warning: naloxone should not be administered to patients who are
physically dependent on (addicted to) narcotics.
Related article: NARCAN.

Naprosyn (*Syntex*) is a proprietary, non-steroidal ANTI-INFLAMMATORY
non-narcotic ANALGESIC, available only on prescription, used to relieve
pain – particularly rheumatic and arthritic pain, and that of acute
gout – and to treat other musculo-skeletal disorders. Produced in the
form of tablets (in two strengths), as a suspension (the potency of the
suspension once diluted is retained for 14 days), and as anal
suppositories, Naprosyn is a preparation of naproxen. In the form of
tablets or suspension it is not recommended for children aged under
five years; the suppositories are not suitable for children.
▲ side-effects: *see* NAPROXEN.

naproxen is a non-steroidal ANTI-INFLAMMATORY non-narcotic ANALGESIC
used to relieve pain – particularly rheumatic and arthritic pain, and
that of acute gout – and to treat other musculo-skeletal disorders. It
is also effective in relieving the pain of menstrual disorders and
difficulties, in preventing recurrent attacks of migraine, and in
reducing high body temperature. Administration (in the form of
naproxen or naproxen sodium) is oral in the form of tablets or as a
dilute suspension, or by anal suppositories.
▲ side-effects: side-effects are relatively uncommon, but may include
gastrointestinal disturbance with nausea; patients may be advised
to take the drug with food or milk. Some patients experience
sensitivity reactions or fluid retention in the tissues (oedema).
Related articles: NAPROSYN; SYNFLEX.

Narcan (*Du Pont*) is a proprietary drug, available only on prescription,
that is most often used to treat the symptoms of acute overdosage of
OPIATES such as morphine. Produced in ampoules for injection, Narcan
is a preparation of naloxone hydrochloride. A weaker form is
available (under the name Narcan Neonatal) for the treatment of
respiratory depression in babies born to mothers who have been given
narcotic analgesics during the birth.
✚ side-effects/warning: *see* NALOXONE.

Naseptin (*ICI*) is a proprietary ANTIBIOTIC, available only on prescription, used to treat staphylococcal infections in and around the nostrils. Produced in the form of a cream for topical application, Naseptin is a preparation of the ANTISEPTIC antibiotic drugs chlorhexidine hydrochloride and neomycin sulphate.
▲/✚ side-effects/warning: *see* CHLORHEXIDINE; NEOMYCIN.

Natuderm (*Burgess*) is a proprietary non-prescription skin emollient (softener and soother), used to treat dry conditions of the skin. Produced in the form of a cream, Natuderm is a preparation of glycerides, sterols and other lipids, water, waxes and GLYCEROL.

Nebcin (*Lilly*) is a proprietary ANTIBIOTIC, used to treat serious infections. Produced in ampoules (in two strengths) for injection, Nebcin is a preparation of the aminoglycoside tobramycin.
▲/✚ side-effects/warning: *see* TOBRAMYCIN.

Nebuhaler (*Astra*) is a large volume inhaler device for use with the BRONCHODILATOR Bricanyl or the inhaled CORTICOSTEROID Pulmicort. It helps young asthmatic children overcome problems they may have with using ordinary inhalers.

Negram (*Sterling Research*) is a proprietary ANTIBIOTIC agent, available only on prescription, used to treat infections of the urinary tract. Produced in the form of tablets and as a sugar-free suspension for dilution (the potency of the suspension once diluted is retained for 14 days), Negram is a preparation of the antimicrobial drug nalidixic acid. It should not be used in children under the age of three months.
▲/✚ side-effects/warning: *see* NALIDIXIC ACID.

Neo-Cortef (*Upjohn*) is a proprietary compound ANTIBIOTIC available only on prescription, used to treat bacterial infections in the outer ear and inflammation in the eye. Produced in the form of ear- or eye-drops and as an ointment, Neo-Cortef is a compound preparation of the antibiotic aminoglycoside neomycin sulphate with the CORTICOSTEROID hydrocortisone acetate.
▲/✚ side-effects/warning: *see* HYDROCORTISONE; NEOMYCIN.

Neo-Lidocaton is a proprietary preparation of the local ANAESTHETIC lignocaine, used in cartridges for dental surgery.
▲/✚ side-effects/warning: *see* LIGNOCAINE.

Neo-Mercazole (*Nicholas*) is a proprietary preparation of the drug carbimazole, available only on prescription, used to treat the effects of an excess of thyroid hormones in the bloodstream (thyrotoxicosis). It works by inhibiting the formation of the hormone thyroxine in the thyroid gland, and is produced in the form of tablets (in two strengths, under the names Neo-Mercazole 5 and Neo-Mercazole 20).
▲/✚ side-effects/warning: *see* CARBIMAZOLE.

neomycin is a broad-spectrum ANTIBIOTIC drug that is effective in treating topical bacterial infections. Too toxic to be used in intravenous or intramuscular administration, it is sometimes used to reduce the levels of bacteria in the colon prior to intestinal surgery or examination, or in the case of liver failure. Even prolonged or widespread topical application may eventually lead to sensitivity reactions. Administration (most often in the form of neomycin sulphate) is oral as tablets or in solution, or topical as nose-drops, ear-drops, eye-drops, ear ointment, eye ointment or nasal spray.

▲ side-effects: prolonged use may eventually lead to temporarily impaired kidney function, malabsorption from the intestines, or to deafness. Prolonged use to treat the outer ear may lead to fungal infection.

✚ warning: neomycin should not be administered to patients with the neuromuscular disease myasthenia gravis. Intervals between doses should be increased for patients with impaired kidney function.
Related articles: AUDICORT; BETNESOL-N; DERMOVATE-NN; DEXA-RHINASPRAY; GRANEODIN; GREGODERM; MINIMS; MYCIGUENT; NEO-CORTEF; NEOSPORIN; NIVEMYCIN; PREDSOL-N; STIEDEX; VISTA-METHASONE N.

Neosporin (*Calmic*) is a proprietary ANTIBIOTIC, available only on prescription, used to treat bacterial infections in the eye. Produced in the form of eye-drops, Neosporin is a compound preparation of the antiseptic antibiotics neomycin sulphate, polymyxin B sulphate and gramicidin.

▲/✚ side-effects/warning: *see* NEOMYCIN; POLYMYXIN B.

neostigmine is an anticholinesterase drug that has the effect of increasing the activity of the neurotransmitter (acetylcholine) that transmits the neural instructions of the brain to the skeletal muscles. It works by inhibiting the "switching-off" of the neural impulses by the breakdown of acetylcholine by enzymes. Its main use is therefore in the treatment of the neuromuscular disease myasthenia gravis (which causes extreme muscle weakness amounting even to paralysis); it is also commonly used to counter the effects of muscle relaxants administered during surgical operations. Occasionally the drug is alternatively used as a parasympathomimetic to stimulate intestinal motility and so promote defecation. Administration is oral in the form of tablets, or by injection.

▲ side-effects: there may be nausea and vomiting, diarrhoea and abdominal cramps, and an excess of saliva in the mouth. Overdosage may cause gastrointestinal disturbance, an excess of bronchial mucus, sweating, faecal and urinary incontinence, vision disorders, nervous agitation and muscular weakness.

✚ warning: neostigmine should not be administered to patients with intestinal or urinary blockage; it should be administered with caution to those with epilepsy, asthma, parkinsonism, low blood pressure (hypotension) or a slow heart rate.

Nepenthe (*Evans*) is a proprietary narcotic ANALGESIC which, because it is a preparation of the OPIATES anhydrous morphine and opium tincture, is on the controlled drugs list. Used to relieve severe pain, especially during the final stages of terminal malignant disease, it is produced in the form of a syrup for dilution (the potency of the syrup

once diluted is retained for four weeks) and in ampoules for injection.
Nepenthe solution is not recommended for children aged under 12
months; the injection is not recommended for children aged under six
years.
▲/✚ side-effects/warning: *see* MORPHINE.

Nephramine (*Boots*) is a proprietary nutritional supplement for
patients unable to feed or be fed via the alimentary canal. Not a
complete diet, however, Nephramine is a selection of essential amino
acids in a form suitable for intravenous infusion.

Nerisone (*Schering*) is a proprietary CORTICOSTEROID preparation,
available only on prescription, used to treat serious non-infective
inflammatory skin conditions, such as eczema. Produced in the form
of a cream, as an oily cream and as an ointment, Nerisone is a
preparation of the steroid diflucortolone valerate. A stronger form is
also available in the form of an oily cream and an ointment (under
the name Nerisone Forte), which is not recommended for children
aged under four years. Nerisone is not commonly used in childhood.

Nestargel (*Nestlé*) is a proprietary non-prescription nutritional
preparation, used to thicken foods for patients who suffer from
vomiting and regurgitation. Produced in the form of a powder,
Nestargel contains calcium lactate and carob seed flour.

Netillin (*Kirby-Warrick*) is a proprietary form of the aminoglycoside
ANTIBIOTIC netilmicin sulphate, available only on prescription. Used to
treat any of many serious bacterial infections, it is produced in
ampoules (in three strengths) for injection.
▲/✚ side-effects/warning: *see* NETILMICIN.

netilmicin is a broad-spectrum ANTIBIOTIC, one of the aminoglycosides
used (singly or in combination with other types of antibiotic) to treat
any of many serious bacterial infections. Administration is by
injection.
▲ side-effects: there may be temporary kidney dysfunction; some
patients experience deafness.
✚ warning: netilmicin should not be administered to patients with
the neuromuscular disease myasthenia gravis. Intervals between
doses should be increased for patients with impaired kidney
functions.
Related article: NETILLIN.

Neulente (*Wellcome*) is a proprietary non-prescription preparation of
highly purified beef INSULIN zinc suspension, used to treat and
maintain diabetic patients. It is produced in vials for injection.

Neuphane (*Wellcome*) is a proprietary non-prescription preparation of
highly purified beef isophane INSULIN, used to treat and maintain
diabetic patients. It is produced in vials for injection.

Neusulin (*Wellcome*) is a proprietary non-prescription preparation of highly purified beef neutral INSULIN, used to treat and maintain diabetic patients. It is produced in vials for injection.

niclosamide is a synthetic ANTHELMINTIC drug used to rid the body of an infestation of tapeworms. Administration is oral as tablets.
▲ side-effects: there may be gastrointestinal disturbance.
✚ warning: side-effects are minimal, but in case the tapeworms are multiplying some doctors prefer to prescribe an additional ANTI-EMETIC for patients to take on waking. The dose should be administered on a relatively empty stomach, and be followed by a purgative after about two hours.
Related article: YOMESAN.

Nidazol (*Steinhard*) is a proprietary ANTIBIOTIC, available only on prescription, used to treat infections caused by anaerobic bacteria and protozoal organisms, and to provide asepsis during surgery. Produced in the form of tablets, Nidazol is a preparation of the amoebicidal drug metronidazole.
▲/✚ side-effects/warning: *see* METRONIDAZOLE.

Niferex (*Tillotts*) is a proprietary, non-prescription IRON preparation, used to treat iron-deficiency anaemia. Produced in the form of tablets and as an elixir for dilution (the potency of the elixir once diluted is retained for 14 days), Niferex is a polysaccharide-iron complex. An additional preparation in the form of capsules is available (under the name Niferex-150) which is not recommended for children.
▲/✚ side-effects/warning: *see* POLYSACCHARIDE-IRON COMPLEX.

Night Nurse (*Beecham Health Care*) is a proprietary non-prescription cold relief preparation produced in the form of capsules. It contains the ANALGESIC paracetamol, ALCOHOL, the ANTITUSSIVE dextromethorphan and the ANTIHISTAMINE promethazine, which has a marked sedative activity.
▲/✚ side-effects/warning: *see* DEXTROMETHORPHAN; PARACETAMOL; PROMETHAZINE HYDROCHLORIDE.

nitrazepam is a comparatively mild HYPNOTIC drug, one of the benzodiazepines used primarily as a TRANQUILLIZER for patients with insomnia, and in whom a degree of sedation during the daytime is acceptable. It is sometimes used to control infantile spasms, which is a rare but serious form of epilepsy. While nitrazepam may control the fits it has no effect on the intellectual deterioration which may accompany infantile spasms (unlike ACTH and corticosteroid therapy). Administration is oral in the form of tablets, as capsules, or as a suspension (mixture).
▲ side-effects: concentration and speed of reaction are affected. There is commonly drowsiness and dry mouth; there may also be sensitivity reactions. Prolonged use may lead to tolerance and a form of dependence (in which there may be insomnia that is worse than before).

nitrofurantoin is an ANTIBACTERIAL that is used particularly to treat inflammation and infections of the urinary tract. It is especially useful in treating kidney infections that prove to be resistant to other forms of therapy. Administration is oral in the form of tablets, as capsules, or as a suspension.

▲ side-effects: there may be nausea and vomiting. Some patients experience tingling in the fingers and toes, or a rash. Rarely, there is allergic liver damage, pulmonary infiltration or peripheral neuropathy.

✚ warning: nitrofurantoin should not be administered to patients with impaired kidney function, or who are aged under one month. The drug is ineffective in patients whose urine is alkaline.
Related articles: FURADANTIN; MACRODANTIN; URANTOIN.

nitrophenol is an ANTIFUNGAL drug used in topical application to treat skin infection (such as athlete's foot). Administration is as an alcohol-based paint, using a special applicator.

Nivaquine (*May & Baker*) is a proprietary ANTIMALARIAL drug, available only on prescription, used primarily in combination with other drugs for the prevention and treatment of malaria. Produced in the form of tablets, as a syrup for dilution (the potency of the elixir once diluted is retained for 14 days), and in ampoules for injection (during emergency treatment only), Nivaquine is a preparation of chloroquine sulphate.

▲/✚ side-effects/warning: *see* CHLOROQUINE.

Nivemycin (*Boots*) is a proprietary form of the aminoglycoside ANTIBIOTIC neomycin sulphate, available only on prescription, used to reduce bacterial levels in the intestines before surgery. Nivemycin is produced in the form of tablets and as an elixir.

▲/✚ side-effects/warning: *see* NEOMYCIN.

Nizoral (*Janssen*) is a proprietary ANTIFUNGAL drug, available only on prescription, used to treat both systemic and skin-surface fungal infections. Produced in the form of tablets, as a suspension, and as a water-miscible cream for topical application, Nizoral is a preparation of the IMIDAZOLE ketoconazole.

▲/✚ side-effects/warning: *see* KETOCONAZOLE.

Noratex (*Norton*) is a proprietary non-prescription skin emollient (softener and soother), used to treat nappy rash and bedsores. Produced in the form of a cream, it contains wool fat, ZINC OXIDE, KAOLIN and talc.

✚ warning: wool fat causes sensitivity reactions in some patients.

Norcuron (*Organon-Teknika*) is a proprietary SKELETAL MUSCLE RELAXANT of the type known as competitive or non-depolarizing; it is used during surgical operations, but only after the patient has been rendered unconscious. Available only on prescription, and produced in ampoules for injection, Norcuron is a preparation of vecuronium bromide.

✚ warning: see VECURONIUM BROMIDE.

Nordox (*Norton*) is a proprietary broad-spectrum ANTIBIOTIC, available only on prescription, used to treat infections of many kinds, such as acne. Produced in the form of capsules, Nordox is a preparation of the TETRACYCLINE doxycycline. It should not be used in children under 12 years.
▲/✚ side-effects/warning: *see* DOXYCYCLINE.

Normasol (*Schering*) is a proprietary non-prescription saline solution, used to clean burns and minor wounds. Produced in the form of a sterile solution, Normasol is a preparation of sodium chloride (saline). An ophthalmic form is also available (under the trade name Normasol Undine) for the washing out of harmful substances and foreign bodies from the eye.

Nuelin (*Riker*) is a proprietary non-prescription BRONCHODILATOR, used to treat asthmatic bronchospasm. Produced in the form of tablets (not recommended for children aged under seven years), as sustained-release tablets (in two strengths under the names Nuelin SA and Nuelin SA 250; not recommended for children aged under six years), and as a syrup for dilution (the potency of the liquid once diluted is retained for 14 days; not recommended for children aged under two years), Nuelin is a preparation of the xanthine drug theophylline.
▲/✚ side-effects/warning: *see* THEOPHYLLINE.

Nurofen (*Crookes Healthcare*) is a proprietary non-prescription non-narcotic ANALGESIC containing ibuprofen.
▲/✚ side-effects/warning: *see* IBUPROFEN.

Nutracel (*Travenol*) is a proprietary form of high-energy nutritional supplement, available only on prescription, intended for infusion into patients who are unable to take food via the alimentary tract such as after total gastrectomy. Produced in two strengths (under the trade names Nutracel 400 and Nutracel 800), it is a preparation of GLUCOSE with MAGNESIUM CHLORIDE and several other mineral salts.

Nutramigen (*Bristol-Myers*) is a proprietary non-prescription milk substitute. Nutritionally complete, it is intended for patients who suffer from milk protein intolerance. Produced in the form of a powder, Nutramigen is a preparation of protein, carbohydrate, fat (corn oil), vitamins and minerals, and is lactose-, fructose- and gluten-free.

Nutranel (*Roussel*) is a proprietary non-prescription dietary supplement. It is intended for patients who suffer from malabsorption of food (for example following gastrectomy). Produced in the form of a powder, Nutranel is a preparation of protein, fat, carbohydrate, vitamins, minerals and trace elements and is low in lactose. It is not suitable as the sole source of nutrition for children, and is unsuitable for infants aged under 12 months.

Nutraplus (*Alcon*) is a proprietary non-prescription skin emollient (softener and soother), used to treat dry skin. Produced in the form of a cream in a water-miscible basis, Nutraplus is a preparation of the hydrating substance urea.

Nutrauxil (*KabiVitrum*) is a proprietary non-prescription dietary supplement. It is intended for patients who suffer from overall dietary insufficiency (as with anorexia nervosa) or from intractable malabsorption of food in the digestive tract. Produced in the form of a liquid feed, Nutrauxil is a preparation of protein, carbohydrate, fat (sunflower oil), vitamins and minerals, and is lactose- and electrolyte-low and gluten-free. It is not suitable as the sole source of nutrition for children aged under five years, but nutritionally is all that anyone else might need.

Nybadex (*Cox*) is a proprietary anti-inflammatory and ANTIFUNGAL compound, available only on prescription, used to treat skin inflammations in which infection is thought to be present. It is produced in the form of a dilute emulsifying ointment for topical application, and contains the CORTICOSTEROID hydrocortisone with the ANTIBIOTIC nystatin, the antifoaming agent dimethicone and the ANTISEPTIC benzalkonium chloride.

▲/✚ side-effects/warning: *see* HYDROCORTISONE; NYSTATIN.

Nystadermal (*Squibb*) is a proprietary CORTICOSTEROID cream, available only on prescription, used for topical application on areas of inflamed skin, particularly in cases of eczema that have failed to respond to less powerful drugs. Nystadermal is a preparation of the steroid triamcinolone acetonide and the ANTIBIOTIC nystatin. It is not commonly used in childhood.

▲/✚ side-effects/warning: *see* NYSTATIN; TRIAMCINOLONE ACETONIDE.

Nystaform (*Bayer*) is a proprietary ANTIFUNGAL preparation, available only on prescription, used in topical application to treat fungal (particularly yeast) infections. Produced in the form of a cream and an anhydrous ointment, Nystaform is a preparation of the ANTIBIOTIC drug nystatin and one of two forms of the ANTISEPTIC chlorhexidine.

▲/✚ side-effects/warning: *see* CHLORHEXIDINE; NYSTATIN.

Nystaform-HC (*Bayer*) is a proprietary CORTICOSTEROID compound, available only on prescription, used to treat skin inflammations in which fungal and bacterial infections are suspected. Produced in the form of a water-miscible cream and an anhydrous ointment, Nystaform-HC is a preparation of the corticosteroid hydrocortisone, the ANTIFUNGAL drug nystatin, and one of two forms of the (mildly antibacterial) ANTISEPTIC chlorhexidine.

▲/✚ side-effects/warning: *see* CHLORHEXIDINE; HYDROCORTISONE; NYSTATIN.

Nystan (*Squibb*) is the name of a proprietary group of ANTIFUNGAL preparations, available only on prescription, used to treat fungal infections (such as candidiasis, thrush). All are forms of the ANTIBIOTIC nystastin. Preparations for oral administration include tablets, a suspension, granules for reconstitution with water to form a solution,

NYSTATIN

and pastilles (for treating mouth infections). A water-miscible cream, gel, ointment and dusting-powder are available for the topical treatment of fungal skin infections.

▲/✚ side-effects/warning: *see* NYSTATIN.

nystatin is an ANTIFUNGAL ANTIBIOTIC drug, effective both in topical application and when taken orally, primarily used specifically to treat the yeast infection candidiasis (thrush). Less commonly, it is used to treat other fungal infections, particularly in and around the mouth. Administration is in many forms: tablets, a suspension, a solution, pastilles, a cream, a gel, an ointment and a dusting-powder.

✚ warning: the full course of treatment must be completed, even if symptoms disappear earlier; recurrence of infection is common when treatment is withdrawn too hastily.

Related articles: DERMOVATE-NN; GREGODERM; MULTILIND; NYSTAFORM; NYSTAN; NYSTATIN-DOME; TERRA-CORTRIL; TINADERM-M.

Nystatin-Dome (*Bayer*) is a proprietary ANTIFUNGAL preparation, available only on prescription, used to treat intestinal candidiasis (thrush) and oral infections. Produced in the form of a suspension, Nystatin-Dome is a preparation of the ANTIBIOTIC nystatin.

▲/✚ side-effects/warning: *see* NYSTATIN.

Octovit (*Smith, Kline & French*) is a proprietary non-prescription mineral-and-VITAMIN compound, used particularly as an IRON supplement (containing ferrous sulphate). Produced in the form of tablets, Octovit contains – apart from iron – calcium, magnesium and zinc, together with thiamine (vitamin B₁), riboflavine (vitamin B₂), PYRIDOXINE (vitamin B₆), cyanocobalamin (vitamin B₁₂), nicotinamide (of the vitamin B complex), ASCORBIC ACID (vitamin C), CALCIFEROL (vitamin D) and TOCOPHEROL (vitamin E). Octovit should not be used simultaneously with tetracycline antibiotics.
▲/✚ side-effects/warning: *see* FERROUS SULPHATE.

Ocusol (*Boots*) is a proprietary ANTIBACTERIAL, available only on prescription, used to treat eye infections. Produced in the form of eye-drops, Ocusol is a preparation of the sulphonamide sulphacetamide sodium together with the astringent-cleanser ZINC SULPHATE.

Oilatum (*Stiefel*) is a proprietary non-prescription skin emollient (softener and soother) in the form of a water-based cream containing arachis oil and povidone. Under the same name there is a bath emulsion containing liquid paraffin and wool alcohols, for use as a emollient soaking medium.

ointments is a general term for a group of essentially greasy preparations that are anhydrous and insoluble in water and so do not wash off. Such unguents are used as bases for many therapeutic preparations for topical application (particularly in the treatment of dry lesions or of ophthalmic complaints). Most have a form of paraffin as their base; a few contain lanolin and wool alcohols, to which a small number of patients may be sensitive.

olive oil is used therapeutically – always warmed beforehand – to soften earwax prior to syringeing the ears, or to treat the brown, flaking skin that commonly appears on the heads of very young infants (cradle cap).

Omnopon (*Roche*) is a proprietary OPIATE narcotic ANALGESIC, a controlled drug which is a preparation of papaveretum, used primarily as premedication before surgery, but also to relieve severe pain. It is produced in the form of tablets and in ampoules for injection.
▲/✚ side-effects/warning: *see* PAPAVERETUM.

Omnopon-Scopolamine (*Roche*) is a proprietary combination of Omnopon and the powerful alkaloid SEDATIVE hyoscine (also known as scopolamine in the USA). It is a controlled drug, and is used primarily as premedication before surgery. It is produced in ampoules for injection.

Oncovin (*Lilly*) is a proprietary form of the VINCA ALKALOID vincristine sulphate, available only on prescription, used to treat acute leukaemia, lymphoma and certain tumours. It is produced in ampoules or as a powder for reconstitution, in both cases for injection.
▲/✚ side-effects/warning: *see* VINCRISTINE SULPHATE.

One-alpha (*Leo*) is a proprietary form of the VITAMIN D analogue alfacalcidol, available only on prescription. It is a powerful preparation and tends only to be used in chronic renal failure or in situations where the more conventional vitamin D preparations have failed. It is produced in the form of capsules (in two strengths) and as drops (with a diluent to adjust concentration).

Ophthaine (*Squibb*) is a proprietary form of local ANAESTHETIC eye-drops, available only on prescription, commonly used during ophthalmic procedures and consisting of a preparation of proxymetacaine hydrochloride.

Ophthalmadine (*SAS Pharmaceuticals*) is a proprietary preparation, available only on prescription, used to treat Herpes simplex infections of the eye. Containing a mild solution of the antiviral agent idoxuridine, it is produced in the form of eye-drops for use during the day, and eye ointment for use overnight.
▲/✚ side-effects/warning: *see* IDOXURIDINE.

opiates are a group of drugs derived from opium, that depress certain functions of the central nervous system. In this way, they can relieve pain (and inhibit coughing). They are also used to treat diarrhoea. Therapeutically, the most important opiate is probably morphine which, with its synthetic derivative heroin (diamorphine), is a narcotic ANALGESIC; all are potentially habituating (addictive).
▲/✚ side-effects/warning: *see* BUPRENORPHINE; CODEINE PHOSPHATE; DEXTROMORAMIDE; DIAMORPHINE; DIHYDROCODEINE TARTRATE; METHADONE; MORPHINE; PAPAVERETUM; PENTAZOCINE; PETHIDINE.

Opticrom (*Fisons*) is an ANTI-INFLAMMATORY preparation available only on prescription, used to treat forms of conjunctivitis caused by allergic reactions. Produced in the form of eye-drops and eye ointment, Opticrom contains sodium cromoglycate.
▲/✚ side-effects/warning: *see* SODIUM CROMOGLYCATE.

Optricrom aqueous (*Fisons*) is a proprietary preparation of the drug sodium cromogluacate, available only on prescription. Produced in the form of eye drops, it is used to treat allergic conjunctivitis.

Optimine (*Kirby-Warrick*) is a proprietary non-prescription form of the ANTIHISTAMINE drug azatadine maleate, used to relieve the symptoms of allergic reactions such as hay fever and urticaria. Produced in the form of tablets and as a syrup for dilution, Optimine is not recommended for children aged under 12 months.
▲/✚ side-effects/warning: *see* AZATADINE MALEATE.

Opulets (*Alcon*) is the name of a proprietary brand of eye-drops which consists of a variety of different drugs. Opulets Chloramphenicol is used to treat bacterial infections in the eye and contains the ANTIBIOTIC chloramphenicol. Opulets Atropine contains the ANTICHOLINERGIC atropine sulphate and is used to dilate the pupils and paralyse the eye muscles. Opulets Cyclopentolate contains the anticholinergic cyclopentolate hydrochloride and is used to dilate the pupils and paralyse the eye muscles. Opulets Pilocarpine contains the parasympathomimetic pilocarpine hydrochloride and is used to treat glaucoma. Opulets Benoxinate contains oxybuprocaine hydrochloride and has a local ANAESTHETIC effect on the eyeballs. Opulets Saline contains sodium chloride and is used as an eye-wash. Opulets Fluorescein contains fluorescein sodium and is a stain for highlighting foreign bodies on the surface of the eye. With the exception of Opulets Saline and Opulets Fluorescein, all these preparations are available only on prescription.

▲/✚ side-effects/warning: *see* ATROPINE SULPHATE; CHLORAMPHENICOL; CYCLOPENTOLATE HYDROCHLORIDE; FLUORESCEIN SODIUM; PILOCARPINE HYDROCHLORIDE; OXYBUPROCAINE HYDROCHLORIDE.

Orabase (*Squibb*) is a proprietary non-prescription ointment, used to protect sores and ulcers in and on the mouth, or in the vicinity of a stoma (an outlet on the skin surface following the surgical curtailment of the intestines). Produced in the form of paste, Orabase's active constituent is CARMELLOSE SODIUM.

Orahesive (*Squibb*) is a proprietary non-prescription preparation, used to protect sores and ulcers in and on the mouth, or in the vicinity of a stoma (an outlet on the skin surface following the surgical curtailment of the intestines). Produced in the form of powder, Orahesive's active constituent is carmellose sodium.

Oralcer (*Vitabiotics*) is a proprietary non-prescription ANTISEPTIC preparation, used to treat infections and ulcers in the mouth. Produced in the form of lozenges, Oralcer contains clioquinol and ascorbic acid (vitamin C).
▲/✚ side-effects/warning: *see* CLIOQUINOL.

Oraldene (*Warner-Lambert*) is a proprietary non-prescription ANTISEPTIC preparation, used to treat sores and ulcers in the mouth. Produced in the form of a mouth-wash, Oraldene's active constituent is HEXETIDINE.

Oramorph (*Boehringer Ingelheim*) is a proprietary oral solution of the powerful narcotic ANALGESIC morphine. Oramorph is not recommended for children under one year of age.
▲/✚ side-effects/warning: *see* MORPHINE.

Orbenin (*Beecham*) is a proprietary ANTIBIOTIC, available only on prescription, used to treat bacterial infections, and especially staphylococcal infections that prove to be resistant to penicillin. Produced in the form of capsules (in two strengths), as a syrup for dilution, and as powder for reconstitution as injections, Orbenin's active constituent is cloxacillin.
▲/✚ side-effects/warning: *see* CLOXACILLIN.

orciprenaline is a BETA-RECEPTOR STIMULANT, and acts as a BRONCHODILATOR. Consequently it is used to treat respiratory problems associated with such conditions as asthma. Nowadays the more specific beta-receptor stimulants salbutamol and terbutaline are more commonly used.

▲ side-effects: increased heart rate and tremor are common.

Related article: ALUPENT.

Orovite (*Bencard*) is a proprietary non-prescription VITAMIN preparation that is not available from the National Health Service. It is used to treat vitamin deficiencies after illness, infection or operation. Produced in the form of tablets and as an elixir, Orovite contains thiamine (vitamin B$_1$), riboflavine (vitamin B$_2$), PYRIDOXINE (vitamin B$_6$), nicotinamide (of the B complex) and ASCORBIC ACID (vitamin C). There is also a granular form (issued under the name Orovite 7) that includes retinol (vitamin A) with CALCIFEROL (vitamin D), produced in sachets for solution in water.

Osmitrol (*Travenol*) is a diuretic drug available only on prescription. It is used to lower pressure within the head (intracranial pressure) when brain swelling is present. Produced in the form of fluid for intravenous infusion (in three strengths). Osmitrol is a preparation of mannitol.

▲/✚ side-effects/warning: *see* MANNITOL.

Osmolite (*Abbott*) is a bland, proprietary, non-prescription, gluten- and lactose-free liquid that is a complete nutritional diet for adult patients (but not for children) who are severely undernourished (such as with anorexia nervosa) or who are suffering from some problem with the absorption of food. Produced in cans, Osmolite contains protein, carbohydrate, fat, vitamins and minerals. It is not suitable for children aged under 12 months.

Ostersoy (*Farley*) is a proprietary non-prescription soya milk. It is intended for children with cows' milk intolerance or who are intolerant of the milk sugar lactose. Produced in the form of a powder for reconstitution Ostersoy is a preparation of soya protein, carbohydrate, fat (vegetable oil), vitamins and minerals, and it is gluten-, lactose- and sucrose-free.

Otosporin (*Calmic*) is a proprietary ANTIBIOTIC preparation, available only on prescription, used to treat infections and inflammation in the outer ear. Produced in the form of ear-drops, Otosporin contains the CORTICOSTEROID hydrocortisone, the ANTIBIOTIC neomycin sulphate and polymyxin B sulphate.

▲/✚ side-effects/warning: *see* HYDROCORTISONE; NEOMYCIN SULPHATE; POLYMYXIN B SULPHATE.

Otrivine (*Ciba*) is a proprietary SYMPATHOMIMETIC nasal DECONGESTANT, available only on prescription, and produced in the form of drops and spray. Otrivine Paediatric drops (at half the strength) are available for children. Otrivine's active constituent is xylometazoline hydrochloride.

Otrivine-Antistin (*Zyma*) is a proprietary non-prescription
ANTIHISTAMINE drug, used to treat allergic and inflammatory
ophthalmic conditions. Produced in the form of eye-drops, Otrivine-
Antistin contains antazoline and xylometazoline hydrochloride. It is
not recommended for children aged under two years. Otrivine-
Antistin is produced also by Ciba in the form of nose-drops and as a
nasal spray, neither of which is available from the National Health
Service.
▲/✚ side-effects/warning: *see* ANTAZOLINE.

oxatomide is an ANTIHISTAMINE, used to treat hay fever, urticaria
(nettle rash) and various other allergic conditions. Administration is
oral in the form of tablets. It is not recommended for children aged
under five years.
▲ side-effects: there may be headache, dry mouth, gastrointestinal
disturbances and/or visual disturbances. High dosage may lead to
increased appetite and consequent weight gain.
Related article: TINSET.

oxybuprocaine is a widely-used local ANAESTHETIC particularly used in
ophthalmic treatments. In the form of oxybuprocaine hydrochloride, it
is administered as eye-drops.
▲ side-effects: there may be initial stinging on application.
Related articles: MINIMS BENOXINATE; OPULETS.

oxymetazoline is a VASOCONSTRICTOR, a potent SYMPATHOMIMETIC used
primarily as a nasal decongestant. It works by constricting the blood
vessels of the nose, thus in turn constricting the nasal mucous
membranes. Administration is in the form of nose-drops or nasal
spray.
▲ side-effects: there may be local irritation.
✚ warning: prolonged use may result in tolerance, leading to even
worse nasal congestion. Oxymetazoline should be administered
with caution to children aged under three months.
Related article: AFRAZINE.

Oxymycin (*DDSA Pharmaceuticals*) is a proprietary ANTIBIOTIC,
available only on prescription, used to treat many microbial
infections, such as severe acne vulgaris. Produced in the form of
tablets, Oxymycin's active constituent is the TETRACYCLINE
oxytetracycline dihydrate. It should not be used in children under 12
years.
▲/✚ side-effects/warning: *see* OXYTETRACYCLINE.

oxytetracycline is a broad-spectrum ANTIBIOTIC used to treat many
serious infections, particularly those of the urogenital organs and
skin or membrane surfaces, and of the respiratory passages. It may
also be used to treat acne, although it is not suitable for children
aged under 12 years. Administration is oral in the form of tablets or
syrup.

▲ side-effects: there may be nausea and vomiting, with diarrhoea; hypersensitivity reactions may occur, as may photosensitivity (sensitivity of the skin and eyes to light), but both are rare.

✚ warning: oxytetracycline should not be administered to patients who have kidney failure. Some bacterial strains have now become resistant.

Related articles: BERKMYCEN; IMPERACIN; OXYMYCIN; TERRA-CORTRIL; TERRAMYCIN; UNIMYCIN.

Paldesic (*RP Drugs*) is a proprietary non-prescription form of the non-narcotic ANALGESIC paracetamol. It is produced in the form of a syrup and is intended for hospital use only.
▲/✚ side-effects/warning: *see* PARACETAMOL.

Palfium (*MCP Pharmaceuticals*) is a proprietary narcotic ANALGESIC which, because it is a preparation of the OPIATE dextromoramide, is on the controlled drugs list. Used to relieve severe pain, especially during the final stages of terminal malignant disease, it is produced in the form of tablets (in two strengths), ampoules (in two strengths) for injection, and anal suppositories (which are not recommended for children).
▲/✚ side-effects/warning: *see* DEXTROMORAMIDE.

Paludrine (*ICI*) is a proprietary non-prescription drug used in the prevention of malaria (*see* ANTIMALARIAL). Produced in the form of tablets, Paludrine is a preparation of proguanil hydrochloride.
▲/✚ side-effects/warning: *see* PROGUANIL.

Pameton (*Winthrop*) is a proprietary non-prescription non-narcotic ANALGESIC, not available from the National Health Service, used to treat pain (especially for patients likely to overdose) and to reduce high body temperature. Produced in the form of tablets, Pameton is a compound preparation of paracetamol and the amino acid methionine (a paracetamol overdose antidote). It is not recommended for children aged under six years.
▲/✚ side-effects/warning: *see* METHIONINE; PARACETAMOL.

Panadeine (*Winthrop*) is a proprietary non-prescription compound ANALGESIC, not available from the National Health Service, used to treat pain and to reduce high body temperature. Produced in the form of tablets, and as effervescent tablets (under the name Panadeine Soluble), it is a preparation of paracetamol and codeine (a combination known as co-codamol), and is not recommended for children aged under seven years. A stronger form is available only on prescription – but not from the National Health Service (under the name Panadeine Forte) – and is not recommended for children.
▲/✚ side-effects/warning: *see* CODEINE PHOSPHATE; PARACETAMOL.

Panadol (*Winthrop*) is a proprietary non-prescription non-narcotic ANALGESIC. Used to treat pain and to reduce high body temperature, it is produced in the form of tablets (of two kinds), as effervescent tablets (under the name Panadol Soluble), and as an elixir for dilution (the potency of the elixir once diluted is retained for 14 days). It is not available from the National Health Service. In all forms Panadol is a preparation of paracetamol, and is not recommended for children aged under three months.
▲/✚ side-effects/warning: *see* PARACETAMOL.

Pancrease (*Ortho-Cilag*) is a proprietary non-prescription form of pancreatic enzymes, used to treat enzymatic deficiency in such conditions as cystic fibrosis and chronic inflammation of the pancreas. Pancrease is produced in the form of capsules.

P

Pancrex (*Paines & Byrne*) is a proprietary non-prescription form of pancreatic enzymes, used to treat enzymatic deficiency in cystic fibrosis. Pancrex is produced in the form of granules, but (under the name Pancrex V) there are also versions available as a powder, as capsules (in two strengths, the weaker under the name Pancrex V"125"), and as tablets (in two strengths, the stronger under the name Pancrex V Forte).

pancuronium bromide is a SKELETAL MUSCLE RELAXANT used primarily under general anaesthesia for medium-duration paralysis. Administration is by injection.

▲ side-effects: paralysis is rapid in onset following injection.

✚ warning: the onset of the paralysis may be accompanied by temporarily increased heart rate: caution should be exercised in relation to patients for whom this might present difficulty. Dosage should be reduced for patients who suffer from impaired kidney function or who are obese.
Related article: PAVULON.

Panoxyl 2.5 (*Stiefel*) is a proprietary, non-prescription, topical preparation for the treatment of acne. Produced in the form of an aqueous gel, Panoxyl 2.5 is a solute preparation of the KERATOLYTIC benzoyl peroxide. A stronger version is produced also in the form of an aqueous gel and additionally as a gel in an alcohol base (under the name Panoxyl 5). And an even stronger preparation is available as an aqueous gel, as a gel in an alcohol base, and as a wash lotion in a detergent base (under the name Panoxyl 10).

▲/✚ side-effects/warning: *see* BENZOYL PEROXIDE.

papaveretum is a compound preparation of alkaloids of opium, about half of which is made up of MORPHINE, the rest consisting of codeine, noscapine and papaverine. It is used as a narcotic ANALGESIC primarily during or following surgery, but also as a SEDATIVE prior to an operation. Administration is oral in the form of tablets, or by injection. All proprietary preparations containing papaveretum are on the controlled drugs list: the drug is potentially addictive.

▲ side-effects: there may be constipation and urinary retention, shallow breathing and cough suppression; there may also be nausea and vomiting, and drowsiness. Injections may cause pain and tissue damage at the site. Tolerance and dependence (addiction) occur readily.

✚ warning: papaveretum should not be administered to patients who are suffering from head injury or intracranial pressure; it should be administered with caution to those with asthma, impaired kidney or liver function, hypotension (low blood pressure) or hypothyroidism (underactivity of the thyroid gland), or who have a history of drug abuse.
Related articles: OMNOPON; OMNOPON-SCOPOLAMINE.

paracetamol is a non-narcotic ANALGESIC used to treat all forms of mild to moderate pain; although it is also effective in reducing high body temperature, it has no capacity for relieving inflammation. In many

P

ways it is similar to ASPIRIN — except that it does not cause gastric irritation. It may (in high overdosage) cause liver damage. Administration is oral in the form of tablets, capsules or a liquid.

▲ side-effects: there are few side effects if dosage is low; overdosage may result in liver dysfunction.

✚ warning: paracetamol should be administered with caution to patients with impaired liver function.

Related articles: CAFADOL; CALPOL; CO-DYDRAMOL; DISPROL; FORTAGESIC; MEDISED; MEDOCODENE; MIGRALEVE; PALDESIC; PAMETON; PANADEINE; PANADOL; PARACODOL; PARACLEAR; PARADEINE; PARAHYPON; SALZONE; SOLPADEINE; UNIGESIC.

Paraclear (*Sussex Pharmaceuticals*) is a proprietary non-prescription non-narcotic ANALGESIC produced in the form of soluble tablets. It contains paracetamol.

▲/✚ side-effects/warning: *see* PARACETAMOL.

Paracodol (*Fisons*) is a proprietary non-prescription compound ANALGESIC that is not available from the National Health Service. Used to treat muscular and rheumatic pain, and produced in the form of tablets for effervescent solution, it is a preparation of paracetamol and codeine phosphate (a combination itself known as co-codamol) and is not recommended for children aged under six years.

▲/✚ side-effects/warning: *see* CODEINE PHOSPHATE; PARACETAMOL.

Paradeine (*Scotia*) is a proprietary non-prescription compound ANALGESIC that is not obtainable from the National Health Service. Used to treat muscular and rheumatic pain, and produced in the form of tablets, Paradeine is a preparation of paracetamol and codeine phosphate, together with the LAXATIVE phenolphthalein.

▲/✚ side-effects/warning: *see* CODEINE PHOSPHATE; PARACETAMOL; PHENOLPHTHALEIN.

paraffin is a hydrocarbon derived from petroleum. Its main therapeutic use is as a base for ointments (in the form of yellow or white soft paraffin). As a mineral oil, liquid paraffin is used as an effective laxative (although prolonged use may have unpleasant side-effects) and as an eye ointment in cases of tear deficiency.

see LIQUID PARAFFIN.

Parahypon (*Calmic*) is a proprietary non-prescription compound ANALGESIC that is not available from the National Health Service. Used to relieve most types of pain, and produced in the form of tablets, Parahypon is a preparation of paracetamol and codeine phosphate with the stimulant caffeine. It is not recommended for children aged under six years.

▲/✚ side-effects/warning: *see* CAFFEINE; CODEINE PHOSPHATE; PARACETAMOL.

paraldehyde is a strong-smelling and fast-acting SEDATIVE. It is primarily used in the treatment of severe and continuous epileptic seizures (status epilepticus), and is administered generally by

P

injection although it is sometimes administered via the rectum in the form of an enema.

▲ side-effects: a rash is not uncommon. The injections may be painful.

✚ warning: paraldehyde should be administered with caution to patients with lung disease or impaired liver function. Keep away from rubber, plastics or fabric.

Paraplatin (*Bristol-Myers*) is a proprietary CYTOTOXIC drug, available only on prescription, used to treat certain types of solid tumour. Produced in the form of powder for reconstitution as a medium for injection, Paraplatin is a preparation of the CISPLATIN derivative carboplatin.

▲/✚ side-effects/warning: *see* CARBOPLATIN.

Parvolex (*Duncan, Flockhart*) is a proprietary form of the amino acid acetylcysteine, available only on prescription, used in emergencies to treat paracetamol overdosage and so to try to limit liver damage. It is produced in ampoules for injection.

▲/✚ side-effects/warning: *see* ACETYLCYSTEINE.

Pavacol-D (*Boehringer Ingelheim*) is a proprietary non-prescription cough mixture. It is a sugar-free preparation of the opiates papaverine hydrochloride and pholcodine for solution with the sugar-substitute sorbitol (the potency of the mixture once diluted is retained for 14 days). It is not recommended for children aged under 12 months.

▲/✚ side-effects/warning: *see* PHOLCODINE.

Pavulon (*Organon-Teknika*) is a proprietary SKELETAL MUSCLE RELAXANT of the type known as competitive or non-depolarizing. Available only on prescription, it is used during surgical operations, but only after the patient has been rendered unconscious. Produced in ampoules for injection, Pavulon is a preparation of pancuronium bromide.

▲/✚ side-effects/warning: *see* PANCURONIUM BROMIDE.

Paxadon (*Steinhard*) is a proprietary non-prescription VITAMIN B supplement that is not available from the National Health Service. Used to treat vitamin deficiency and associated symptoms, Paxadon is a preparation of PYRIDOXINE hydrochloride (vitamin B_6). It is produced in the form of tablets.

▲/✚ side-effects/warning: *see* PYRIDOXINE.

Paxofen (*Steinhard*) is a proprietary ANTI-INFLAMMATORY non-narcotic ANALGESIC, available only on prescription, used to treat the pain of rheumatic and other musculo-skeletal disorders. Produced in the form of tablets (in three strengths), Paxofen is a preparation of ibuprofen.

▲/✚ side-effects/warning: *see* IBUPROFEN.

Pecram (*Zyra*) is a proprietary non-prescription BRONCHODILATOR, used to treat asthma. Produced in the form of sustained release tablets, Percram is a preparation of aminophylline.

▲/✚ side-effects/warning: *see* AMINOPHYLLINE.

Ped-El (*KabiVitrum*) is a preparation of additional electrolytes and trace elements for use in association with Vamin (proprietary) amino acid solutions for intravenous nutrition. Available only on prescription, Ped-El is intended primarily for paediatric use. *see* VAMIN.

*pediculicidal drugs kill lice of the genus *Pediculus*, which infest either the body or the scalp − or both − and cause intense itching. Scratching tends only to damage the skin surface, and may eventually cause weeping lesions or bacterial infection on top. Best known and most used pediculicides include malathion and carbaryl; the once commonly used lindane is now no longer recommended for lice on the scalp because resistant strains have emerged. Administration is topical, generally in the form of a lotion; contact between drug and skin should be as long as possible (at least two hours), which is why shampoos are less commonly used.
▲/✚ side-effects/warning: *see* BENZYL BENZOATE; CARBARYL; LINDANE; MALATHION.

Penbritin (*Beecham*) is a proprietary form of the broad-spectrum penicillin ampicillin, available only on prescription. It is used most commonly to treat infections of the respiratory passages and the middle ear. Penbritin is produced in the form of capsules (in two strengths), as tablets for children, as a syrup (in two strengths, for dilution; the potency of the syrup once diluted is retained for seven days), as a children's suspension for use with a pipette, and as powder for reconstitution as a solution for injections.
▲/✚ side-effects/warning: *see* AMPICILLIN.

Pendramine (*Degussa*) is a proprietary non-steroidal ANTI-INFLAMMATORY drug, available only on prescription, used to relieve the pain and to halt the progress of severe rheumatoid arthritis. The drug may also be used as a long-term chelating agent to treat poisoning by the metals copper or lead (especially in metabolic disorders like Wilson's disease). Produced in the form of tablets (in two strengths), Pendramine is a preparation of the penicillin-derivative penicillamine.
▲/✚ side-effects/warning: *see* PENICILLAMINE.

Penetrol (*Crookes Healthcare Products UK*) is a proprietary non-prescription preparation for the relief of catarrh. Produced in the form of an inhalant and as lozenges, it contains menthol, eucalyptus and peppermint oils.
▲/✚ side-effects/warning: *see* PEPPERMINT OIL.

penicillamine is a breakdown product of penicillin that is an extremely effective CHELATING AGENT: it binds various metals (and mineral substances) as it passes through the body before being excreted in the normal way. It is thus used to treat various forms of metallic poisoning − notably copper poisoning in Wilson's disease, lead and mercury poisoning − and can also be used to assist in the treatment of severe rheumatoid arthritis or juvenile chronic arthritis,

P

especially when anti-inflammatory analgesics (such as aspirin) have
proved unsuccessful; in the treatment of chronic hepatitis once the
acute phase is over; and in the treatment of biliary cirrhosis.
Administration is oral in the form of tablets.

▲ side-effects: there may be nausea, but this can be minimized by
taking the drug before food or on going to bed. Between the sixth
and twelfth weeks of treatment there is commonly a loss of the
sense of taste. There is commonly also a rash. Some patients
experience extreme weight loss, mouth ulcers, muscle weakness,
fluid retention and/or blood disorders.

✚ warning: penicillamine should not be administered to patients with
the serious skin disorder lupus erythematosus; it should be
administered with caution to those with impaired kidney function,
or some forms of hypertension (high blood pressure), who are
taking any form of immunosuppressant drug, or who are sensitive
to penicillin. Patients should be warned that treatment may take
up to 12 weeks for any effect to become apparent, and up to six
months to achieve its full therapeutic effect. Regular and frequent
blood counts and urine analyses are essential.
Related articles: DISTAMINE; PENDRAMINE.

penicillin G is a term for the ANTIBIOTIC more commonly known as
benzylpenicillin.
see BENZYLPENICILLIN.

penicillin V is a term for the ANTIBIOTIC more commonly known as
phenoxymethylpenicillin.
see PHENOXYMETHYLPENICILLIN.

penicillin VK is a term for the potassium salt of the ANTIBIOTIC more
commonly known as phenoxymethylpenicillin.
see PHENOXYMETHYLPENICILLIN.

penicillinases are enzyme-like substances produced by some bacteria
that commonly inhibit or completely neutralize the antibacterial
activity of many forms of PENICILLIN. Treatment of infections caused by
bacteria that produce penicillinases has generally therefore to be
undertaken with other forms of antibiotic.

penicillins are ANTIBIOTIC drugs that work by interfering with the
synthesis of bacterial cell walls. They are absorbed rapidly by most
(but not all) body tissues and fluids, perfuse through the kidneys, and
are excreted in the urine. One great disadvantage of penicillins is
that many patients are allergic to them − allergy to one means
allergy to them all − and may cause reactions that range from a
minor rash right up to anaphylactic shock, which may be fatal. Very
high dosage may rarely cause brain damage and convulsions, or may
cause abnormally high body levels of sodium or potassium, with
consequent symptoms. Best known and most used penicillins include
benzylpenicillin (penicillin G, the first of the penicillins),
phenoxymethylpenicillin (penicillin V), cloxacillin, flucloxacillin,
amoxycillin and ampicillin. Those taken orally may cause diarrhoea.

✚warning: *see* AMOXYCILLIN; AMPICILLIN; AZLOCILLIN; BACAMPICILLIN HYDROCHLORIDE; BENETHAMINE PENICILLIN; BENZATHINE PENICILLIN; BENZYLPENICILLIN; CARBENICILLIN; CARFECILLIN SODIUM; CICLACILLIN; CLOXACILLIN; FLUCLOXACILLIN; MECILLINAM; METHICILLIN SODIUM; MEZLOCILLIN; PHENETHICILLIN; PHENOXYMETHYLPENICILLIN; PIPERACILLIN; PIVAMPICILLIN; PIVMECILLINAM; PROCAINE PENICILLIN; TALAMPICILLIN HYDROCHLORIDE; TICARCILLIN.

Penidural (*Wyeth*) is a proprietary ANTIBIOTIC, available only on prescription, used to treat many forms of infection. Produced in the form of a suspension for dilution (the potency of the suspension once diluted is retained for 14 days), as drops for children, and in vials for injection (under the name Penidural-LA), Penidural is a preparation of benzathine penicillin.
▲/✚ side-effects/warning: *see* BENZATHINE PENICILLIN.

pentamidine is an ANTI-PROTOZOAL drug that is used to treat pneumonia caused by the protozoan micro-organism *Pneumocystis carinii* in patients whose immune system has been suppressed (either following transplant surgery or because of a condition such as AIDS). It is not ordinarily available in the United Kingdom.

pentazocine is a powerful narcotic ANALGESIC used to treat moderate to severe pain. Much like MORPHINE in effect and action, it is less likely to cause dependence. Administration is oral in the form of capsules or tablets, topical in the form of anal suppositories, or by injection. Treatment by injection has a stronger effect than oral treatment. The proprietary form is on the controlled drugs list.
▲side-effects: there is sedation and dizziness, with nausea; injection may lead to hallucinations. There is often also constipation. Tolerance and dependence (addiction) may result from prolonged treatment.
✚warning: pentazocine should not be administered to patients with high blood pressure (hypertension), heart failure, respiratory depression or head injury, who are taking any other narcotic analgesic, or have kidney or liver damage. Patients should be warned that hallucinations and other disturbances in thought and sensation may occur, especially following administration by injection.
Related article: FORTRAL.

peppermint oil is used to relieve the discomfort of abdominal colic and distension of severe indigestion or flatulence. It is thought to work by direct action on the smooth muscle of the intestinal walls. Administration is oral in the form of capsules.
▲side-effects: there may be heartburn and local irritation.
✚warning: peppermint oil should not be administered to patients who suffer from paralytic ileus or ulcerative colitis; a very few patients are allergic to it.
Related articles: COLPERMIN; TERCODA.

Periactin (*Merck, Sharp & Dohme*) is a proprietary non-prescription ANTIHISTAMINE, used both to treat the symptoms of allergic disorders

P

such as hay fever and as a tonic for stimulating appetite. Produced in the form of tablets and as a syrup for dilution (the potency of the syrup once diluted is retained for 14 days), Periactin is a preparation of cyproheptadine hydrochloride, and is not recommended for children aged under two years.

▲/✚ side-effects/warning: *see* CYPROHEPTADINE HYDROCHLORIDE.

Perifusin (*Merck*) is a proprietary fluid nutritional preparation, available only on prescription. Produced in the form of a solution for intravenous infusion into patients who cannot be fed via the alimentary canal because of conditions such as coma or prolonged disorders of the gastrointestinal tract, Perifusin is a preparation of amino acids with electrolytes.

Persantin (*Boehringer Ingelheim*) is a proprietary preparation of the drug dipyridamole, available only on prescription, used as an additional treatment with anticoagulants or aspirin in the prevention of thrombosis, especially during or following surgical procedure. It works by inhibiting the adhesiveness of blood platelets so that they stick neither to themselves nor to the walls of valves or tubes surgically inserted. The drug is produced in the form of tablets (in two strengths) and in ampoules for injection.

pertussis vaccine (or whooping cough VACCINE) is a suspension of dead pertussis bacteria (*Bordetella pertussis*) that is injected to cause the body's own defence mechanisms to form antibodies and thus provide immunity. It is available on prescription by itself, but it is most commonly administered as one element in the triple vaccination procedure involving diphtheria-pertussis-tetanus (DPT) vaccine. The vaccine remains the subject of some controversy over the number of children who may or may not have been brain-damaged by inoculation. It would in any case be extremely difficult to attribute such damage definitively to the use of the vaccine. It has been estimated that permanent brain damage might be expected to occur in 1 in 300,000 vaccinations. However, the likelihood of catching whooping cough and developing brain damage as a result is much higher. Furthermore, there is an occasional death associated with whooping cough. As is usual with the triple vaccination, administration is by a series of three injections.

✚ warning: in general, pertussis vaccine should not be administered to children who suffer a severe local or general reaction to the initial dose, or who have a history of brain damage at birth or of cerebral irritation or seizures. It should be administered with extreme caution to children whose first degree relatives have a history of seizures or who appear to have any form of neurological disorder.

see also DIPHTHERIA-PERTUSSIS-TETANUS (DPT) VACCINE.

pethidine is a narcotic ANALGESIC used primarily for the relief of moderate to severe pain. Its effect is rapid and short-lasting, so its sedative properties are made use of only as a premedication prior to surgery or to enhance the effects of other anaesthetics during or following surgery. Administration (as pethidine hydrochloride) is oral in the form of tablets, or by injection. Proprietary forms are on the controlled drugs list. Occasionally it is used in combination with chlorpromazine prior to painful procedures. The combination provides good pain relief and sedation because chlorpromazine potentiates the effect of pethidine (and other opiates).

▲ side-effects: shallow breathing, urinary retention, constipation and nausea are all fairly common; tolerance and dependence (addiction) are possible. There may also be drowsiness and pain at the site of injection.

✚ warning: pethidine should not be administered to patients with head injury or intracranial pressure; it should be administered with caution to those with impaired kidney or liver function, asthma, depressed respiration, insufficient secretion of thyroid hormones (hypothyroidism) or low blood pressure (hypotension). *Related article:* PETHILORFAN.

Pethilorfan (*Roche*) is a proprietary narcotic ANALGESIC that is on the controlled drugs list; it is used to treat moderate to severe pain, particularly in childbirth. Produced in ampoules for injection, Pethilorfan is a preparation of pethidine hydrochloride with the respiratory stimulant levallorphan tartrate.

▲/✚ side-effects/warning: *see* PETHIDINE.

Petrolagar (*Wyeth*) is a proprietary non-prescription LAXATIVE that is not available from the National Health Service. Produced in the form of a sugar-free emulsion, Petrolagar is a preparation of two forms of liquid paraffin.

Pevaryl (*Ortho-Cilag*) is a proprietary non-prescription ANTIFUNGAL drug, used in topical application to treat fungal infections on the skin such as nail infections, and particularly in the genital areas. Produced in the form of a cream, a lotion and a spray-powder in an aerosol unit, Pevaryl is a preparation of econazole nitrate.

▲/✚ side-effects/warning: ECONAZOLE NITRATE.

Phenergan (*May & Baker*) is a proprietary non-prescription ANTIHISTAMINE, used to treat the symptoms of allergies such as hay fever and for emergency treatment of reactions to drugs or injected substances. It is produced in the form of tablets (in two strengths), as an elixir for dilution (the potency of the elixir once diluted is retained for 14 days), neither of which is recommended for children aged under six months, and (only on prescription) in ampoules for injection, which is not recommended for children aged under five years. Phenergan is a preparation of promethazine hydrochloride. Under the name Phenergan Compound Expectorant, a compound linctus is also available, but not from the National Health Service, which consists of a preparation of promethazine hydrochloride and several LAXATIVE constituents; it too is not recommended for children aged under five years. Phenergan is occasionally used as a sedative in childhood.

▲/✚ side-effects/warning: *see* PROMETHAZINE HYDROCHLORIDE.

phenethicillin is a penicillin-type ANTIBIOTIC that is used both to treat bacterial infection and to prevent it. Administration (as a potassium salt) is oral in the form of capsules or a dilute syrup.

▲ side-effects: there may be sensitivity reactions ranging from a minor rash to urticaria and joint pains, diarrhoea and (occasionally) to high temperature or anaphylactic shock.

✚ warning: phenethicillin should not be administered to patients who are known to be allergic to penicillins; it should be administered with caution to those with impaired kidney function.
Related article: BROXIL.

phenindamine tartrate is an ANTIHISTAMINE used to treat the symptoms of allergic conditions such as hay fever and urticaria. It has only a mildly depressant action on the brain and so is less sedating than most antihistamines, and may in fact cause slight stimulation of the central nervous system. Administration is oral in the form of tablets.

▲ side-effects: concentration and speed of thought and movement may be affected; there may be nausea, headache, and/or weight gain, dry mouth, gastrointestinal disturbances and visual problems.

pheniramine maleate is an ANTIHISTAMINE used to treat the symptoms of allergic conditions such as hay fever and urticaria. Administration is oral in the form of tablets.

▲ side-effects: concentration and speed of thought and movement may be affected; there may be nausea, headache, and/or weight gain, dry mouth, gastrointestinal disturbances and visual problems.
Related article: DANERAL SA.

phenobarbitone is a powerful BARBITURATE, used as an ANTICONVULSANT in the prevention of recurrent epileptic seizures. Its use may cause behavioural disturbances (such as hyperactivity) in children. It is not used as commonly as it once was in older children, but it is still prescribed a great deal for fits in the newborn period. Blood level tests can be performed to optimize the dosage. Administration (as phenobarbitone or phenobarbitone sodium) is oral in the form of tablets and an elixir, or by injection. All proprietary preparations containing phenobarbitone are on the controlled drugs list.

▲ side-effects: there is drowsiness and lethargy; sometimes there is also depression, muscle weakness and/or sensitivity reactions in the form of skin rashes or blood disorders. Juvenile patients may experience psychological disturbance.

✚ warning: phenobarbitone should not be administered to patients with porphyria. It should be administered with caution to those with impaired kidney or liver function, or who have respiratory disorders. Withdrawal of treatment should be gradual.

phenol, or carbolic acid, is a very early DISINFECTANT still much used for the cleaning of wounds or inflammation (such as boils and abscesses), the maintenance of hygiene in the mouth, throat or ear, and as a preservative in injections. Administration is topical in solutions, lotions, creams and ointments.

✚warning: phenol is highly toxic if swallowed in concentrated form.

phenolphthalein is a LAXATIVE that works by irritating the intestinal walls. Its use is now rare because of an association with blood disorders that affect the composition of the urine, with sensitivity reactions, and with a duration of effect that may continue for several days as the chemical is recycled through the liver. Proprietary preparations that contain phenolphthalein all also contain either other forms of laxative or an antacid.
Related article: AGAROL.

phenothiazine derivatives (or phenothiazines) are a group of drugs that are chemically related but are not restricted to a single mode of activity. Many are ANTIPSYCHOTIC drugs, including some of the tranquillizers best known and most used – such as chlorpromazine, promazine, thioridazine, fluphenazine and trifluoperazine. Some of these are used also as ANTI-EMETICS. Others – such as piperazine – are ANTHELMINTICS.
▲/✚ side-effects/warning: *see* CHLORPROMAZINE; PIPERAZINE; PROCHLORPERAZINE.

phenoxymethylpenicillin, or penicillin V, is a widely-used ANTIBIOTIC, particularly effective in treating tonsillitis, infection of the middle ear, and some skin infections, and to prevent the onset of rheumatic fever. Administration (as a potassium salt sometimes called phenoxymethylpenicillin VK) is oral in the form of tablets or liquids.
▲ side-effects: there may be sensitivity reactions ranging from a minor rash to urticaria and joint pains, and (occasionally) to high temperature or anaphylactic shock.
✚warning: phenoxymethylpenicillin should not be administered to patients known to be allergic to penicillins; it should be administered with caution to those with impaired kidney function.
Related articles: APSIN VK; CRYSTAPEN V; DISTAQUAINE V-K; ECONOCIL VK; STABILLIN V-K; V-CIT-K.

phenylbutazone is an ANTI-INFLAMMATORY non-narcotic ANALGESIC which, because of its sometimes severe side-effects, is used solely in the treatment of progressive fusion of the synovial joints of the spine (ankylosing spondylitis) under medical supervision in hospitals. Even for that purpose, it is used only when other therapies have failed. Treatment then, however, may be prolonged. Administration is oral in the form of tablets.
▲ side-effects: there may be gastrointestinal disturbances, nausea, vomiting, and allergic reactions such as a rash. Less often, there is inflammation of the glands of the mouth, throat and neck; pancreatitis, nephritis or hepatitis; or headache and visual disturbances. Rarely, there is severe fluid retention (which may eventually in susceptible patients precipitate heart failure) or serious and potentially dangerous blood disorders.
✚warning: phenylbutazone should not be administered to patients with cardiovascular disease, thyroid disease, or inpaired liver or

kidney function; who are pregnant; or who have a history of stomach or intestinal haemorrhaging.
Related articles: BUTACOTE; BUTAZOLIDIN; BUTAZONE.

phenylephrine is a VASOCONSTRICTOR and a SYMPATHOMIMETIC drug. It is sometimes used in the form of a spray or drops to clear nasal congestion; as eye-drops to dilate the pupil and facilitate ophthalmic examination; or as a constituent in some proprietary preparations produced to treat bronchospasm in conditions such as asthma.
▲ side-effects: topical application may promote the appearance of a form of dermatitis. As nasal drops or spray, excessive use may lead to tolerance and worse congestion than previously.
✚ warning: phenylephrine should not be administered to patients with severe hypertension (high blood pressure), or from overactivity of the thyroid gland (hyperthyroidism).
Related articles: BETNOVATE; BRONCHODILATOR; DIMOTANE EXPECTORANT; DIMOTAPP; DUO-AUTOHALER; HAYPHRYN; MEDIHALER-DUO; MINIMS; SOFRAMYCIN.

phenytoin is an ANTICONVULSANT drug that is also an ANTI-ARRHYTHMIC. It is consequently used both to treat the severer forms of epilepsy (not including petit mal), and to regularize the heartbeat (especially following the administration of a heart stimulant). Administration (as phenytoin or phenytoin sodium) is oral in the form of tablets, chewable tablets, capsules and a suspension, or by injection.
▲ side-effects: the skin and facial features may coarsen during prolonged treatment; there may also be acne, enlargement of the gums, and/or growth of excess hair. Some patients enter a state of confusion. Nausea and vomiting, headache, blurred vision, blood disorders and insomnia may occur.
✚ warning: monitoring of concentration of the drug in the blood plasma is preferable in the initial treatment of epilepsy in order to establish an optimum dosage. Withdrawal should be gradual. Drug interactions are common.
Related articles: EPANUTIN; EPANUTIN READY MIXED PARENTERAL.

pHiso-Med (*Winthrop*) is a proprietary non-prescription DISINFECTANT used as a soap or shampoo substitute in acne and seborrhoeic conditions, for bathing mothers and babies in maternity units to prevent cross infection, and for pre-operative hand and skin cleansing. Produced in the form of a solution, pHiso-Med is a preparation of chlorhexidine gluconate.
✚ warning: sensitivity may occur.

pholcodine is an OPIATE that is used as an ANTITUSSIVE constituent in cough linctuses or syrups. Although its action on the cough centre of the brain resembles that of other opiates, it has no ANALGESIC effect.
▲ side-effects: there is commonly constipation. High or prolonged dosage may lead to respiratory depression.
Related articles: EXPULIN; GALENPHOL; PAVACOL-D; PHOLCOMED.

Pholcomed (*Medo*) is a proprietary brand of ANTITUSSIVES used to treat an irritable and unproductive cough. Produced in the form of a

sugar-free linctus for use by diabetics (in two strengths, under the names Pholcomed-D and Pholcomed Forte Diabetic) (only Pholcomed D is available from the National Health Service), Pholcomed is a compound of the ANTITUSSIVE pholcodine and the MUSCLE RELAXANT papaverine hydrochloride, both of which are OPIATES. The Forte linctuses are not recommended for children.
▲/✚ side-effects/warning: *see* PHOLCODINE.

Pholcomed Expectorant (*Medo*) is a proprietary non-prescription ANTITUSSIVE, not available from the National Health Service, being a compound preparation of the EXPECTORANT guaiphenesin and the SYMPATHOMIMETIC methylephedrine hydrochloride.

Phosphate-Sandoz (*Sandoz*) is a proprietary non-prescription phosphate supplement, which may be required in addition to vitamin D in patients with vitamin D-resistant rickets. Produced in the form of tablets, Phosphate-Sandoz is a preparation of sodium acid phosphate, sodium bicarbonate and potassium bicarbonate.

Phyllocontin Continus (*Napp*) is a proprietary non-prescription BRONCHODILATOR, used to treat asthma. Produced in the form of sustained-release tablets (in three strengths, the weakest labelled for children, the strongest labelled Forte), Phyllocontin Continus is a preparation of aminophylline. The two stronger forms of tablets are not recommended for children, and the paediatric tablets are not recommended for children aged under 12 months.
▲/✚ side-effects/warning: *see* AMINOPHYLLINE.

Physeptone (*Calmic*) is a proprietary narcotic ANALGESIC that is on the controlled drugs list. Used to treat severe pain, and produced in the form of tablets and in ampoules for injection, Physeptone is a preparation of the OPIATE methadone hydrochloride.
▲/✚ side-effects/warning: *see* METHADONE.

physostigmine is a vegetable alkaloid (derived from calabar beans) used in dilute solution in the form of eye-drops to treat glaucoma or to contract the pupil of the eye after it has been dilated through the use of ANTICHOLINERGICS such as ATROPINE for the purpose of ophthalmic examination. It works by improving drainage in the tiny channels of the eye processes. It is, however, potentially irritant, causing gastrointestinal disturbance and excessive salivation if absorbed, and is most commonly used in combination with other drugs, particularly PILOCARPINE.

Phytex (*Pharmax*) is a proprietary non-prescription ANTIFUNGAL drug, used to treat fungal infections in the skin and nails. Produced in the form of a paint for topical application, Phytex is a preparation of various natural acids, including salicylic acid, together with methyl salicylate.
▲/✚ side-effects/warning: Hypersensitivity reactions may occur.

Phytocil (*Radiol*) is a proprietary non-prescription ANTIFUNGAL drug, used in topical application, to treat skin infections, especially

P

athlete's foot. Produced in the form of a cream, and a powder in a sprinkler tin, Phytocil is a compound preparation that includes several minor antifungal constituents, including salicylic acid.
▲/✚ side-effects/warning: Hypersensitivity may occur.

phytomenadione is the technical term for vitamin K, a fat-soluble vitamin essential to the production of clotting factors in the blood, and to the metabolism of the proteins necessary for the calcification of bone. Good food sources include vegetable oils, liver, pork meat and green vegetables. Therapeutically, phytomenadione is administered to make up deficiency – especially in newborn babies whose intestines have not had time to obtain the normal bacterial agents that synthesize the vitamin. Administration is oral in the form of tablets, or by intramuscular injection.
Related articles: KONAKION; VITLIPID.

Picolax (*Nordic*) is a proprietary non-prescription LAXATIVE produced in the form of a sugar-free powder for solution. Picolax is a preparation of the stimulant laxative sodium picosulphate and the ANTACID laxative magnesium citrate.
▲/✚ side-effects/warning: *see* SODIUM PICOSULPHATE.

pilocarpine is a parasympathomimetic drug used in dilute solution in the form of eye-drops to treat glaucoma or to contract the pupil of the eye after it has been dilated for the purpose of ophthalmic examination. It works by improving drainage in the channels of the eye processes. It is, however, potentially irritant, causing eyeache and blurred vision, and even gastrointestinal disturbance and excessive salivation is absorbed. As pilocarpine hydrochloride or pilocarpine nitrate, it is commonly used in combination with other drugs, particularly PHYSOSTIGMINE.
Related articles: ISOPTO; MINIMS.

piperacillin is a broad-spectrum penicillin-type ANTIBIOTIC, used to treat many serious or compound forms of bacterial infection, and to prevent infection during or following surgery. Administration is by injection or infusion.
▲ side-effects: there may be sensitivity reactions ranging from a minor rash to urticaria and joint pains, and (occasionally) to high temperature or anaphylactic shock.
✚ warning: piperacillin should not be administered to patients known to be allergic to penicillins; it should be administered with caution to those with impaired kidney function.
Related article: PIPRIL.

piperazine is an ANTHELMINTIC drug, one of the PHENOTHIAZINE derivatives, used to treat infestation by roundworms or threadworms. Treatment should take no longer than seven days; in the treatment of some species a single dose is sufficient. Administration (as piperazine citrate, piperazine hydrate or piperazine phosphate) is oral in the form of tablets, a syrup or a dilute elixir.

▲ side-effects: there may be nausea and vomiting, with diarrhoea; there may also be urticaria. Rarely, there is dizziness and lack of muscular co-ordination.

✚ warning: piperazine should not be administered to patients with liver disease or epilepsy; it should be administered with caution to those with impaired kidney function, neurological disease or psychiatric disorders.

Related articles: ANTEPAR; ASCALIX; PRIPSEN.

Pipril (*Lederle*) is a proprietary broad-spectrum penicillin-type ANTIBIOTIC, available only on prescription, used to treat many serious or compound forms of bacterial infection, and to prevent infection during or following surgery. Produced in the form of a powder in vials (in two strengths) and in an infusion bottle, Pipril is a preparation of piperacillin.

▲/✚ side-effects/warning: *see* PIPERACILLIN.

pirbuterol is a BRONCHODILATOR of the type known as a selective BETA-RECEPTOR STIMULANT, used to treat asthmatic broncho-spasm. It has fewer cardiac side-effects than some others of its type, and is administered orally in the form of capsules, as a syrup or by aerosol inhalation.

▲ side-effects: there may be headache and nervous tension, associated with tingling of the fingertips and a fine tremor of the muscles of the hands. Administration other than by inhalation may cause an increase in the heart rate.

Related article: EXIREL.

Piriton (*Allen & Hanburys*) is a proprietary non-prescription preparation of the ANTIHISTAMINE chlorpheniramine maleate, used to treat allergic conditions such as hay fever and urticaria. It is produced in the form of tablets, as sustained-release tablets ("spandets", not recommended for children), and as a syrup for dilution (the potency of the syrup once diluted is retained for 14 days); it is also produced in ampoules for injection, but in that form is only available on prescription.

▲/✚ side-effects/warning: *see* CHLORPHENIRAMINE.

Pitressin (*Parke-Davis Medical*) is a proprietary preparation of the HORMONE argipressin, which is a synthetic version of vasopressin. Available only on prescription, it is administered primarily to diagnose or to treat pituitary-originated diabetes insipidus, and to treat the haemorrhaging of varicose veins in the oesophagus (the tubular channel for food between throat and stomach). Produced in ampoules for injection (generally in hospitals only).

▲/✚ side-effects/warning: *see* VASOPRESSIN.

pivampicillin is a more active form of the ANTIBIOTIC ampicillin that is converted in the body to ampicillin after absorption. It has similar actions and uses.

▲/✚ side-effects/warning: *see* AMPICILLIN.

Related articles: MIRAXID; PONDOCILLIN.

pivmecillinam hydrochloride is a form of the ANTIBIOTIC mecillinam that can be taken orally. It has similar actions and uses.
▲/✚ side-effects/warning: *see* MECILLINAM.
Related articles: MIRAXID; SELEXID.

pizotifen is an ANTIHISTAMINE structurally related to TRICYCLIC antidepressant drugs. It is used to treat and prevent headaches, particularly those in which blood pressure inside the blood vessels plays a part − such as migraine. Administration is oral in the form of tablets and an elixir.
▲ side-effects: concentration and speed of thought and movement may be affected. There may be drowsiness, dry mouth and blurred vision, with constipation and difficulty in urinating; sometimes there is muscle pain and/or nausea. Patients may put on weight.
✚ warning: pizotifen should not be administered to patients with closed-angle glaucoma or urinary retention.
Related article: SANOMIGRAN.

PK Aid 1 (*Scientific Hospital Supplies*) is a proprietary non-prescription nutritional supplement for patients who suffer from amino acid abnormalities (such as phenylketonuria). It contains essential and non-essential amino acids − except phenylalanine.

Plaquenil (*Sterling Research*) is a proprietary ANTI-INFLAMMATORY drug, available only on prescription, used primarily to treat rheumatoid arthritis and forms of the skin disease lupus erthematosus. Treatment of rheumatoid arthritis may take up to six months to achieve full effect. The drug is also used in the prevention and treatment of malaria. Produced in the form of tablets, Plaquenil is a preparation of hydroxychloroquine sulphate.

Plasma-Lyte (*Travenol*) is the name of a selection of proprietary infusion fluids for the intravenous nutrition of a patient in whom feeding via the alimentary tract is not possible. All contain glucose in the form of dextrose, and water.

Platosin (*Nordic*) is a proprietary CYTOTOXIC drug, available only on prescription, used to treat certain solid tumours. It works by damaging the DNA of newly forming cells and is especially used to treat cancers that are metastatic and have failed to respond to other forms of therapy. Produced in the form of a powder in vials (in three strengths) for injection, and as a powder for reconstitution as a medium for injection, Platosin is a preparation of the drug cisplatin.
▲/✚ side-effects/warning: *see* CISPLATIN.

Plesmet (*Napp*) is a proprietary non-prescription preparation of ferrous glycine sulphate, used as an IRON supplement in the treatment of iron-deficiency anaemia, and produced in the form of a syrup for dilution (the potency of the syrup once diluted is retained for 14 days).
▲/✚ side-effects/warning: *see* FERROUS GLYCINE SULPHATE.

Puserix MMR is a preparation of measles, mumps and rubella VACCINE, and is given in the second year of life.

pneumococcal vaccine is a VACCINE that provides protection against the organism *Pneumococcus*. It consists of a suspension of polysaccharides from a number of capsular types of pneumococci, administered by subcutaneous or intramuscular injection. Like the influenza vaccine, it is intended really only for those people at risk from infection in a community – e.g. children who have had their spleens removed or who have sickle cell disease. Immunity is reckoned to last for about five years.
➕warning: vaccination should not be given to patients who are aged under two years, who have any form of infection, or who are pregnant. It should be administered with caution to those with cardiovascular or respiratory disease. Some patients experience sensitivity reactions, which may be serious. Although protection may last for only five years, revaccination should be avoided because of the risk of adverse reactions.

Pneumovax (*Morson*) is a proprietary form of the pneumococcal vaccine, available only on prescription for the immunization of people for whom the risk of pneumococcal infection is unusually high.
➕warning: see PNEUMOCOCCAL VACCINE.

podophyllin is a non-proprietary compound paint for the topical treatment of varrucas (plantar warts) and warts in the ano-genital region. It is a solute preparation of podophyllum resin, a highly acidic substance.
▲side-effects: application may cause pain (because of the acidity).
➕warning: the paint should not be used on the face. The maximum duration for paint to remain on the skin is six hours: it should then be washed off. Avoid areas of normal skin. Do not attempt to treat a large number or a whole area of warts at any one time: the highly acidic drug may be absorbed.
Related article: POSALFILIN.

podophyllum resin is the highly acidic substance from which podophyllin compound paint is derived. The resin is also a constituent of a proprietary laxative.
▲/➕ side-effects/warning: *see* PODOPHYLLIN.

Point-Two (*Hoyt*) is a proprietary non-prescription form of fluoride supplement for administration in areas where the water supply is not fluoridated, especially to growing children. Produced in the form of a mouth-wash, Point-Two is a preparation of SODIUM FLUORIDE.

poliomyelitis vaccine is a VACCINE available in two types. Poliomyelitis vaccine, inactivated, is a suspension of dead viruses injected into the body for the body to generate antibodies and so become immune. Poliomyelitis vaccine, live, is a suspension of live but attenuated polio viruses (of polio virus types 1, 2 and 3) for oral administration. In the United Kingdom, the live vaccine is the medium of choice, and the administration is generally simultaneous with the administration of the diphtheria-pertussis-tetanus (DPT) vaccine – three times during the first year of life, and a booster

P

at school entry age. The inactivated vaccine remains available for patients for whom there are contra-indications to the use of the live vaccine.

✚warning: poliomyelitis vaccine should not be administered to patients known to have immunodeficiency disorders, who have diarrhoea or cancer, where there is infection.

pol/vac (inact) is an abbreviation for poliomyelitis vaccine, inactivated.
see POLIOMYELITIS VACCINE.

pol/vac (oral) is an abbreviation for poliomyelitis vaccine, live (oral).
see POLIOMYELITIS VACCINE.

P

Polybactrin (*Calmic*) is a proprietary antibiotic, available only on prescription, used either as a powder for reconstitution as a solution for bladder irrigation to prevent bladder and urethral infections, or in the form of a powder spray as a topical treatment for minor burns and wounds. In each case, active constituents are polymyxin B sulphate, neomycin sulphate and bacitracin.

Polycal (*Cow & Gate*) is a proprietary non-prescription nutritional supplement for patients with renal failure, liver cirrhosis, disorders of amino acid metabolism and protein intolerance, and who require a high-energy diet. Produced in the form of a powder for solution, Polycal contains glucose, maltose and polysaccharides.

Polycose (*Abbott*) is a proprietary non-prescription nutritional supplement for patients with renal failure, liver cirrhosis, disorders of amino acid metabolism and protein intolerance, and who require a high-energy, low-fluid diet. Produced in the form of a powder for solution, Polycose contains glucose polymers.

Polyfax (*Calmic*) is a proprietary ANTIBIOTIC drug, available only on prescription, used in topical application to treat infections in the skin and the eye. Produced in the form of an ointment in a paraffin base, and as an eye ointment, Polyfax is a preparation of polymyxin B sulphate and bacitracin zinc.
▲/✚ side-effects/warning: *see* POLYMYXIN B.

polygeline is a special refined, partly degraded, form of the hydrolized animal protein gelatin, used in infusion with saline (sodium chloride) as a means of expanding overall blood volume in patients whose blood volume is dangerously low through shock, particularly in cases of severe burns or septicaemia.
▲ side-effects: rarely, there are hypersensitive reactions.
✚warning: polygeline should not be administered to patients with congestive heart failure, severely impaired kidney function, or certain blood disorders; ideally, blood samples for cross-matching should be taken before administration.

polymyxin B is an ANTIBIOTIC used to treat several forms of bacterial infection. Its use would be more popular were it not so toxic. Because of its toxicity, administration (as polymyxin B sulphate) virtually always has to be topical in the form of solutions (as in eye-drops and ear-drops) or ointments.
▲ side-effects: there may be numbness and tingling in the limbs, blood and protein in the urine, dizziness, breathlessness and overall weakness.
✚ warning: polymyxin B should not be administered to patients with the neuromuscular disease myasthenia gravis; it should be administered with caution to those with impaired kidney function.
Related articles: AEROSPORIN; GREGODERM; MAXITROL; NEOSPORIN; OTOSPORIN; POLYBACTRIN; POLYFAX; POLYTRIM; TERRA-CORTRIL; TRIBIOTIC.

polysaccharide-iron complex is an IRON-rich compound used to restore iron to the blood (where it forms part of haemoglobin) in cases of iron-deficiency anaemia. Once a patient's blood haemoglobin level has reached normal, treatment should nevertheless continue for at least three months to replenish fully the reserves of iron in the body.
▲ side-effects: large doses may cause gastrointestinal upset and diarrhoea; there may be vomiting. Prolonged treatment may result in constipation.
✚ warning: polysaccharide-iron complex should not be administered to patients already taking tetracycline antibiotics.
Related article: NIFEREX.

polystyrene sulphonate resins are used to treat excessively high levels of potassium in the blood, as may occur in renal failure. Administration is oral as a solution, or topical in the form of a retention enema (to be retained for as long as nine hours, if possible). Adequate fluid intake during oral treatment is essential, to prevent impaction of the resins.
▲ side-effects: some patients treated by enema experience rectal ulcers.
✚ warning: resins that contain calcium should be avoided in patients with metastatic cancer or abnormal secretion by the parathyroid glands. Resins that contain sodium should be avoided by patients with congestive heart failure or impaired kidney function.
Related articles: CALCIUM RESONIUM; RESONIUM A.

Polytar Emollient (*Stiefel*) is a proprietary non-prescription brand of preparations used to treat non-infective skin inflammations, including psoriasis and eczema. The standard form is produced as a bath additive, and is a preparation of ANTISEPTICS and natural oils including COAL TAR and ARACHIS OIL. An alcohol-based shampoo is also available (under the name Polytar Liquid), as is a gelatin-based shampoo (under the name Polytar Plus Liquid).

Polytrim (*Wellcome*) is a proprietary ANTIBIOTIC, available only on prescription, used in the form of eye-drops to treat bacterial infections

233

in the eye. Polytrim is a preparation of the drugs trimethoprim and polymyxin B sulphate.
▲/✚ side-effects/warning: *see* POLYMYXIN B; TRIMETHOPRIM.

polyvinyl alcohol is used as a surfactant tear-distributor, administered in the form of eye-drops to patients whose lachrymal apparatus is dysfunctioning. It works by helping the aqueous layer provided by the lachrymal apparatus (tear fluid) to spread across an eyeball on which the normal mucous surface is patchy or missing.
Related articles: HYPOTEARS; LIQUIFILM TEARS; SNO TEARS.

Pondocillin (*Burgess*) is a proprietary ANTIBIOTIC, available only on prescription, used to treat systemic bacterial infections and infections of the upper respiratory tract, of the ear, nose and throat, and of the urinary tracts. Produced in the form of tablets, as a sugar-free suspension, and as granules in sachets, Pondocillin is a preparation of the broad-spectrum PENICILLIN pivampicillin.
▲/✚ side-effects/warning: *see* PIVAMPICILLIN.

Ponstan (*Parke-Davis*) is a proprietary ANTI-INFLAMMATORY non-narcotic ANALGESIC, available only on prescription, used to treat pain in rheumatoid arthritis, osteoarthritis and other musculo-skeletal disorders. Produced in the form of capsules, as tablets, as soluble (dispersible) tablets (under the name Ponstan Dispersible), and as a children's suspension for dilution (the potency of the suspension once diluted is retained for 14 days), Ponstan is a preparation of mefenamic acid. None of these products is recommended for children aged under six months.
▲/✚ side-effects/warning: *see* MEFENAMIC ACID.

Portagen (*Bristol-Myers*) is a proprietary non-prescription milk substitute used to treat patients whose metabolisms have difficulty in absorbing fats and are unable to tolerate lactose, such as in liver cirrhosis and after surgery of the intestine. Portagen is a preparation of proteins, glycerides, sucrose, vitamins and minerals, and is glucose- and lactose-free.

Posalfilin (*Norgine*) is a proprietary non-prescription compound ointment for topical application, intended to treat and remove anogenital warts and varrucas (plantar warts). Posalfilin is a preparation of the KERATOLYTIC salicylic acid and the highly acidic substance podophyllum resin. It should not be used for facial warts.
▲/✚ side-effects/warning: *see* SALICYLIC ACID.

potassium is a metallic element that occurs naturally only in compounds. In the body, a highly sensitive balance is maintained between potassium within the cells and sodium in the fluids outside the cells (although chemically the two elements are very similar). Nerve impulses are transmitted by means of an almost instantaneous transference of potassium and sodium across cell membranes that sets up a momentary electric current. Deficiency or excess of potassium thus interferes with the actions of most nerves, and particularly those of the heart. Fluid loss from the body results in potassium loss – and therapeutically most potassium is administered to make up such losses, especially following the use of some potassium-depleting drugs (such as the THIAZIDE DIURETICS or CORTICOSTEROIDS).

potassium chloride is used primarily as a POTASSIUM supplement to treat conditions of potassium deficiency, especially during or following severe loss of body fluids or treatment with drugs that deplete body reserves. Administration of potassium chloride is oral, or by injection or infusion.
Related articles: BURINEX-K; CENTYL-K; DEXTROLYTE; DIARREST; DIORALYTE; ELECTROSOL; KLOREF; LASIX; LEO-K; MICRO-K; REHIDRAT; RUTHIMOL; SANDO-K; SLOW-K.

potassium citrate administered orally has the effect of making the urine alkaline instead of acid. This is of use in relieving pain in some infections of the urinary tract or the bladder. Administration is in the form of tablets or a non-proprietary liquid mixture.
▲side-effects: there may be mild diuresis. Prolonged high dosage may lead to excessively high levels of potassium in the blood.
✚warning: potassium citrate should be administered with caution to patients with heart disease or impaired kidney function.

potassium hydroxyquinoline sulphate is a drug that has both ANTIBACTERIAL and ANTIFUNGAL properties. It is used mostly as a constituent in anti-inflammatory and antibiotic creams and ointments that also contain corticosteroids, used to treat skin disorders. Rarely, it causes sensitivity reactions.
Related articles: QUINOCORT; QUINODERM; QUINOPED.

potassium permanganate is a general DISINFECTANT used in solution for cleaning burns and abrasions and maintaining asepsis in wounds that are suppurating or weeping.
✚warning: avoid splashing mucous membranes, to which it is an irritant. It also stains skin and fabric.

povidone-iodine is a complex of iodine on an organic carrier, used as an ANTISEPTIC in topical application to the skin and as a mouth wash. Produced in the form of a gel and a solution, it works by slowly releasing the iodine it contains.
▲side-effects: rarely, there may be sensitivity reactions.
Related articles: BETADINE; DISADINE DP; VIDENE.

Pragmatar (*Bioglan*) is a proprietary non-prescription ointment used in topical application to treat chronic eczema and psoriasis. It is a preparation of various mildly KERATOLYTIC and antibiotic agents including SALICYLIC ACID in a water-miscible base.

pralidoxime mesylate is an unusual drug that is used virtually solely in combination with the belladonna alkaloid ATROPINE in the treatment of severe poisoning by organophosphoric compounds (such as those used as insecticides). The drug is particularly effective in

P

reversing the dangerous muscular paralysis that may affect the entire body. Diagnosis is critical, in that the use of atropine and pralidoxime mesylate to treat poisoning by other compounds used as insecticides may have no effect whatever and can be dangerous. Administration is by injection; repeated doses may be required.

▲ side-effects: there is drowsiness, dizziness and visual disturbances, muscular weakness, nausea and headache, and rapid heart and breathing rate.

✚ warning: pralidoxime mesylate should be administered with caution to patients with the neuromuscular disease myasthenia gravis, or impaired kidney function.

Precortisyl (*Roussel*) is a proprietary CORTICOSTEROID preparation, available only on prescription, used to treat inflammation, especially in allergic conditions. It may also be used for systemic corticosteroid therapy. Produced in the form of tablets (in three strengths, the strongest under the name Precortisyl Forte), its active ingredient is the glucocorticoid steroid prednisolone. It is not recommended for children aged under 12 months.

▲/✚ side-effects/warning: *see* PREDNISOLONE.

Pred Forte (*Allergan*) is a porprietary CORTICOSTEROID preparation available only on prescription, used either to treat non-infected inflammatory ear and eye conditions. Produced in the form of eye-drops. Pred Forte is a preparation of prednisolone acetate.

▲/✚ side-effects/warning: *see* PREDNISOLONE.

Prednesol (*Glaxo*) is a proprietary CORTICOSTEROID preparation, available only on prescription, used to treat inflammation, especially in allergic conditions. It may also be used for systemic corticosteroid therapy. Produced in the form of tablets, its active ingredient is the glucocorticoid steroid prednisolone disodium phosphate. It is not recommended for children aged under 12 months.

▲/✚ side-effects/warning: *see* PREDNISOLONE.

prednisolone is a synthetic CORTICOSTEROID, a glucocorticoid used to treat inflammation, especially in allergic conditions. It may also be used for systemic corticosteroid therapy in many conditions, such as asthma. It is used in the nephrotic syndrome (a disease of the kidneys in which protein leaks into the urine) and in such conditions as ulcerative colitis. Administration (as prednisolone, prednisolone acetate, prednisolone sodium phosphate or prednisolone steaglate) is oral in the form of tablets, or topical in the form of creams, lotions and ointments, as anal suppositories and a retention enema, or by injection.

✚ warning: withdrawal of treatment must be gradual if the patient has had a prolonged course.

▲ side-effects: treatment of susceptible patients may engender a euphoria, or a state of confusion or depression. Rarely, there is peptic ulcer. Stunting of growth may occur if a long course of treatment is given. Significant weight gain may occur together

with the development of a moon-shaped face – these effects are reversible on stopping the treatment.
Related articles: DELTACORTRIL; DELTALONE; DELTA-PHORICOL; DELTASTAB; MINIMS; PRECORTISYL; PREDNESOL; PREDSOL; SINTISONE.

prednisone is a synthetic CORTICOSTEROID that is converted in the body to the glucocorticoid PREDNISOLONE, and is used to treat inflammation especially in allergic conditions (particularly those affecting the bronchial passages). Administration is oral in the form of tablets.
▲/✚ side-effects/warning: *see* PREDNISOLONE.
   Related articles: DECORTISYL; ECONOSONE.

Predsol (*Glaxo*) is a proprietary CORTICOSTEROID preparation, available only on prescription, used either to treat ulcerative colitis and inflammations of the rectum and anus, especially in Crohn's disease, or to treat non-infected inflammatory ear and eye conditions.
Produced in the form of a retention enema and anal suppositories, and as ear- or eye-drops, Predsol is a preparation of the glucocorticoid prednisolone sodium phosphate. Ear- and eye-drops that additionally contain the antibiotic neomycin sulphate are also available (under the name Predsol-N).
▲/✚ side-effects/warning: *see* NEOMYCIN; PREDNISOLONE.

Preferid (*Brocades*) is a proprietary CORTICOSTEROID, available only on prescription and used to treat severe non-infective skin inflammations such as eczema. Produced in the form of a water-miscible cream or as an ointment in a paraffin base. Preferid is a preparation of the steroid budesonide.
▲/✚ side-effects/warning: *see* BUDESONIDE.

Pregestimil (*Bristol-Myers*) is a proprietary non-prescription nutritionally complete milk substitute used by patients whose metabolisms are unable to tolerate cows' milk, sucrose or lactose, and who in addition have difficulty in absorbing fats following surgery of the intestine. Produced in the form of a powder, Pregestimil is a preparation of glucose, the milk fat casein, cornoil, modified starch, vitamins and minerals, and is gluten-, sucrose- and lactose-free.

prilocaine is primarily a local ANAESTHETIC, the drug of choice for very many topical or minor surgical procedures, especially in dentistry (because it is absorbed directly through mucous membranes). Administration is (in the form of a solution of prilocaine hydrochloride) by injection or topically as a cream.
✚ warning: prilocaine should not be administered to patients with the neural disease myasthenia gravis; it should be administered with caution to those with heart or liver failure (in order not to cause depression of the central nervous system and convulsions), or from epilepsy. Full facilities for emergency cardio-respiratory resuscitation should be on hand during anaesthetic treatment.
Related article: EMLA.

primaquine is an ANTIMALARIAL drug used to administer the coup de grace to benign tertian forms of malaria following initial treatment with the powerful drugs CHLOROQUINE and/or amodiaquine. Administration is oral in the form of tablets.

▲ side-effects: there may be nausea and vomiting, anorexia and jaundice. Rarely, there are blood disorders or depression of the bone-marrow's capacity for forming new blood cells.

✚ warning: a blood count is essential before administration to check that a patient has sufficient blood levels of a specific enzyme, without which the presence of the drug may cause blood disorders. Primaquine should be administered with caution to patients who are pregnant.

primidone is an ANTICONVULSANT drug used in the treatment of all forms of epilepsy (except absence seizures). It is converted in the body to the BARBITURATE phenobarbitone, and its actions and effects are thus identical to those of that drug. It is not commonly used nowadays.

▲/✚ side-effects/warning: *see* PHENOBARBITONE.
Related article: MYSOLINE.

Primperan (*Berk*) is a proprietary ANTINAUSEANT, available only on prescription, used to treat nausea and vomiting, especially in gastrointestinal disorders, during treatment for cancer with cytotoxic drugs or radiotherapy, or in association with migraine. Produced in the form of tablets, as a sugar-free syrup for dilution (the potency of the syrup once diluted is retained for 14 days) and in ampoules for injection, Primperan is a preparation of metoclopramide hydrochloride. It is not recommended for children aged under five years.

▲/✚ side-effects/warning: *see* METOCLOPRAMIDE.

Prioderm (*Napp*) is a proprietary non-prescription drug used to treat infestations of the scalp and pubic hair by lice (pediculosis), or of the skin by the itch-mite (scabies). Produced in the form of a lotion in an alcohol base, and as a cream shampoo, Prioderm is a preparation of the insecticide malathion.

▲/✚ side-effects/warning: *see* MALATHION.

Pripsen (*Reckitt & Colman*) is a proprietary non-prescription ANTHELMINTIC, used to treat infections by threadworm and roundworm. Produced in the form of an oral powder, Pripsen is a preparation of the phenothiazine derivative piperazine phosphate with various stimulant LAXATIVES, and is not recommended for children aged under three months.

▲/✚ side-effects/warning: *see* PIPERAZINE.

Pro-Banthine (*Gold Cross*) is a proprietary ANTICHOLINERGIC antispasmodic drug, available only on prescription, used to assist in the treatment of gastrointestinal disorders arising from muscular spasm of the intestinal walls. It is also sometimes used to treat children for bedwetting or who wet during the day because they have

irritable bladders. Produced in the form of tablets, Pro-Banthine is a preparation of propantheline bromide.
▲/✚ side-effects/warning: *see* PROPANTHELINE BROMIDE.

procaine is a local ANAESTHETIC that is now seldom used. Once popular, it has been overtaken by anaesthetics that are longer-lasting and better absorbed through mucous membranes. Because of this poor absorption it cannot be used as a surface anaesthetic. It remains available, however, and may be used for regional anaesthesia or by infiltration, usually in combination with adrenaline. Administration (as procaine hydrochloride) is by injection.
▲ side-effects: rarely, there are sensitivity reactions − which may be serious.
✚ warning: the metabolite of procaine inhibits the action on the body of sulphonamide drugs.

procaine penicillin is a penicillin-type ANTIBIOTIC that is a derivative of benzylpenicillin. It is primarily used in long-lasting (depot) injections. Administration is by intramuscular injection.
▲/✚ side-effects/warning: *see* BENZYLPENICILLIN.

prochlorperazine is a phenothiazine derivative used as an ANTIPSYCHOTIC drug in the treatment of psychosis (such as schizophrenia); as an ANXIOLYTIC in the short term treatment of anxiety; and as an ANTI-EMETIC in the prevention of nausea caused by gastrointestinal disorder, by chemotherapy and radiotherapy in the treatment of cancer, by motion within a vehicle, or by the vertigo that results from infection of the middle or inner ear. Administration (as prochlorpromazine maleate or prochlorpromazine mesylate) is oral in the form of tablets, sustained-release capsules and syrups, topical in the form of anal suppositories, or by injection.
▲ side-effects: concentration and speed of thought and movement may be affected. High doses may cause neuromuscular disorders, especially in children. This side-effect can sometimes be alarming and therefore the medication should not be used unnecessarily in childhood.
Related articles: STEMETIL; VERTIGON.

Proctofibe (*Roussel*) is a proprietary non-prescription LAXATIVE that is not available from the National Health Service. A bulking agent − which works by increasing the overall mass of faeces within the rectum, so stimulating bowel movement − Proctofibe is a preparation of grain fibre and citrus fibre. Produced in the form of tablets, it is not recommended for children aged under three years, and counselling is advised before use.

proflavine cream is a non-proprietary formulation that includes beeswax, wool fat, liquid paraffin and some mild antibacterial agents; it is used in topical application as a dressing for minor skin infections, burns and abrasions.
✚ warning: wool fat causes sensitivity reactions in some patients.

proguanil is an ANTIMALARIAL drug used to try to prevent the contraction of malaria by travellers in tropical countries. Its effectiveness is not guaranteed, and the traveller is advised to take measures as far as possible to avoid being bitten by mosquitoes. Administration (as proguanil hydrochloride) is oral in the form of tablets.

▲ side-effects: there may be mild gastric disorder.

✚ warning: proguanil should be administered with caution to patients who suffer from impaired kidney function.

Related article: PALUDRINE.

promethazine hydrochloride is a powerful ANTIHISTAMINE that also has HYPNOTIC and ANTITUSSIVE properties. Consequently, although it is used to treat the symptoms of allergic conditions (such as hay fever and urticaria, but additionally including the emergency treatment of anaphylactic shock), it is used also to induce sleep in the treatment of insomnia or as a premedication prior to surgery, and as a cough suppressant in cough linctuses. It may also be used as an ANTI-EMETIC in the prevention of nausea due to motion sickness or to ear infection. Its effect is comparatively long-lasting. Administration is oral in the form of tablets and a dilute elixir, or by injection.

▲ side-effects: concentration and speed of thought and movement may be affected. There may be headache, drowsiness and dry mouth, with gastrointestinal disturbances. Some patients experience blurred vision and/or sensitivity reactions on the skin.

Related articles: MEDISED; PHENERGAN.

promethazine theoclate is a salt of the powerful ANTIHISTAMINE promethazine, used primarily to prevent nausea and vomiting caused by motion sickness or infection of the ear. Promethazine theoclate is slightly longer-acting than the hydrochloride, but otherwise is similar in every respect.

▲/✚ side-effects/warning: *see* PROMETHAZINE HYDROCHLORIDE.

Related article: AVOMINE.

Propaderm (*Allen & Hanburys*) is a proprietary brand of CORTICOSTEROID preparations, available only on prescription, used in topical application to treat severe non-infective skin inflammation such as eczema, especially in patients whose conditions have not responded to less powerful corticosteroids. Produced in its standard form of a cream and ointment, Propaderm is a preparation of the powerful steroid beclomethasone dipropionate. An ointment additionally containing the ANTIBACTERIAL drug chlortetracycline hydrochloride (under the name Propaderm-A) is available for infective skin inflammation, and a cream and an ointment additionally containing the iodine-rich ANTISEPTIC clioquinol (under the name Propaderm-C) are also available.

▲/✚ side-effects/warning: *see* BECLOMETHASONE DIPROPIONATE; CHLORTETRACYCLINE; CLIOQUINOL.

propantheline bromide is an ANTICHOLINERGIC drug used to assist in the treatment of gastrointestinal disorders that involve muscle spasm

of the intestinal wall. It is also used to treat bedwetting in children and may also be used to treat daytime wetting, which is related to an irritable bladder. Administration is oral in the form of tablets.
▲ side-effects: there is commonly dry mouth and thirst.
Related article: PRO-BANTHINE.

propofol is a general ANAESTHETIC used specifically for the initial induction of anaesthesia; it is not used for the maintenance of anaesthesia throughout a surgical procedure. Recovery after treatment is rapid and without any hangover effect. Administration is by injection.
▲ side-effects: there may sometimes be pain on injection, which can be overcome by prior administration of suitable premedication (such as a narcotic analgesic). Urine may turn green.
Related article: DIPRIVAN.

propranolol is a BETA-BLOCKER, used primarily to regularize the heartbeat and to treat and prevent angina pectoris (heart pain) and hypertension in adults. It may additionally be used to relieve the symptoms of excess thyroid hormones in the bloodstream (thyrotoxicosis), or of migraine, and it is also often used to relieve anxiety (particularly if there is tremor or palpitations). Administration (as propranolol hydrochloride) is oral in the form of tablets and sustained-release capsules, or by injection.
✚ warning: propranolol should not be administered to patients with asthma.
▲ side-effects: the heart rate is slowed; there may also be bronchospasm (causing asthma-like symptoms), gastrointestinal disturbances, and tingling or numbness in the fingers and toes.
Related articles: ANGILOL; BEDRANOL.

propylthiouracil is a drug that prevents the production or secretion of the HORMONE thyroxine by the thyroid gland, so treating an excess in the blood of thyroid hormones and the symptoms that it causes (thyrotoxicosis). Treatment may be on a maintenance basis over a long period (dosage adjusted to optimum effect) or may be merely preliminary to surgical removal of the thyroid gland. Administration is oral in the form of tablets.
▲ side-effects: an itching rash may indicate a need for alternative treatment. There may also be nausea and headache; occasionally there is jaundice or hair loss. Rarely, there may be a tendency to haemorrhage.

Prosigmin (*Roche*) is a proprietary preparation of neostigmine, available only on prescription. The drug prolongs the action of the natural neurotransmitter acetylcholine, and can thus be used both in the diagnosis of disorders of the neurotransmission process caused by disease such as myesthesia gravis or by drug treatments (through a comparison of its effect with the effect of its absence), and as an antidote to muscle relaxants and anaesthetics which block the action of the neurotransmitter (in which case, atropine should be administered simultaneously). It is produced in ampoules (in two strengths) for injection (in the form of neostigmine methylsulphate) and as tablets (as neostigmine bromide).

▲/✚ side-effects/warning: *see* NEOSTIGMINE.

Prosobee (*Bristol-Myers*) is a proprietary food product that is nutritionally a complete diet, for use by patients whose metabolic processes are unable to tolerate milk or lactose. Produced in the form of a liquid concentrate, it is a preparation of protein (soya protein), carbohydrate (corn syrup solids), fat (soya oil, coconut oil), VITAMINS, minerals and trace elements, and is gluten-, sucrose-, fructose- and lactose-free. Prosobee is also produced as a powder containing protein (soya protein), carbohydrate (corn syrup solids), fat (coconut oil, corn oil), and vitamins and minerals, that is also gluten-, sucrose-, fructose- and lactose-free.

Prosparol (*Duncan, Flockhart*) is a proprietary nutritional preparation for patients requiring a high energy, low fluid and low electrolyte diet. Produced in the form of an emulsion, Prosparol is a preparation of ARACHIS OIL in water.

Prostin VR (*Upjohn*) is a proprietary hormonal drug, available only on prescription, used to maintain newborn babies born with heart defects while preparations are made for corrective surgery in intensive care. Produced in ampoules for injection or infusion, Prostin VR is a preparation of the prostaglandin alprostadil (prostaglandin E1).

▲/✚ side-effects/warning: *see* ALPROSTADIL.

pseudoephedrine is a VASOCONSTRICTOR, a SYMPATHOMIMETIC drug that is also a BRONCHODILATOR, used mainly as a nasal decongestant. In all respects its actions and effects are identical to those of the closely-related drug ephedrine hydrochloride.

▲/✚ side-effects/warning: *see* EPHEDRINE HYDROCHLORIDE.

Related articles: BENYLIN DECONGESTANT; DIMOTANE PLUS; DIMOTANE WITH CODEINE; GALPSEUD; SUDAFED.

Psoriderm (*Dermal*) is a proprietary ANTISEPTIC used to treat non-infective skin conditions such as psoriasis. Produced in the form of a cream, a scalp lotion (used as a shampoo) and a bath emulsion, Psoriderm's active constituent is coal tar.

PsoriGel (*Alcon*) is a proprietary ANTISEPTIC used to treat non-infective skin conditions such as psoriasis and chronic eczema. Produced in the form of a gel, PsoriGel is a preparation of coal tar solution in an emollient alcohol base.

Psorin (*Thames*) is a proprietary, non-prescription compound preparation used in topical application to treat chronic and mild forms of the troublesome skin disorder psoriasis. Produced in the form of an ointment in an emollient base, Psorin is a combination of dithranol, salicylic acid and coal tar.

▲/✚ side-effects/warning: *see* RIMITEROL.

Pulmadil (*Riker*) is a proprietary BRONCHODILATOR, available only on prescription, used to treat bronchospasm in patients with asthma. Produced in a metered-dosage aerosol, and in metered-dosage cartridges (under the name Pulmadil Puto), Pulmadil is a preparation of the SYMPATHOMIMETIC rimiterol hydrobromide.
▲/✚ side-effects/warning: *see* RIMITEROL.

Pulmicort (*Astra*) is a proprietary CORTICOSTEROID preparation, available only on prescription, used to prevent the inflammatory symptoms of bronchial asthma. Produced in a metered-dosage aerosol (in two strengths, the weaker labelled for children and named Pulmicort LS), Pulmicort is a preparation of budesonide.
▲/✚ side-effects/warning: *see* BUDESONIDE.

Puri-Nethol (*Wellcome*) is a proprietary CYTOTOXIC drug, available only on prescription, used to treat acute leukaemia, especially in children. It works by combining with new-forming cells in a way that prevents normal cell replication. Produced in the form of tablets, Puri-Nethol is a preparation of mercaptopurine.

Pyopen (*Beecham*) is a proprietary ANTIBIOTIC, available only on prescription, used mainly to treat infections of the urinary tract and respiratory tract. Produced in the form of a powder for reconstitution as a medium for injection, Pyopen is a preparation of the PENICILLIN carbenicillin.
▲/✚ side-effects/warning: *see* CARBENICILLIN.

pyrazinamide is an ANTIBACTERIAL that is one of the major forms of treatment for tuberculosis, and particularly tuberculous meningitis. It is used generally in combination (to cover resistance and for maximum effect) with other drugs such as ISONIAZID or RIFAMPICIN. Treatment lasts for between 6 and 18 months, depending on the severity of the condition and on the specific drug combination. Administration is oral in the form of tablets.
▲ side-effects: there may be symptoms of liver malfunction, including high temperature, severe weight loss and jaundice. There may be nausea and vomiting, sensitivity reactions such as urticaria, and/or blood disorders.
✚ warning: it should be administered with caution to patients with impaired liver function, diabetes or gout. Regular checks on liver function are essential.
Related article: ZINAMIDE.

pyridostigmine is a drug that has the effect of increasing the activity of the neurotransmitters which transmit the neural instructions of the brain to the muscles. It works by inhibiting the "switching off" of the neural impulses as they pass from one nerve cell to another, therefore increasing transmission. Its main use is in the treatment of the neuromuscular disease myasthenia gravis (which causes extreme muscle weakness amounting even to paralysis); it is also used to reverse the effects of muscle relaxants administered during surgical operations. Occasionally the drug is used to stimulate intestinal motility and so promote defecation. Administration is oral in the form of tablets, or by injection.

▲ side-effects: there may be nausea and vomiting, diarrhoea and abdominal cramps, and an excess of saliva in the mouth. Overdosage may cause gastrointestinal disturbance, an excess of bronchial mucus, sweating, faecal and urinary incontinence, vision disorders, excessive dreaming, nervous agitation and muscular weakness.

✚ warning: pyridostigmine bromide should not be administered to patients with intestinal or urinary blockage; it should be administered with caution to those with epilepsy, asthma, hypotension (low blood pressure) or a slow heart rate.
Related article: MESTINON.

pyridoxine is the chemical name for vitamin B_6, a VITAMIN that is essential in the diet for the metabolism of amino acids and the maintenance of body cells. Good food sources include fish, liver, peas and beans, yeast and whole grains. A deficiency – rare in the Western world but which may occur due to certain drug treatments, such as with isoniazid – may dispose a patient towards nerve or blood disorders, and in children might eventually cause convulsions. Therapeutically, it is administered to make up a vitamin deficiency (and especially if that deficiency has resulted in neuritis or anaemia).
Related articles: ABIDEC; ALLBEE WITH C; BC 500; DALIVIT; KETOVITE; OCTOVIT; OROVITE; PAXADON.

pyrimethamine is an ANTIMALARIAL drug used primarily to prevent contraction of malaria by travellers in tropical countries. However, if the disease is contracted, the drug is effective in treating forms of malaria that are resistant to treatment with the more commonly-prescribed drug chloroquine, and additionally prevents most relapses of benign tertiary forms. Pyrimethamine can also be used to treat the protozoal infection toxoplasmosis. Administration is oral in the form of tablets.

▲ side-effects: suppression of the bone-marrow's capacity for forming new blood cells occurs with prolonged treatment. There may be rashes.

✚ warning: pyrimethamine should be administered with caution to patients with impaired liver or kidney function, or who are taking folic acid supplements (for example, during pregnancy). High doses require regular blood counts.
Related articles: DARAPRIM; FANSIDAR; MALOPRIM.

pyrithione zinc shampoos are ANTIMICROBIAL scalp preparations used to treat dandruff.

Quellada (*Stafford-Miller*) is a proprietary non-prescription preparation of the antiparasitic lindane, used to treat infestation of the skin of the trunk and limbs by itch-mites (scabies) or by lice (pediculosis). It is also used to treat hair lice infestations. Produced in the form of a lotion, it is also available as a shampoo (under the name Quellada Application PC). Neither is recommended for children aged under one month. Children under six months should be treated only under medical supervision. Both are for external use only.
▲/✚ side-effects/warning: *see* LINDANE.

Questran (*Bristol-Myers*) is a proprietary ANTIDIARRHOEAL RESIN, available only on prescription. It is used to relieve itching in liver disease. Produced in the form of powder in sachets, Questran is a preparation of cholestyramine. It is not recommended for children aged under six years.
▲/✚ side-effects/warning: *see* CHOLESTYRAMINE.

Quinaband (*Seton*) is a proprietary non-prescription form of bandaging impregnated with ZINC OXIDE, CALAMINE and CLIOQUINOL, used to treat and dress ulcers, burns and scalds. (Further bandaging is required to keep it in place.)

quinine is an alkaloid of cinchona which was for years used as the main treatment for malaria. Now synthetic and less toxic drugs – such as chloroquine and proguanil – have replaced it almost entirely, although it is still used (in the form of quinine sulphate or quinine hydrochloride) in cases that prove to be resistant to the newer drugs or for emergency cases in which large doses are necessary. Administration is oral in the form of tablets, or by injection.
▲ side-effects: toxic effects – corporately called cinchonism – include nausea, headache and abdominal pain, visual disturbances, ringing in the ears (tinnitus), a rash and confusion. Some patients may experience visual disturbances and temporary blindness, others may undergo further sensitivity reactions.

Quinocort (*Quinoderm*) is a proprietary ANTIFUNGAL and ANTIBACTERIAL STEROID preparation, available only on prescription, used to treat inflammation, particularly when associated with fungal infections. Produced in the form of vanishing cream for topical application, Quinocort is a combination of the steroid hydrocortisone and the antifungal, antibacterial and deodorant potassium hydroxyquinoline sulphate.
▲/✚ side-effects/warning: *see* HYDROCORTISONE; POTASSIUM HYDROXYQUINOLINE SULPHATE.

Quinoderm (*Quinoderm*) is a proprietary, non-prescription, topical preparation for the treatment of acne. Produced in the form of a cream (in two strengths in an astringent vanishing cream basis) and a lotion-gel (in two strengths in an astringent creamy basis), Quinoderm is a combination of the keratolytic benzoyl peroxide and the antifungal, antibacterial and deodorant potassium hydroxyquinoline sulphate. Another form is available, only on

Q

prescription, to treat severe and inflamed acne (under the name
Quinoderm with Hydrocortisone). As its name suggests, this
additionally contains the CORTICOSTEROID hydrocortisone; it too is
produced in an astringent vanishing cream basis.

▲/✚ side-effects/warning: *see* BENZOYL PEROXIDE; HYDROCORTISONE;
POTASSIUM HYDROXYQUINOLINE SULPHATE.

Quinoped (*Quinoderm*) is a proprietary non-prescription topical
ANTIFUNGAL preparation for the treatment of skin infections such as
athlete's foot. Produced in the form of a cream in an astringent basis,
Quinoped is a compound of the KERATOLYTIC benzoyl peroxide and the
antifungal ANTIBACTERIAL and deodorant potassium hydroxyquinoline
sulphate.

▲/✚ side-effects/warning: *see* BENZOYL PEROXIDE; POTASSIUM
HYDROXYQUINOLINE SULPHATE.

Rapitard MC (*Novo*) is a proprietary non-prescription preparation of highly purified beef-with-pork INSULIN, used to treat and maintain diabetic patients. Rapitard MC is produced in the form of vials for regular injection.

R.B.C. (*Rybar*) is a proprietary non-prescription ANTIHISTAMINE, used to treat skin irritation (itching and nettle rash), stings and bites, and sunburn. Produced in the form of a cream, R.B.C. contains the antihistamine antazoline hydrochloride, the antiseptic CETRIMIDE, CALAMINE and camphor.

Rehidrat (*Searle*) is a proprietary non-prescription oral rehydration solution, used to treat patients suffering from dehydration and sodium depletion caused by acute diarrhoea, gastro-enteritis and various other conditions that lead to salt and water deficiency. Produced in the form of a (lemon-, lime- or orange-flavoured) powder in sachets for reconstitution with water for drinking, Rehidrat contains a mixture of salts and sugars: SODIUM CHLORIDE, POTASSIUM CHLORIDE, SODIUM BICARBONATE, citric acid, GLUCOSE, sucrose and fructose.

Relaxit (*Pharmacia*) is a proprietary non-prescription form of micro-enema administered rectally to soften the faeces and promote bowel movement, particularly to relieve cases of persistent constipation. Produced in the form of single-dose disposable packs with a nozzle, Relaxit is a compound preparation that includes sodium citrate. For children aged under three years there are special instructions for the use of this enema.

Rennie (*Nicholas Kiwi*) is a proprietary non-prescription ANTACID produced in the form of tablets. It contains calcium carbonate and magnesium carbonate.
▲/✚ side-effects/warning: *see* MAGNESIUM CARBONATE.

reproterol hydrochloride is a BRONCHODILATOR, a SYMPATHOMIMETIC that relaxes spasms in bronchial smooth muscle and so is useful in treating all forms of asthma. Administration is oral in the form of tablets, as a dilute elixir which must be diluted (and is then potent for 14 days); topical in the form of an inhalant spray; or as a respirator solution.
▲ side-effects: there may be nausea and vomiting, flushing and sweating, restlessness, and a tremor. High dosage may cause an increase in the heart rate, with high blood pressure.
Related article: BRONCHODIL.

Resonium-A (*Winthrop*) is a proprietary non-prescription ion exchange resin used to treat high blood levels of POTASSIUM, particularly in patients who develop renal failure. It is produced in the form of a powdered resin, consisting of a preparation of sodium polystyrene sulphonate.

resorcinol is an astringent drug that in topical application causes skin to peel (it is a KERATOLYTIC) and relieves itching (it is antipruritic); it is most used in ointments and lotions to treat acne or remove dandruff.

✚ warning: prolonged usage, leading to absorption, may cause underactivity of the thyroid gland (hypothyroidism) with resultant symptoms (myxoedema) and eventual convulsions.
Related article: ESKAMEL.

Retcin (*DDSA Pharmaceuticals*) is a proprietary ANTIBIOTIC, available only on prescription, used to treat many types of bacterial infections, especially in patients who are allergic to penicillin-type antibiotics. Produced in the form of tablets, Retcin is a preparation of the erythromycin.

▲/✚ side-effects/warning: *see* ERYTHROMYCIN.

Rheomacrodex (*Pharmacia*) is a proprietary form of the plasma substitute dextran, available only on prescription, used in infusion with either saline (sodium chloride) or glucose to make up a deficiency in the overall volume of blood in a patient, to improve blood flow or to prevent thrombosis (blood clots) following surgery. It is produced in flasks (bottles) for infusion.

▲/✚ side-effects/warning: *see* DEXTRAN.

Rhinocort (*Astra*) is a proprietary nasal spray, available only on prescription, used to treat nasal congestion caused by allergy. Consisting of a preparation of the CORTICOSTEROID budesonide, it is produced in an aerosol with a nasal adaptor for metered inhalation.

▲/✚ side-effects/warning: *see* BUDESONIDE.

ribavirin, also known as tribavirin, is an ANTIVIRAL drug that may be used to treat a winter-time viral respiratory infection called bronchiolitis, particularly in infants with underlying disorders which would make them liable to a more serious illness. It is given, in hospital, as a continuous aerosol for inhalation usually into a head box, and treatment usually lasts for a minimum of three days.

Rifadin (*Merrell*) is a proprietary ANTITUBERCULAR drug, available only on prescription, generally used in combination with other antitubercular drugs. It may also be used to treat leprosy in dapsone-resistant cases. Produced in the form of capsules (in two strengths), as a syrup, and in the form of a powder for reconstitution as a medium for intravenous infusion, Rifadin is a preparation of the ANTIBIOTIC rifampicin.

▲/✚ side-effects/warning: *see* RIFAMPICIN.

rifampicin is an ANTIBIOTIC that is one of the major forms of treatment for tuberculosis. Even so, it is used generally in combination (to cover resistance and for maximum effect) with other antitubercular drugs such as ISONIAZID or STREPTOMYCIN. Treatment lasts for between 6 and 18 months depending on severity and on the specific drug combination, but the use of rifampicin tends to imply the shorter duration. The drug is also effective in the treatment of leprosy in cases where the usual antileprotic drug DAPSONE has failed. Rifampicin may also be used to treat close contacts of patients with bacterial meningitis in order to prevent them developing a serious illness. Administration is oral in the form of capsules, tablets or a syrup, or by injection or infusion.

▲ side-effects: there are often gastrointestinal problems involving nausea, vomiting, diarrhoea and weight loss; many patients also undergo the symptoms of flu, which may also lead to breathlessness. Rarely, there is kidney failure, liver dysfunction, jaundice, alteration in the composition of the blood and/or discoloration of the urine, saliva and other body secretions. Sensitivity reactions, such as a rash or urticaria, can occur.

✚ warning: rifampicin should be administered with caution to those with impaired liver function. One other effect of the drug is that soft contact lenses may become discoloured.

Related articles: RIFADIN; RIFINAH; RIMACTANE; RIMACTAZID.

R

Rifinah (*Merrell*) is a proprietary ANTITUBERCULAR drug, available only on prescription, used to treat tuberculosis. Produced in the form of tablets (in two strengths, under the trade names Rifinah 150 and Rifinah 300), Rifinah is a combined preparation of rifampicin and isoniazid.

▲/✚ side-effects/warning: *see* ISONIAZID; RIFAMPICIN.

Rikospray Silicone (*Riker*) is a proprietary non-prescription barrier skin protectant, used to treat bedsores and nappy rash, or to protect and sanitize a stoma (an outlet on the skin surface following the surgical curtailment of the intestines). Produced in a pressurized aerosol pack for spray application, Rikospray Silicone is a preparation of the ANTIBIOTIC cetylpyridinium chloride together with the astringent antiperspirant aluminium dihydroxyallantoinate in a water repellent basis containing the antifoaming agent dimethicone.

Rimactane (*Ciba*) is a proprietary ANTITUBERCULAR drug, available only on prescription, used in combination with other antitubercular drugs. Produced in the form of capsules (in two strengths), as a syrup and in the form of a powder for reconstitution as a medium for intravenous infusion, Rimactane is a preparation of the ANTIBIOTIC rifampicin.

▲/✚ side-effects/warning: *see* RIFAMPICIN.

Rimactazid (*Ciba*) is a proprietary ANTITUBERCULAR drug, available only on prescription, used singly or in combination with other antitubercular drugs. It may also be used to treat certain other bacterial infections. Produced in the form of tablets (in two strengths, under the names Rimactazid 150 and Rimactazid 300), Rimactazid is a combined preparation of the ANTIBIOTICS rifampicin and isoniazid.

▲/✚ side-effects/warning: *see* ISONIAZID; RIFAMPICIN.

Rimevax (*Smith, Kline & French*) is a proprietary VACCINE against measles (rubeola), available only on prescription. It is a powdered preparation of live but attenuated measles viruses for administration with a diluent by injection to provide active immunization. Rimevax is not recommended for children aged under 12 months.

▲ side-effects: there may be inflammation at the site of injection. Rarely, there may be high temperature, headache, a rash, swelling of the lymph glands, pain in the joints and/or a cough. Very rarely, there are allergic reactions, and in a few patients convulsions have followed the high fever.

✚ warning: rimevax should not be administered to patients with any infection, particularly tuberculosis and other infections of the airways; who are markedly allergic to eggs (the viruses are cultured in chick-embryo tissue); who have known immune-system abnormalities, including leukemia; who are known to be allergic to neomycin; or who are already taking corticosteroid drugs, cytotoxic drugs or undergoing radiation treatment. It should be administered with caution to those with epilepsy (especially children) or any other condition potentially involving convulsive fits, and those who have recently had a blood transfusion.

Rimifon (*Roche*) is a proprietary ANTITUBERCULAR drug, available only on prescription, used in combination with other antitubercular drugs. Produced in ampoules for injection, Rimifon is a preparation of the ANTIBIOTIC isoniazid.

▲/✚ side-effects/warning: *see* ISONIAZID.

rimiterol is a BRONCHODILATOR, a BETA-RECEPTOR STIMULANT SYMPATHOMIMETIC that is useful in treating asthma. Administration (in the form of rimiterol hydrobromide) is topical in the form of an inhalant spray.

▲ side-effects: there may be nausea and vomiting, flushing and sweating, and a tremor. Overdosage may cause an increase in the heart rate, with high blood pressure.

Related article: PULMADIL.

Rite-Diet (*Welfare Foods*) is a brand of special foods for special diets. For patients who require a gluten-free diet there are sweet biscuits and crackers, digestive biscuits, savoury biscuits, bread, bread with soya bran, high-fibre bread, a bread mix, and a flour mix. For patients on a low-protein diet there is macaroni, spaghetti (in two sizes), a flour mix, a bread mix, bread, bread with soya bran, bread without salt, white bread with added fibre, sweet biscuits, crackers, cream-filled biscuits and cream wafers. Most of these are also available specially prepared for patients on a combined gluten-free low-protein diet. Finally, for patients on a low-sodium diet, there is another form of bread.

Rivotril (*Roche*) is a proprietary ANTICONVULSANT, available only on prescription, used to treat epilepsy. It is produced in the form of tablets (in two strengths) and in ampoules (with diluent) for injection, and is a preparation of the BENZODIAZEPINE clonazepam.

▲/✚ side-effects/warning: *see* CLONAZEPAM.

Roccal (*Winthrop*) is a proprietary non-prescription DISINFECTANT, used to cleanse the skin before operations, to cleanse wounds and to sterilize dressings. Produced in the form of a solution, Roccal is a preparation of benzaldonium chloride. A concentrated form is available (under the name Roccal Concentrate 10X) for the preparation of the same solution, using purified water. Roccal should not be used with soap.

rose bengal is a form of dye which (in solution), when placed in contact with the cornea of the eye, makes obvious any lesion or foreign body (particularly on the conjunctiva and the cornea). Administration is thus ordinarily in the form of eye-drops.
Related article: MINIMS.

Rotahaler (*A&H*) is a dry powder inhaler device used to deliver either the BRONCHODILATOR VENTOLIN, or the inhaler CORTICOSTEROID BECOTIDE. The powder is contained in capsules called rotacaps that are broken open within the Rotahaler and then inhaled. This type of inhaler is easier to use than a standard metered-dosed aerosol inhaler.

rubella vaccine is a VACCINE against German measles (rubella) that is medically recommended for pre-pubertal girls between the ages of 10 and 14, because German measles during pregnancy constitutes a serious risk to the foetus. Vaccination should not take place if the patient is pregnant or likely to become pregnant within the following three months, because initially the vaccine can have similar effects to German measles. The vaccine is prepared as a freeze-dried suspension of live but attenuated viruses grown in cell cultures; administration is by injection.

rub/vac is an abbreviation for rubella vaccine.
see RUBELLA VACCINE.

Rynacrom (*Fisons*) is a proprietary non-prescription preparation used to treat allergic nasal congestion. Produced in the form of a nasal spray (with a metered-dose pump), as nasal drops, and in cartridges for nasal insufflation, Rynacrom is a preparation of sodium cromoglycate. A similar nasal spray additionally containing the ANTIHISTAMINE xylometazoline hydrochloride is also available (under the name Rynacrom Compound).
▲/✚ side-effects/warning: *see* SODIUM CROMOGLYCATE.

Salactol (*Dermal*) is a proprietary non-prescription compound preparation in the form of a paint for topical application, intended to remove warts (particularly verrucas) and hardened skin. With its own special applicator, Salactol's major active constituent is the ANTIBACTERIAL KERATOLYTIC salicylic acid.

▲/✚ side-effects/warning: *see* SALICYLIC ACID.

Salatac (*Dermal*) is a proprietary non-prescription compound preparation in the form of a gel for topical application, intended to remove warts (particularly varrucas) corns and calluses. With its own applicator Salatac's major active constituient is the ANTIBACTERIAL KERATOLYTIC salicylic acid.

▲/✚ side-effects/warning: *see* SALICYLIC ACID.

Salazopyrin (*Pharmacia*) is a proprietary preparation, available only on prescription, used primarily to treat ulcerative colitis. Because the drug also has ANTI-INFLAMMATORY properties, it is additionally used to treat rheumatoid arthritis (although there are some haematological side-effects). Produced as tablets (in two forms, one enteric-coated under the name Salazopyrin EN-tablets), as suppositories, and as a retention enema in a disposable pack, Salazopyrin is a preparation of the SULPHONAMIDE sulphasalazine.

▲/✚ side-effects/warning: *see* SULPHASALAZINE.

salbutamol is a SYMPATHOMIMETIC BRONCHODILATOR, of the type known as a selective BETA-RECEPTOR STIMULANT, used to treat asthmatic bronchospasm. It has fewer cardiac side-effects than some others of its type, and is administered orally in the form of tablets, as sustained-release tablets, as a sugar-free liquid, and as an inhalant cartridge or by nebulization; it is also administered by injection or infusion. Inhalers available for use with salbutamol include the ROTAHALER, the DISKHALER and AEROLIN AUTOHALER in addition to the ordinary aerosol inhaler. The aerosol inhaler can be used together with a spacer device called a VOLUMATIC in quite young children.

▲ side-effects: there may be headache and nervous tension, associated with tingling of the fingertips and a fine tremor of the hands. Administration other than by inhalation may cause an increase in the heart rate; infusion may lower blood potassium levels. If salbutamol is injected, there may be pain in the injection site. *Related articles:* ASMAVEN; COBUTOLIN; VENTIDE; VENTOLIN.

salicylic acid is an ANTIFUNGAL drug that is used to treat minor skin infections such as athlete's foot. Administration is topical, in the form of a solution, a collodion (paint or gel), as an ointment − or, in combination with precipitated sulphur, as an ointment or a cream − as a shampoo, and even in an impregnated adhesive plaster.

▲ side-effects: side-effects are rare, confined largely to the effects of too widescale an application (*see below*) and to sensitivity reactions.

✚ warning: in applying salicylic acid topically, areas of healthy skin and the anogenital region should be avoided. Application to large areas is also inadvisable (absorption through the skin may lead to gastrointestinal disturbance and tinnitus − ringing in the ears).

Related articles: ANTHRANOL; CUPLEX; DITHROLAN; DUOFILM; IONIL T; KERALYT; PHYTEX; PHYTOCIL; PRAGMATAR; PSORIN; SALACTOL; VERRUGON.

Salzone (*Wallace*) is a proprietary non-prescription preparation of the non-narcotic ANALGESIC paracetamol, used to treat pain anywhere in the body. It is produced in the form of an elixir for dilution (the potency of the elixir once diluted is retained for 14 days).
▲/✚ side-effects/warning: *see* PARACETAMOL.

Sandimmun (*Sandoz*) is a proprietary preparation of the powerful immunosuppressant cyclosporin, available only on prescription, used to prevent tissue rejection following donor grafting or transplant surgery, specifically in bone-marrow, liver, kidney, pancreas, heart, or heart-and-lung transplant operations. It is administered as an oral solution.
▲/✚ side-effects/warning: *see* CYCLOSPORIN.

Sandocal (*Sandoz*) is a proprietary non-prescription calcium supplement, used to make up depleted calcium levels, and to treat calcium-deficient conditions such as osteomalacia and rickets; it may also be helpful when taken during pregnancy or when breast-feeding. Produced in the forms of tablets, Sandocal's active constituents include CALCIUM (in the form of calcium lactate and calcium gluconate), potassium bicarbonate and sodium bicarbonate. It should be avoided in patients with renal impairment.
▲/✚ side-effects/warning: *see* CALCIUM GLUCONATE; CALCIUM LACTATE.

Sandoglobulin (*Sandoz*) is a proprietary preparation of human normal immunoglobulin (HNIG) available only on prescription, used in infusion to correct immunoglobulin deficiency in children with defects of immunoglobulin manufacture. This would render such patients susceptible to infection. It is also used to treat certain forms of *thrombocytopanaemia* (a condition characterized by easy bruising and caused by a low platelet count in the patient's blood).
✚warning: see HNIG.

Sando-K (*Sandoz*) is a proprietary non-prescription POTASSIUM supplement, used to make up deficient blood levels of potassium. Produced in the form of tablets for effervescent solution in water, it contains POTASSIUM CHLORIDE and potassium bicarbonate, and is not recommended for children.

Sanomigran (*Sandoz*) is a proprietary preparation of the ANTIHISTAMINE pizotifen, a drug related to some of the antidepressants. It is used to treat headaches, particularly migraine. Available only on prescription, and produced in the form of tablets (in two strengths), and as a sugar-free elixir, Sanomigran is not recommended for children aged under five years.
▲/✚ side-effects/warning: *see* PIZOTIFEN.

Savloclens (*ICI*) is a proprietary non-prescription ANTISEPTIC used to prevent infection of wounds and burns. Produced in the form of

S

sachets of sterile solution, Savloclens is a compound preparation of the disinfectants chlorhexidine gluconate and cetrimide. It is generally available only in hospitals.

▲/✚ side-effects/warning: *see* CETRIMIDE; CHLORHEXIDINE.

Savlodil (*ICI*) is a proprietary non-prescription ANTISEPTIC used to prevent infection of wounds and burns. Produced in the form of sachets of sterile solution, Savlodil is a compound preparation of the disinfectants chlorhexidine gluconate and cetrimide. (It is a weaker preparation than the similar Savloclens.)

▲/✚ side-effects/warning: *see* CETRIMIDE; CHLORHEXIDINE.

Savlon Hospital Concentrate (*ICI*) is a proprietary non-prescription ANTISEPTIC used to prevent infection of wounds and burns, and to prepare skin prior to surgery. Produced in the form of sachets of sterile solution, Savlon Hospital Concentrate is a compound preparation of the disinfectants chlorhexidine gluconate and cetrimide, and may be used in dilute form.

▲/✚ side-effects/warning: *see* CETRIMIDE; CHLORHEXIDINE.

*scabicidal drugs are used to treat infestations by itch-mites (Sarcoptes scabiei). The female mite tunnels into the top surface of the skin in order to lay eggs, causing severe irritation as she does so. Newly-hatched mites, also causing irritation with their secretions, then pass easily from person to person on direct contact. Treatment is (almost always) with local applications of LINDANE or BENZYL BENZOATE in the form of a cream: these kill the mites. Every member of an infected household should be treated, and clothing and bedding should also be disinfested.

Scoline (*Duncan Flockhart*) is a proprietary SKELETAL MUSCLE RELAXANT, available only on prescription, that has an effect for only five minutes, and is thus used − following the initial injection of an intravenous BARBITURATE in order to control pain − for short, complete and predictable paralysis (mostly during diagnostic or surgical procedures). Produced in ampoules for injection, Scoline is a preparation of suxamethonium chloride.

▲/✚ side-effects/warning: *see* SUXAMETHONIUM CHLORIDE.

Scopoderm TTS (*Ciba*) is a proprietary preparation of the alkaloid drug hyoscine, used as an ANTI-EMETIC for travel sickness. It is produced in the form of self-adhesive dressing which release hyoscine when in contact with the skin. It is not recommended for children aged under ten years.

▲ side-effects: see HYOSCINE.

✚ warning: patients should wash their hands often after handling the dressing and should only use one at a time.

scopolamine is another name (most commonly used in the United States) for the powerful alkaloid drug hyoscine.

see HYOSCINE.

Sea-Legs (*Bioceuticals*) is a proprietary non-prescription anti-motion sickness preparation. It contains the ANTIHISTAMINE meclozine.
▲/✚ side-effects/warning: *see* MECLOZINE.

Securopen (*Bayer*) is a proprietary ANTIBIOTIC of the penicillin type, available only on prescription, used primarily to treat infections of the urinary tract, upper respiratory tract, and septicaemia. Produced in the form of powder in vials for reconstitution as a medium for infusion, Securopen is a preparation of azlocillin.
▲/✚ side-effects/warning: *see* AZLOCILLIN.

*sedatives are drugs that calm and soothe, relieving anxiety and nervous tension, and disposing towards drowsiness. They are used particularly for premedication prior to surgery. Many are hypnotic drugs (such as BARBITURATES) used in doses lower than those administered to induce sleep. The term TRANQUILLIZER is more commonly used of the sedatives (such as BENZODIAZEPINES) that do not tend to cause dependence (addiction).

Select-A-Jet Dopamine (*International Medication Systems*) is a potent proprietary preparation of the SYMPATHOMIMETIC drug dopamine hydrochloride, used to treat cardiogenic shock. It is produced as a liquid in vials for dilution and infusion.
▲/✚ side-effects/warning: *see* DOPAMINE.

selenium sulphide is a substance thought to act as an antidandruff agent, and used accordingly as the active constituent in some shampoos.
✚warning: selenium sulphide, or preparations containing it, should not be used within 48 hours of a hair colorant or a permanent wave.

Selexid (*Leo*) is a proprietary ANTIBIOTIC of the penicillin type, available only on prescription, used to treat many forms of infection, but particularly salmonellosis and infections of the urinary tract. Produced in the form of tablets and as a suspension (in sachets), Selexid is a preparation of the drug pivmecillinam hydrochloride.
▲/✚ side-effects/warning: *see* PIVMECILLINAM HYDROCHLORIDE.

Selexidin (*Leo*) is a proprietary ANTIBIOTIC of the penicillin type, available only on prescription, used to treat many forms of infection, but particularly those of the intestines and the urinary tract. Produced in the form of a powder for reconstitution as a medium for injections, Selexidin is a preparation of the drug mecillinam.
▲/✚ side-effects/warning: *see* MECILLINAM.

Selsun (*Abbott*) is a proprietary non-prescription shampoo containing selenium sulphide, a substance thought to act as an antidandruff agent. Selsun should not be used within 48 hours of a hair colorant or a permanent wave.

Semitard MC (*Novo*) is a proprietary non-prescription preparation of highly purified pork INSULIN zinc suspension, used to treat

S

and maintain diabetic patients. It is produced in vials for injection.

senna is a powerful stimulant LAXATIVE which acts by increasing the muscular activity of the intestinal walls. It is still in fairly common use, but may take between 8 and 12 hours to have any relieving effect on constipation. Senna preparations also may be administered to evacuate the bowels before an abdominal X-ray or prior to endoscopy or surgery.

✚ warning: senna preparations should not be administered to patients who suffer from intestinal blockage.

▲ side-effects: the urine may be coloured red; it may cause abdominal cramp. Very prolonged use should be avoided.

Related articles: AGIOLAX; SENOKOT.

Senokot (*Reckitt & Colman*) is a proprietary LAXATIVE containing preparations of senna derivatives (sennosides), used to treat constipation or administered to prepare patients for X-ray, endoscopy or surgery. Non-prescription preparations are produced in the form of granules or as a syrup for dilution (the potency of the syrup once dilute is retained for 14 days). Senokot in tablet form is available only on prescription. It is not recommended in any form for children aged under 2 years.

▲/✚ side-effects/warning: *see* SENNA.

Septrin (*Wellcome*) is a proprietary SULPHONAMIDE, available only on prescription, used to treat bacterial infections, especially of the urinary tract. Produced in the form of tablets (in three strengths), as soluble (dispersible) tablets, as a suspension (in two strengths for dilution (the potency of either suspension once diluted is retained for 14 days), and in ampoules for injection or (following dilution) infusion, Septrin is a preparation of the compound drug co-trimoxazole, made up of the sulphonamide sulphamethoxazole with the ANTIBACTERIAL agent trimethoprim.

▲/✚ side-effects/warning: *see* CO-TRIMOXAZOLE.

Setlers (*Beecham Health Care*) is a proprietary non-prescription ANTACID containing calcium carbonate and magnesium carbonate.

▲/✚ side-effects/warning: *see* MAGNESIUM CARBONATE.

silver nitrate is a salt that has astringent and ANTISEPTIC properties and is useful in topical application. It is still used, in mild solution as eye drops, to prevent eye infection caused by gonorrhoea in the newborn in certain parts of the world. Silver nitrate is also used to treat a weeping umbilical cord. In this case it is often used on the end of a stick for accurate application.

✚ warning: silver nitrate is toxic if ingested; prolonged application discolours the skin (and fabrics). Solutions should be protected from light.

silver sulphadiazine is a compound preparation of silver with the SULPHONAMIDE sulphadiazine. In the form of a cream for topical application, it thus has broad-spectrum ANTIBACTERIAL capability as well as the astringent and ANTISEPTIC qualities of the silver, and is used primarily to treat skin infections and to protect wounds, burns and bedsores.

▲ side-effects: side-effects are rare, but there may be sensitivity reactions including rashes.

✚ warning: silver sulphadiazine should not be administered to patients who are allergic to sulphonamides; it should be administered with caution to those with impaired function of the liver or kidneys.
Related article: FLAMAZINE.

simple eye ointment is a bland, sterile formulation of liquid paraffin and wool fat, used both as a night-time eye lubricant (in conditions that cause dry eyes) and to soften the crusts of infections of the eyelids (blepharitis).

✚ warning: wool fat may cause sensitivity reactions in some patients.

simple linctus is a non-proprietary formulation of fairly standard constituents that together make an ANTITUSSIVE as good as many proprietary ones. The constituents include citric acid, anise water, amaranth solution and chloroform spirit.

simple ointment is a bland, sterile formulation of liquid paraffin, wool fat and stearyl alcohol, used as a household ointment for topical application on minor wounds and burns, and areas of dry or cracked skin.

✚ warning: wool fat may cause sensitivity reactions in some patients.

Sintisone (*Farmitalia Carlo Erba*) is a proprietary CORTICOSTEROID preparation, available only on prescription, used to treat inflammation (particularly rheumatoid arthritis and inflammatory skin diseases) and to suppress the symptoms of allergy (particularly those of asthma). Produced in the form of tablets, Sintisone is a preparation of the cortisone-derivative prednisolone.

▲/✚ side-effects/warning: *see* PREDNISOLONE.

Siopel (*Care*) is a proprietary non-prescription barrier cream used to treat and dress itching skin and skin infections, nappy rash and bedsores, or to protect and sanitize a stoma (an outlet on the skin surface following the surgical curtailment of the intestines). It contains the ANTISEPTIC cetrimide and the antifoaming agent dimethicone.

*skeletal muscle relaxants act on voluntary (skeletal) muscles of the body. Some are used during operations to aid surgery (e.g. tubocurarine) and act by interfering with the actions of the neurotransmitter acetylcholine at sites between nerve and muscle. Others used in the treatment of painful muscle spasms act within the central nervous system (e.g. DIAZEPAM). Drugs of this class are quite distinct from SMOOTH MUSCLE RELAXANTS.

Slo-Phyllin (*Lipha*) is a proprietary non-prescription BRONCHODILATOR, used to treat asthmatic bronchospasm. Produced in the form of sustained-release capsules, Slo-Phyllin is a preparation of the xanthine drug theophylline. The capsules come in three different strengths. All contain little white pellets. The capsules can either be swallowed whole or broken open over food so that the pellets are mixed with certain foods and then swallowed. Slo-Phyllin is not recommended for children aged under two years.
▲/✚ side-effects/warning: *see* THEOPHYLLINE.

Slow-Fe (*Ciba*) is a proprietary non-prescription IRON supplement, used to treat iron deficiency in the bloodstream. Produced in the form of sustained-release tablets, Slow-Fe is a preparation of ferrous sulphate. It is not recommended for children aged under 12 months.
▲/✚ side-effects/warning: *see* FERROUS SULPHATE.

Slow-K (*Ciba*) is a proprietary non-prescription POTASSIUM supplement, used to make up a blood deficiency of potassium (as may occur in patients with severe diarrhoea, or in patients being treated with diuretics). Produced in the form of sustained-release tablets, Slow-K is a preparation of potassium chloride.

Slow Sodium (*Ciba*) is a proprietary non-prescription preparation of sodium chloride, used as a dietry supplement in patients who have mild degrees of sodium depletion. It is produced in the form of sustained release tablets, and therefore it is only suitable for older children.
▲/✚ side-effects/warning: *see* SODIUM CHLORIDE.

Sno Phenicol (*Smith & Nephew*) is a proprietary ANTIBIOTIC used to treat bacterial infections. It is a preparation of the drug chloramphenicol.
▲/✚ side-effects/warning: *see* CHLORAMPHENICOL.

Sno Tears (*Smith & Nephew*) is a proprietary non-prescription form of synthetic tears administered in drops to lubricate the surface of the eye in patients whose lachrymal glands or ducts are dysfunctioning. It is a preparation of polyvinyl alcohol.

sodium aurothiomalate is the form in which the metallic element gold may be prescribed to treat severe forms of rheumatoid arthritis. Unlike ANTI-INFLAMMATORY non-narcotic ANALGESICS, however, gold works slowly so that full effects are achieved only after four or five months. Improvement then is significant, not only in the reduction of joint inflammation but also in associated inflammations. Administration is by intramuscular injection.
▲ side-effects: about one in every twenty patients experiences severe reactions, especially blood disorders; in all patients there may be skin reactions, mouth ulcers, the accumulation of fluid in the tissues (oedema) and/or neural effects in the extremities.
✚ warning: sodium aurothiomalate should not be administered to patients who suffer from certain blood disorders; regular blood

counts during treatment are essential. It should be administered with caution to those with impaired function of the liver or kidneys, eczema or colitis. Weekly test doses should be administered to establish changing levels of tolerance within the body; treatment under such monitoring — unless relapse occurs — may then continue for life.
Related article: MYOCRISIN.

sodium bicarbonate is an ANTACID used for the rapid relief of indigestion and acid stomach. For this purpose it is readily available in the form of powder (for solution), as tablets or as a mixture (liquid). Sodium bicarbonate is also sometimes used in infusion to relieve conditions of severe metabolic acidosis — when the acidity of body fluids is badly out of balance with the alkalinity as may occur in diabetic coma.
▲ side-effects: following the intake of sodium bicarbonate as an antacid, belching is virtually inevitable through the liberation of carbon dioxide.
✚ warning: sodium bicarbonate should not be taken by patients with impaired kidney function, or who are on a low-sodium diet. Prolonged use is to be avoided, or the cramps and muscular weakness of alkalosis may occur.

sodium calciumedetate is a CHELATING AGENT, an antidote to poisoning by lead. It works by forming chemical complexes, binding (and so neutralizing) metal ions to the drug which can then be excreted safely in the usual fashion. Administration is by injection or by topical application in the form of a cream (on areas of skin that have become broken or sensitive through contact with the metal).
▲ side-effects: there may be nausea and/or cramp. Overdosage causes kidney damage.
✚ warning: sodium calciumedetate should be administered with caution to patients with impaired kidney function.
Related article: LEDCLAIR.

sodium chloride is a vital constituent of the human body, in both blood and tissues, and is the major form in which the mineral element sodium appears. (Sodium is involved in the balance of extracellular fluids, maintains electrical potentials in the nervous system, and is essential for the functioning of the muscles.) Sodium chloride, or salt, is contained in many foods; too much salt in the diet may lead to the accumulation of fluids in the tissues (oedema) and/or high blood pressure (hypertension). Therapeutically, sodium chloride is widely used as saline solution (0.9%) or as dextrose saline (to treat dehydration and shock), as a medium with which to effect bladder irrigation (specifically to dissolve blood clots), as a sodium supplement in patients with low sodium levels, as a mouth-wash, and for topical application in solution as a cleansing lotion.
▲ side-effects: overdosage may lead to high blood pressure (hypertension), and the accumulation of fluid within the tissues (oedema).
✚ warning: sodium chloride should be administered with caution

S

to patients with heart failure, high blood pressure (hypertension), fluid retention, or impaired kidney function.

sodium cromoglycate is a drug used to prevent recurrent asthma attacks. How it works is not fully understood though it seems to prevent release of inflammatory mediators, but its effect is particularly marked in allergic conditions. It is used solely prophylactically: the drug has no remedial value in acute attacks. Advice to this effect − that administration must be regular whether symptoms are present or not − is generally given by the prescribing doctor. Administration is usually in the form of inhalation, either from an aerosol or nebulizer, or from a spinhaler (which is a form of dry powder inhaler).

▲ side-effects: there may be coughing accompanied by temporary bronchospasm. Inhalation of the dry powder preparation may cause irritation of the throat.

✚ warning: dosage is adjusted to the requirements of individual patients (but administration is generally three or four times a day). *Related article:* INTAL.

sodium fluoride is the normal form of fluoride in toothpastes and added to many water supplies to assist in the prevention of tooth decay. Because many water authorities now add fluoride to their region's drinking-water, sodium fluoride should be administered therapeutically only in relation to levels each patient would naturally be receiving anyway. Administration is oral in the form of tablets, as drops, as a gel, or as a mouth-wash.

▲ side-effects: some patients eventually notice white flecks on their teeth; overdosage may cause yellow-brown discoloration.

✚ warning: in general, sodium fluoride is normally prescribed only in areas where the water is not fluoridated at source. *Related articles:* EN-DE-KAY; FLUOR-A-DAY LAC; FLUORIGARD; POINT-TWO; ZYMAFLUOR.

sodium fusidate is a narrow-spectrum ANTIBIOTIC used most commonly in combination with other antibiotics to treat staphylococcal infections − especially skin infections, abscesses and infections of bone − that prove to be resistant to penicillin. Administration is oral in the form of tablets and as a suspension, or by infusion.

▲ side-effects: there may be nausea with vomiting; a rash may occur. Some patients experience temporary kidney dysfunction.

✚ warning: regular monitoring of liver function is essential during treatment. *Related article:* FUCIDIN.

sodium hypochlorite solutions are used as DISINFECTANTS for cleansing abrasions, burns and ulcers. They differ only in concentration. Non-proprietary solutions are available in 8% and 1% (chlorine) concentrations; both must be diluted before use, for normal skin can tolerate no more than 0.5% available chlorine in topical application.

sodium ironedetate is a form in which IRON can be made available to the body, an iron supplement used to treat iron deficiency and associated anaemia. Administration is oral in the form of a sugar-free elixir.
▲ side-effects: large doses may cause gastrointestinal upset and diarrhoea; there may be vomiting. Prolonged treatment may result in constipation.
✚ warning: sodium ironedetate should not be administered to patients already taking tetracycline antibiotics.
Related article: SYTRON.

sodium picosulphate is a stimulant LAXATIVE which works by direct action within the intestinal walls of the colon. Prescribed to relieve constipation and to prepare patients for X-ray, endoscopy or surgery, the drug is administered orally in the form of an elixir or a solution.
▲ side-effects: prolonged use may eventually precipitate the onset of atonic non-functioning colon.
✚ warning: sodium picosulphate should not be administered to patients who suffer from intestinal blockage; it should be administered with caution to children.
Related articles: LAXOBERAL; PICOLAX.

sodium valproate is an ANTICONVULSANT drug used to treat both major and minor forms of epilepsy. Administration is oral in the form of tablets and as a liquid (or dilute syrup).
▲ side-effects: there may be nausea and gastrointestinal disturbance, increased appetite and consequent weight gain, temporary hair loss, and impaired liver function. If severe vomiting and weight loss occur, treatment should be withdrawn at once.
✚ warning: sodium valproate should not be administered to patients with liver disease; liver function should be monitored for at least the first six months of treatment. The drug may cause some urine tests to be misleading in relation to diabetic patients.
Related article: EPILIM.

Sofradex (*Roussel*) is a proprietary compound ANTIBIOTIC, available only on prescription, used to treat inflammation and infection in the eye or outer ear. Produced in the form of drops and as an ointment, Sofradex is a combination of the CORTICOSTEROID dexamethasone and the broad-spectrum antibiotic framycetin.
▲/✚ side-effects/warning: *see* DEXAMETHASONE; FRAMYCETIN.

Soframycin (*Roussel*) is a proprietary ANTIBIOTIC, available only on prescription, used to treat many forms of infection. Major uses include topical application on the skin, as eye-drops and eye ointment and as a cream for use in the outer ear. Produced for topical application, as drops, as an ointment and as a water-miscible cream, Soframycin in all forms is a preparation of the broad-spectrum antibiotic framycetin sulphate.
▲/✚ side-effects/warning: *see* FRAMYCETIN.

Solivito (*KabiVitrum*) is a proprietary VITAMIN supplement, available only on prescription, used in injection or infusion. It contains almost

S

all forms of VITAMIN B together with ASCORBIC ACID (vitamin C), and is produced in the form of a powder for reconstitution either with water or with glucose (or an equivalent medium).

Soliwax (*Martindale*) is a proprietary non-prescription form of eardrops designed to soften and dissolve ear-wax (cerumen), and commonly prescribed for use at home two nights consecutively before syringeing of the ears in a doctor's surgery. Its solvent constituent is DIOCTYL SODIUM SULPHOSUCCINATE (also called docusate sodium).
✚ warning: soliwax should not be used if there is inflammation in the ear, or where there is any chance that the eardrum has been perforated.

Solpadeine (*Sterling Research*) is a proprietary non-prescription compound ANALGESIC that is not available from the National Health Service. It is used to relieve the pain of headaches, and of rheumatism and other musculo-skeletal disorders. Produced in the form of tablets for effervescent solution. Solpadeine is a combination of paracetamol, codeine phosphate and caffeine.
▲/✚ side-effects/warning: *see* CAFFEINE; CODEINE PHOSPHATE; PARACETAMOL.

Solu-Cortef (*Upjohn*) is a proprietary CORTICOSTEROID preparation, available only on prescription, used to make up natural steroid deficiency, to suppress inflammation or allergic symptoms, or to treat shock. Produced in the form of powder for reconstitution as a medium for injection, Solu-Cortef is a form of hydrocortisone.
▲/✚ side-effects/warning: *see* HYDROCORTISONE.

Solu-Medrone (*Upjohn*) is a proprietary CORTICOSTEROID preparation, available only on prescription, used to suppress inflammation or allergic symptoms, to relieve fluid retention around the brain, or to treat shock. Produced in the form of powder for reconstitution as a medium for injection, Solu-Medrone is a form of methylprednisolone.
▲/✚ side-effects/warning: *see* METHYLPREDNISOLONE.

Solvazinc (*Thames*) is a proprietary non-prescription ZINC supplement used to make up a body deficiency of that mineral. Produced in the form of tablets for effervescent solution, Solvazinc is a preparation of zinc sulphate.
▲/✚ side-effects/warning: *see* ZINC SULPHATE.

somatrem is a synthesized form of human growth HORMONE (HGH, or somatotrophin), prepared by genetic engineering for therapeutic use. It is produced using sequences of DNA to create what is known as a growth hormone of human sequence, and is used to treat dwarfism and other problems of short stature in much the same way as somatropin.
▲/✚ side-effects/warning: *see* SOMATROPIN.

somatropin is a synthetc form of human growth hormone (HGH or somatotrophin) prepared by genetic engineering for therapeutic use.

Its use is indicated in short stature caused by proven growth hormone deficiency and also in a condition called Turner's syndrome (this is a chromosomal disorder affecting girls and resulting in small stature). Since somatotrophin is very expensive, and needs to be given by regular injection until a child stops growing, treatment is only commenced after appropiate investigation to estimate the child's own growth hormone production. Whether growth hormone should be given to children with short stature, who do not have growth hormone deficiency, is a subject of some debate. Treatment is only possible in patients beore the ends of their long bones fuse. Growth stops when this happens. Somatotrophin is administered by regular injections; the interval between injections may vary between two to three injections per week to daily injections.

▲ side-effects: there is a risk of the formation of antibodies against the hormone. Local reactions may occur at the site of injection and therefore the site should be rotated.

✚ warning: it should be administered with caution to diabetics, the dose of insulin may need to be adjusted.

Related article: GENOTROPIN 4IU.

sorbitol is a sweet-tasting carbohydrate that is used as a sugar substitute (particularly by diabetics) and as the carbohydrate in some nutritional supplements administered by injection or infusion.

✚ warning: large oral doses may cause gastrointestinal disturbance.

Spinhaler (*Fisons*) is a dry powder inhaler, used for the inhalation of INTAL capsules. The capsule is pierced within the inhaler and the powder is then inhaled. Such treatment is useful in the prevention of asthma but Intal is of no benefit in treating an actual attack.

Spiretic (*DDSA Pharmaceuticals*) is a proprietary DIURETIC of the type that retains (rather than depletes) potassium in the body. Available only on prescription, it is used to treat fluid retention caused by cirrhosis of the liver, congestive heart failure, high blood pressure (*see* ANTIHYPERTENSIVE) or kidney disease. It is produced in the form of tablets (in two strengths), and is a preparation of the comparatively weak diuretic spironolactone.

▲/✚ side-effects/warning: *see* SPIRONOLACTONE.

Spiroctan (*MCP Pharmaceuticals*) is a proprietary DIURETIC of the type that retains (rather than depletes potassium in the body. Available only on prescription, it is used to treat fluid retention caused by cirrhosis of the liver, congestive heart failure, high blood pressure (*see* ANTIHYPERTENSIVE) or kidney disease. It is produced in the form of tablets (in two strengths) and as capsules, and is a preparation of the comparatively weak diuretic spironolactone.

▲/✚ side-effects/warning: *see* SPIRONOLACTONE.

Spiroctan-M (*MCP Pharmaceuticals*) is a proprietary DIURETIC of the type that retains (rather than depletes) potassium in the body. Available only on prescription, it is used to treat fluid retention caused by cirrhosis of the liver, congestive heart failure, high blood pressure (*see* ANTIHYPERTENSIVE) or kidney disease. It is produced in the form of ampoules for injection, and is transformed to a metabolite of spironolactone.

▲/✚ side-effects/warning: *see* SPIRONOLACTONE.

Spirolone (*Berk*) is a proprietary DIURETIC of the type that retains (rather than depletes) potassium in the body. Available only on prescription, it is used to treat fluid retention caused by cirrhosis of the liver, congestive heart failure, high blood pressure (*see* ANTIHYPERTENSIVE) or kidney disease. It is produced in the form of tablets (in three strengths), and is a preparation of the comparatively weak diuretic spironolactone.

▲/✚ side-effects/warning: *see* SPIRONOLACTONE.

spironolactone is a DIURETIC of the type that retains (rather than depletes) potassium in the body, used primarily to treat fluid retention caused by cirrhosis of the liver, congestive heart failure, high blood pressure (*see* ANTIHYPERTENSIVE) or kidney disease. It is also used to treat the symptoms of an excess of the hormone aldosterone in the blood acting by antagonizing this hormone. Administration is oral in the form of tablets or capsules, or by injection. Comparatively weak by itself, spironolactone is often used in combination with other diuretics that are potassium-depleting (such as frusemide) and potentiates their effect.

▲ side-effects: many patients experience gastrointestinal disturbances. In male patients the breasts may enlarge (gynaecomastia); female patients may have irregular periods. *Related articles:* ALDACTONE; DIATENSEC; LARACTONE; SPIRETIC; SPIROCTAN; SPIROCTAN-M; SPIROLONE.

Stabillin-V-K (*Boots*) is a proprietary preparation of the penicillin-type ANTIBIOTIC phenoxymethylpenicillin, used primarily to treat infections of the head and throat, and some skin conditions. Available only on prescription, it is produced in the form of tablets and as an elixir (in three strengths) for dilution (the potency of the elixir once diluted is retained for seven days).

▲/✚ side-effects/warning: *see* PHENOXYMETHYLPENICILLIN.

Stafoxil (*Brocades*) is a proprietary ANTIBIOTIC, available only on prescription, used to treat bacterial infections, especially staphylococcal infections that prove to be resistant to penicillin. Produced in the form of capsules (in two strengths), Stafoxil is a preparation of flucloxacillin. It is not recommended for children aged under two years.

▲/✚ side-effects/warning: *see* FLUCLOXACILLIN.

Staphcil (*Lederle*) is a proprietary ANTIBIOTIC, available only on prescription, used to treat bacterial infections and especially staphylococcal infections that prove to be resistant to penicillin. Produced in the form of capsules (in two strengths) and in vials for injection, Staphcil is a preparation of flucloxacillin.

▲/✚ side-effects/warning: *see* FLUCLOXACILLIN.

Stemetil (*May & Baker*) is a proprietary ANTI-EMETIC, available only on prescription, used to relieve symptoms of nausea caused by the vertigo and loss of balance experienced in infections of the inner and middle ears, or by cytotoxic drugs in the treatment of cancer. Produced in the form of tablets (in two strengths), as a syrup for dilution (the potency of the syrup once diluted is retained for 14 days), as anal suppositories (in two strengths), and in ampoules for injection, Stemetil is a preparation of the major TRANQUILLIZER prochlorperazine.
▲/✚ side-effects/warning: *see* PROCHLORPERAZINE.

Steribath (*Stuart*) is a proprietary, non-prescription, concentrated solution for use in the bath as a DISINFECTANT and cleansing agent. Its active constituent is a form of iodine.

***steroids** are a class of naturally occurring and synthetic agents whose structure is based on the chemical sterone. In the body they include HORMONES of the adrenal cortex and sex glands (such as oestrogens and progestogens), bile acids and VITAMINS of the D group. Many types of drugs are available based on the steroids, and they are used to treat many types of disorder (including sex-hormone linked disorders, rheumatic pain and certain skin disorders).

Ster-Zac (*Hough*) is the name of three proprietary DISINFECTANT cleansing products. Ster-Zac Powder is a non-prescription dusting powder used to prevent infection in minor wounds and around the umbilical cord; it contains the antiseptic hexachlorophane, the mild astringent zinc oxide, and starch. Ster-Zac Bath Concentrate is a mild solution of the antiseptic triclosan, available without prescription, used to treat staphylococcal skin infections. And Ster-Zac DC Skin Cleanser, available only on prescription, is intended for use instead of soap either for surgeons to scrub up with before undertaking surgical operations, or for patients who suffer from acne and skin infections; it is the antiseptic hexachlorophane in the form of a cream.
▲/✚ side-effects/warning: *see* HEXACHLOROPHANE.

Stesolid (*CP Pharmaceuticals*) is a proprietary preparation of the benzodiazepine diazepam. Produced in the form of tubes (for rectal insertion) and in ampoules for injection. Given rectally diazepam is very rapidly absorbed and is therefore very useful in stopping convulsions when given by this route. Not only can this rectal preparation be used in hospital but it can also be used by parents at home to help stop convulsions if they should occur and be prolonged.
▲/✚ side-effects/warning: *see* DIAZEPAM.

Stiedex (*Stiefel*) is a proprietary CORTICOSTEROID cream, available only on prescription, used for topical application to skin inflammations and allergic skin disorders. It consists of the steroid desoxymethasone (in two strengths, the weaker under the trade name Stiedex LP) in an oily cream base. A third version, additionally containing the ANTIBIOTIC neomycin, is also produced (under the name Stiedex LPN). Neither are commonly used in childhood.
▲/✚ side-effects/warning: *see* DESOXYMETHASONE.

Stomahesive (*Squibb*) is a proprietary non-prescription paste intended for the filling and sealing of skin creases round a stoma (an outlet on the skin surface following the surgical curtailment of the intestines).

Strepsils (*Crookes Healthcare*) are proprietary non-prescription throat lozenges that contain the ANTISEPTICS 2,4-dichlorobenzyl alcohol and amylmetacresol.

streptomycin is an aminoglycoside ANTIBIOTIC now used almost solely for the treatment of tuberculosis, for which it is administered in combination with other antibiotics. Treatment of tuberculosis takes between 6 and 18 months. Administration of streptomycin is by injection.
➕ warning: streptomycin should be administered with extreme caution to patients with impaired kidney function. Regular blood tests can be performed to measure the level of the drug in the blood and thereby check that the correct dosage is being given.
▲ side-effects: there may be hearing difficulties and dysfunction of the kidneys. Prolonged treatment may cause an excess of magnesium in the body.

Stugeron (*Janssen*) is a proprietary non-prescription preparation of the ANTIHISTAMINE cinnarizine, used to treat nausea caused by the vertigo and loss of balance experienced in infections of the middle and inner ears. It is produced in the form of tablets. A stronger version of cinnarizine (produced under the trade name Stugeron Forte) is also used to treat circulatory problems of the extremities; it is rarely used for children.

Sublimaze (*Janssen*) is a narcotic ANALGESIC on the controlled drugs list, primarily used to enhance the effect of a BARBITURATE general ANAESTHETIC, allowing the barbiturate dose to be smaller. Produced in ampoules for injection, Sublimaze is a preparation of the morphine-like fentanyl.
▲/➕ side-effects/warning: *see* FENTANYL.

Sudafed (*Calmic*) is a proprietary non-prescription nasal DECONGESTANT; unlike most decongestants, however, it is produced in the form of tablets (for swallowing), and an elixir for dilution (the potency of the elixir once diluted is retained for 14 days). Both forms are preparations of the ephedrine derivative pseudoephedrine hydrochloride.
▲/➕ side-effects/warning: *see* EPHEDRINE HYDROCHLORIDE.

Sudafed Linctus (*Calmic*) is a proprietary non-prescription cough preparation, produced in the form of linctus for dilution (the potency of the linctus once diluted is retained for four weeks). It is a preparation of the ephedrine derivative psuedoephedrine hydrochloride and the ANTITUSSIVE dextromethorphan hydrobromide. It is not recommended for children aged under two years.
▲/➕ side-effects/warning: *see* EPHEDRINE HYDROCHLORIDE; DEXTROMETHORPHAN.

Sudafed Plus (*Calmic*) is a proprietary non-prescription preparation of the ANTIHISTAMINE tripolidine and the sympathomimetic pseudoephedrine. It is used in allergic conditions of the nose. It is not recommended for children under two years.

▲/✚ side-effects/warning: *see* TRIPOLIDINE; PSEUDOEPHEDRINE.

Sudocrem (*Tosasra*) is a proprietary non-prescription skin emollient (softener and soother) used to treat nappy rash, bedsores and eczema, and sometimes to dress burns. Produced in the form of a cream, its active constituents include zinc oxide, benzyl benzoate and wool fat.

✚ warning: wool fat may cause sensitivity reactions in some patients.

sulconazole nitrate is an ANTIFUNGAL drug, one of the IMIDAZOLES, used to treat skin infections. Administration is by topical application in the form of a water-miscible cream.

▲ side-effects: some patients experience sensitivity reactions, especially skin irritation.

✚ warning: keep well away from the eyes.
Related article: EXELDERM.

Suleo-C (*International Labs*) is a proprietary non-prescription drug used to treat infestations of the scalp and pubic hair by lice. Produced in the form of a lotion and a shampoo, Suleo-C is a preparation of the pediculicide carbaryl.

✚ warning: see CARBARYL.

Suleo-M (*International Labs*) is a proprietary non-prescription drug used to treat infestations of the scalp and pubic hair by lice (pediculosis), or of the skin by the itch-mite (scabies). Produced in the form of a lotion, Suleo-M is a preparation of the insecticide malathion in an alcohol solution.

✚ warning: see MALATHION.

sulfadoxine is an ANTIBACTERIAL, a long-acting SULPHONAMIDE, used solely in combination with PYRIMETHAMINE to prevent or treat malaria.

sulphacetamide is an ANTIBIOTIC, one of the SULPHONAMIDES, used (in solution) primarily in the form of eye-drops and eye ointment to treat local bacterial infections. Ophthalmic administration is most commonly in the form of drops during the daytime, and as ointment for overnight treatment.

sulphadiazine is an ANTIBIOTIC, one of the more potent SULPHONAMIDES, once widely used to treat bacterial infections. Administration is oral in the form of tablets, or by infusion.

▲ side-effects: there may be nausea and vomiting, with skin disorders; changes in the composition of the blood may occur.

✚ warning: sulphadiazine should not be administered to patients with liver or kidney failure, or certain disorders of the blood, or who are aged under six weeks; it should be administered with caution to those with impaired kidney function or sensitivity to light. Adequate fluid intake is essential.
Related article: SULPHATRIAD.

S

sulphadimidine is an ANTIBIOTIC, one of the SULPHONAMIDES, used to treat bacterial infections − particularly infections of the urinary tract − and to prevent meningococcal meningitis in patients at high risk from infection. Among the least toxic of the sulphonamides, sulphadimidine is especially useful in the treatment of children. Administration is oral in the form of tablets, or by injection.
▲ side-effects: there may be nausea and vomiting, with skin disorders; changes in the composition of the blood may occur.
✚ warning: sulphadimidine should not be administered to patients who suffer from liver or kidney failure, or certain disorders of the blood, or who are aged under six weeks; it should be administered with caution to those with impaired kidney function or sensitivity to light. Adequate fluid intake is essential.
Related article: SULPHAMEZATHINE.

sulphafurazole is an ANTIBACTERIAL, one of the SULPHONAMIDES, used to treat bacterial infections − particularly infections of the urinary tract. Administration is oral in the form of tablets or as a syrup.
▲ side-effects: there may be nausea and vomiting, with skin disorders; changes in the composition of the blood may occur.
✚ warning: sulphafurazole should not be administered to patients with liver or kidney failure, or from certain disorders of the blood, or who are aged under six weeks; it should be administered with caution to those with impaired kidney function ot sensitivity to light. Adequate fluid intake is essential.

sulphamethoxazole is an ANTIBACTERIAL, one of the SULPHONAMIDES, that in combination with the antibacterial agent TRIMETHOPRIM − forming a compound drug called co-trimoxazole − is in widespread use to treat many infections, especially infections of the urinary tract. Rarely, sulphamethoxazole is used by itself in the treatment of urinary infections; administration is oral in the form of tablets, and patients should be advised to increase fluid intake during treatment.
see CO-TRIMOXAZOLE.

Sulphamezathine *(ICI)* is a proprietary ANTIBACTERIAL, available only on prescription, used to treat bacterial infections − particularly bacillary dysentery and infections of the urinary tract − and to prevent meningococcal meningitis in patients at high risk from infection. Produced in ampoules for injection, Sulphamezathine is a preparation of the SULPHONAMIDE sulphadimidine.
▲/✚ side-effects/warning: *see* SULPHADIMIDINE.

sulphasalazine is an ANTIBACTERIAL, used primarily to induce a remission of the symptoms of ulceration of the intestinal wall (generally in the colon) and, having induced it, to maintain it. Because the drug also has anti-inflammatory properties, it is additionally used to treat rheumatoid arthritis (although there are some haematological side-effects). Administration is oral in the form of (enteric-coated or plain) tablets, or in suppositories, or as a retention enema. Some of the side-effects can be serious.
▲ side-effects: side-effects are common with higher doses. There may be nausea with vomiting and other gastrointestinal disturbance;

S

headache, vertigo, ringing in the ears (tinnitus) and high temperature; and a rash. A change in the composition of the blood may cause a form of anaemia and a discoloration of the urine and of the tear-fluid lubricating the eyes. Even more seriously, there may be inflammation of the pancreas or of the heart.

✚warning: sulphasalazine should not be administered to patients known to be sensitive to salicylates (aspirin-type drugs) or to sulphonamides; it should be administered with caution to those with liver or kidney disease. Adequate fluid intake must be maintained.

Related article: SALAZOPYRIN.

Sulphatriad (*May & Baker*) is a proprietary compound ANTIBACTERIAL, available only on prescription, used to treat various forms of bacterial infection. Produced in the form of tablets, Sulphatriad is a combination of the three SULPHONAMIDES sulphadiazine, sulphamerazine and sulphathiazole.

▲/✚ side-effects/warning: *see* SULPHADIAZINE.

sulphonamides (or sulpha drugs) are derivatives of a red dye called sulphanilamide that have the property of preventing the growth of bacteria. Most are administered orally and are rapidly absorbed in the stomach and small intestine, are short-acting, and thus may have to be taken several times a day. Their quick progress through the body and excretion in the urine makes them particularly suited to the treatment of urinary infections. One or two sulphonamides are long-acting (and may be used to treat diseases such as malaria or leprosy), and another one or two are poorly absorbed (for which reason they were until recently used to treat intestinal infections). Best known and most used sulphonamides include sulphadiazine, sulphadimidine and sulphafurazole. Sulphonamides tend to cause side-effects – particularly nausea, vomiting, diarrhoea and headache – some of which (especially sensitivity reactions) may become serious; bone-marrow damage may result from prolonged treatment. As a general rule, patients being treated with sulphonamides should try to avoid exposure to sunlight. As antibacterial agents they are distinct from ANTIBIOTICS, and in some cases the one class of drug may be substituted for the other when there are adverse side-effects.

see SULFADOXINE; SULPHACETAMIDE; SULPHADIAZINE; SULPHADIMIDINE; SULPHAFURAZOLE; SULPHAMETHOXAZOLE; SULPHASALAZINE.

sulphones are closely related to the SULPHONAMIDES, have much the same therapeutic action, and are thus used for much the same purposes. They are particularly successful in preventing the growth of the bacteria responsible for leprosy, malaria and tuberculosis. Best known and (possibly) most used is dapsone.

see DAPSONE.

sulphur is a non-metallic element thought to be active against external parasites and fungal infections of the skin. Its common use in creams, ointments or lotions for treating skin disorders such as acne, dermatitis and psoriasis would appear to have little scientific basis.

suxamethonium chloride is a SKELETAL MUSCLE RELAXANT that has an effect for only five minutes, and is thus used − following the initial injection of an intravenous BARBITURATE − for short, complete and predictable paralysis (mostly during diagnostic or surgical procedures). Recovery is spontaneous. Administration is by injection or infusion.

▲ side-effects: blood levels of potassium rise temporarily under treatment. There may be muscle pain afterwards. Repeated doses may cause prolonged muscle paralysis.

✚ warning: suxamethonium chloride should not be administered to patients with severe liver disease or severe burns. Premedication is usually with atropine. During treatment, the paralysis is irreversible.

Related articles: ANECTINE; SCOLINE.

*sympathomimetics are drugs that have effects mimicking those of the sympathetic nervous system in some cases by releasing noradrenaline from nerves. There are two main types that act directly, although several sympathomimetics belong to both types. Alpha-adrenergic sympathomimetics (such as phenylephrine) are VASOCONSTRICTORS and are particularly used in nasal decongestants. Beta-adrenergic sympathomimetics (such as salbutamol, *see* BETA-RECEPTOR STIMULANTS) are frequently SMOOTH MUSCLE RELAXANTS, particularly on bronchial smooth muscle, and are used especially as BRONCHODILATORS.

see ADRENALINE; DOBUTAMINE HYDROCHLORIDE; DOPAMINE; EPHEDRINE HYDROCHLORIDE; FENOTEROL; ISOPRENALINE; ORCIPRENALINE SULPHATE; PHENYLEPHRINE; PIRBUTEROL; REPROTEROL; RIMITEROL; SALBUTAMOL; TERBUTALINE.

Synacthen (*Ciba*) is a proprietary form of a HORMONE that stimulates the adrenal gland into functioning to produce corticosteroid hormones (corticotrophin). This may be useful therapeutically but in fact Synacthen is primarily used to test adrenal gland function. Synacthen consists of a preparation of tetracosactrin, and it is produced in ampoules for injection.

▲/✚ side-effects/warning: *see* TETRACOSACTRIN.

Synalar (*ICI*) is a series of proprietary CORTICOSTEROID ointments and creams, available only on prescription, for topical application on skin infections or inflammation. All contain the steroid fluocinolone acetonide. The standard form is a 0.025% solution, in both ointment and cream. Synalar Cream 1:10 is a cream (only) consisting of a 0.0025% solution; Synalar Cream 1:4 is a cream (only) consisting of a 0.00625% solution. Synalar C is both ointment and cream as the standard version, but with the addition of the ANTIFUNGAL agent CLIOQUINOL. Synalar N is both ointment and cream as the standard version, but with the addition of the ANTIBIOTIC agent NEOMYCIN. There is also a similar gel with which to massage the scalp; its content is the same as the standard ointment and cream.

▲/✚ side-effects/warning: *see* FLUOCINOLONE ACETONIDE.

Synflex (*Syntex*) is a proprietary non-narcotic ANALGESIC, available only on prescription, used to treat migraine and menstrual and inflammatory pain, and pain following surgery. Produced in the form of tablets, it is a preparation of the non-steroidal ANTI-INFLAMMATORY drug naproxen sodium.
▲/✚ side-effects/warning: *see* NAPROXEN.

Synkavit (*Roche*) is a proprietary non-prescription form of the water-soluble VITAMIN K substitute menadiol sodium phosphate. It is as good as the real vitamin (phytomenadione) in making up vitamin deficiency and thus ensuring properly effective blood clotting. It is produced in the form of tablets and in ampoules for injection.
✚warning: see MENADIOL SODIUM PHOSPHATE.

Synogist (*Townendale*) is a proprietary non-prescription medicated shampoo containing an ANTIBIOTIC, used to treat conditions of the scalp associated with bacterial or fungal infection (particularly of the sebaceous glands).
✚warning: keep the shampoo away from the eyes.

Syntaris (*Syntex*) is a proprietary nasal spray, available only on prescription, used to treat the symptoms of nasal allergy (such as hay fever). Consisting of a preparation of the CORTICOSTEROID flunisolide, it is produced in a bottle with a pump and applicator. It is not recommended for children aged under five years.

Synthamin (*Travenol*) is a proprietary series of nutritional supplements for infusion into patients unable to take food via the alimentary canal. They are all a preparation of amino acids; most also contain electrolytes. Available only on prescription, each should be administered only by qualified personnel.

Syntopressin (*Sandoz*) is a proprietary preparation of lypressin, one of the derivatives of the antidiuretic HORMONE vasopressin. Available only on prescription, it is used to treat pituitary-originated diabetes insipidus, and is produced in the form of a nasal spray.
▲/✚ side-effects/warning: *see* VASOPRESSIN.

Syraprim (*Wellcome*) is a proprietary ANTIBIOTIC drug, available only on prescription, used to treat bacterial infections, particularly those of the urinary tract. Produced in the form of tablets (in two strengths) and in ampoules for injection, Syraprim is a preparation of the antibacterial agent trimethoprim.
▲/✚ side-effects/warning: *see* TRIMETHOPRIM.

Sytron (*Parke-Davis*) is a proprietary non-prescription iron supplement, used to make up IRON deficiency (and so treat anaemia). Produced in the form of a sugar-free elixir for dilution (the potency of the elixir once diluted is retained for 14 days), it consists of sodium ironedetate.

S

Tagamet (*Smith, Kline & French*) is a proprietary preparation of the drug cimetidine, available only on prescription, used to treat pepticulcers, it is also useful for treating severe acid reflux and to relieve heartburn. It works by reducing the secretion of gastric acids. It is produced in the form of tablets (in three strengths), as a syrup for dilution (the potency of the syrup once dilute is retained for 28 days), in ampoules for injection, and in bags for infusion. It is not recommended for children aged under 12 months.
▲/✚ side-effects/warning: *see* CIMETIDINE.

talampicillin is a broad-spectrum penicillin-type ANTIBIOTIC, a derivative of AMPICILLIN, used to treat severe bacterial infections (such as respiratory infection, infection of the middle ear, and infections of the urinary tract). Administration is oral in the form of tablets and as a dilute syrup.
▲ side-effects: there may be sensitivity reactions. Some patients experience diarrhoea.
✚ warning: talampicillin should not be administered to patients known to be sensitive to penicillins; it should be administered with caution to those with any allergy at all, or to those with impaired kidney function.
Related article: TALPEN.

Talpen (*Beecham*) is a proprietary ANTIBIOTIC of the penicillin type, available only on prescription, used to treat severe bacterial infections (such as respiratory infection, infection of the middle ear, and infections of the urinary tract). Produced in the form of tablets, and as a syrup for dilution (the potency of the syrup once dilute is retained for seven days), Talpen is a preparation of the ampicillin-derivative talampicillin.
▲/✚ side-effects/warning: *see* TALAMPICILLIN.

Tambocor (*Riker*) is a proprietary ANTIARRHYTHMIC drug, available only on prescription, used to treat various forms of heartbeat irregularities. Produced in the form of tablets, and in ampoules for injection, Tambocor is a preparation of the local ANAESTHETIC LIGNOCAINE analogue flecainide acetate.
▲/✚ side-effects/warning: *see* FLECAINIDE ACETATE.

Tarband (*Seton*) is a proprietary non-prescription form of impregnated bandaging incorporating ZINC PASTE and COAL TAR, used to dress conditions of chronic eczema and psoriasis. Further bandaging is required to hold it in place.
✚ warning: it should not be used to cover broken or inflamed skin.
▲ side-effects: there may be skin sensitivity. The dressing may stain skin and hair (and fabric).

Tarcortin (*Stafford-Miller*) is a proprietary cream, available only on prescription, for topical application to conditions of chronic eczema and psoriasis and other dermatoses. It is a compound of the CORTICOSTEROID hydrocortisone with the cleansing agent COAL TAR.
▲/✚ side-effects/warning: *see* HYDROCORTISONE.

Tavegil (*Sandoz*) is a proprietary non-prescription ANTIHISTAMINE used to treat allergic conditions such as hay fever, dermatitis and urticaria, or sensitivity reactions to drugs. Produced in the form of tablets, and as a sugar-free elixir for dilution (the potency of the elixir once dilute is retained for 14 days), Tavegil is a preparation of clemastine fumarate.
▲/✚ side-effects/warning: *see* CLEMASTINE.

Tears Naturale (*Alcon*) is a proprietary non-prescription form of synthetic tear-fluid, produced in the form of drops, used to make up for a deficiency in the lachrymal apparatus of the eye. It is a compound of the plasma substitute DEXTRAN with the artificial tears liquid hypromellose.

Teejel (*Napp*) is a proprietary non-prescription gel containing both an ANTISEPTIC and an ANALGESIC, used to treat mouth ulcers, sore gums or inflammation of the tongue. The gel is intended to be massaged in gently. It consists of a compound of the analgesic choline salicylate with the antiseptic cetalkonium chloride (both in solution). It is not recommended for children aged under four months.

Tegretol (*Geigy*) is a proprietary preparation of the ANTICONVULSANT drug carbamazapine, available only on prescription, used to treat most forms of epilepsy (but not minor attacks). It is produced in the form of tablets (in three strengths) and as a sugar-free liquid for dilution (the potency of the liquid once dilute is retained for 14 days).
▲/✚ side-effects/warning: *see* CARBAMAZEPINE.

Tegretol Retard (*Geigy*) is a proprietary preparation of the ANTICONVULSANT drug carbamazapine, available only on prescription. It is used to treat major forms of epilepsy. Tegretol Retard tablets result in continuous release of carbamazapine and this may cause less fluctuation of the blood level than with ordinary tablets. It is produced in the form of tablets in two strengths.
▲/✚ side-effects/warning: *see* CARBAMAZEPINE.

Temgesic (*Reckitt & Colman*) is a proprietary narcotic ANALGESIC, available only on prescription, and is on the controlled drugs list. It is used to treat all forms of pain. Produced in the form of tablets to be retained under the tongue, and in ampoules for injection, it is a preparation of the OPIATE buprenorphine hydrochloride.
▲/✚ side-effects/warning: *see* BUPRENORPHINE.

Tensilon (*Roche*) is a proprietary preparation of the anticholinesterase drug edrophonium chloride, available only on prescription. The drug prolongs the action of the natural neurotransmitter acetylcholine, and can thus be used both in the diagnosis of disorders of the neurotransmission process caused by disease or by drug treatments (through a comparison of its effect with the effect of its absence), and as an antidote to muscle relaxants which block the action of the neurotransmitter (in which case, atropine should be administered simultaneously). It is mainly used to help diagnose myasthenia gravis. It is produced in ampoules for injection.

▲/✚ side-effects/warning: *see* EDROPHONIUM CHLORIDE.

terbutaline is a BETA-RECEPTOR STIMULANT and BRONCHODILATOR that is especially useful in treating all forms and stages of asthma. In younger children terbutaline can be given as an aerosol using a spacer device called a nebuhaler. It can also be given as a powder, inhaled through a device through a called a Turbohaler. Administration is also in the form of tablets, sustained-release tablets or a dilute syrup, as an inhalant via an aerosol or nebuliser, or by injection or infusion.

▲ side-effects: there may be a tremor. High dosage may cause an increase in the heart rate.

Related articles: BRICANYL; MONOVENT.

Tercoda (*Sinclair*) is a proprietary non-prescription cough elixir that is not available from the National Health Service. Active constituents include codeine phosphate and the EXPECTORANT terpin hydrate.

▲/✚ side-effects/warning: *see* CODEINE PHOSPHATE.

Tercolix (*Vestric*) is a proprietary non-prescription cough elixir that is not available from the National Health Service. Active constituents include codeine phosphate and menthol and the EXPECTORANT terpin hydrate.

▲/✚ side-effects/warning: *see* CODEINE PHOSPHATE.

terfenadine is a relatively new ANTIHISTAMINE used to treat the symptoms of allergic disorders. Unlike most, it has little sedative effect. Administration is oral in the form of tablets or as a dilute suspension.

▲ side-effects: side-effects are comparatively uncommon, but there may be headache.

Related article: TRILUDAN.

terlipressin is a derivative of the antidiuretic HORMONE VASOPRESSIN, and is similarly a VASOCONSTRICTOR. It is used primarily to halt bleeding from varicose veins in the oesophagus − the part of the alimentary tract between the throat and the stomach. Administration is by intravenous injection.

▲ side-effects: there may be nausea, cramp, and an urge to defecate; some patients experience sensitivity reactions. If the vasoconstriction affects the coronary arteries, there may be heartbeat irregularities.

✚ warning: terlipressin should not be administered to patients with chronic kidney disease or vascular disease; it should be administered with caution to those with epilepsy, asthma, migraine or heart failure.

Related article: GLYPRESSIN.

Terra-Cortril (*Pfizer*) is the name of several CORTICOSTEROID preparations that are also ANTIBIOTIC, available only on prescription, used for local or topical application to treat skin disorders in which bacterial or other infection is also implicated. The standard form, produced as an ointment and as a spray in an aerosol, combines the steroid hydrocortisone and the TETRACYCLINE antibiotic oxytetracycline. Terra-Cortril Ear Suspension also contains the antibiotic polymyxin B sulphate. Terra-Cortril Nystatin is a cream that is a combination of hydrocortisone and oxytetracycline with the ANTIFUNGAL agent nystatin.

▲/✚ side-effects/warning: *see* HYDROCORTISONE; NYSTATIN; OXYTETRACYCLINE; POLYMYXIN B.

Terramycin (*Pfizer*) is a proprietary ANTIBIOTIC, available only on prescription, used to treat bacterial and other infections. Produced in the form of capsules and tablets, it is a preparation of the TETRACYCLINE oxytetracycline hydrochloride. It is not recommended for children aged under 12 years.

▲/✚ side-effects/warning: *see* OXYTETRACYCLINE.

Tertroxin (*Glaxo*) is a proprietary preparation of the thyroid HORMONE triiodothyronine (in the form of liothyronine sodium), available only on prescription, used to make up hormonal deficiency (hypothyroidism) and thus to treat the associated symptoms (myxoedema). It is produced in the form of tablets.

▲/✚ side-effects/warning: *see* LIOTHYRONINE SODIUM.

tetanus vaccine stimulates the formation in the body of the appropriate antitoxin – that is, an antibody produced in response to the presence of the toxin of the tetanus bacterium, rather than to the presence of the bacterium itself. Its effectiveness is improved by being adsorbed on to a mineral carrier (such as aluminium hydroxide or calcium phosphate). Its most common form of administration is as one constituent of the triple vaccine against diphtheria, whooping cough (pertussis) and tetanus (the DIPHTHERIA-PERTUSSIS-TETANUS, or DPT, vaccine), administered during early life, although it is administered by itself at any age for those at special risk, or administered as a double vaccine with the DIPHTHERIA VACCINE for those who wish not to be given the whooping cough vaccine. Administration is by injection.

Tetavax (*Merieux*) is a proprietary preparation of adsorbed TETANUS VACCINE, produced in syringes and vials for injection.

tet/vac/ads is an abbreviation for the kind of tetanus vaccine that is adsorbed on to a mineral carrier for injection.
see TETANUS VACCINE.

tet/vac/ft is an abbreviation for tetanus vaccine formol toxoid, the plain vaccine (that is not adsorbed on to a carrier).
see TETANUS VACCINE.

Tetrabid-Organon (*Organon*) is a proprietary broad-spectrum ANTIBIOTIC, available only on prescription, used to treat many forms of infection including pustular acne. Produced in the form of sustained-

release capsules, it is a preparation of the TETRACYCLINE tetracycline hydrochloride. It is not suitable for children aged under 12 years.
▲/✚ side-effects/warning: *see* TETRACYCLINE.

Tetrachel (*Berk*) is a proprietary broad-spectrum ANTIBIOTIC, available only on prescription, used to treat many forms of infection including pustular acne. Produced in the form of capsules and tablets, it is a preparation of the TETRACYCLINE tetracycline hydrochloride. It is not suitable for children aged under 12 years.
▲/✚ side-effects/warning: *see* TETRACYCLINE.

tetrachloroethylene is an ANTHELMINTIC drug used to treat infestations by hookworms (parasitic worms that attach to the inner wall of the small intestine, feeding not only on the passing food-mass but also on blood from the intestine wall).
▲ side-effects: there may be nausea and headache, with drowsiness.

tetracosactrin is a synthetic HORMONE that acts on the adrenal glands to release CORTICOSTEROIDS, especially HYDROCORTISONE. Like its natural equivalent corticotrophin, tetracosactrin is useful in the treatment of allergic disorders, inflammation and especially asthma. It may also be used to test adrenal function.
▲ side-effects: if treatment is prolonged there may be high blood pressure (hypertension), sodium and water retention (oedema) leading to weight gain, loss of blood potassium and muscle weakness.

tetracycline is a broad-spectrum ANTIBIOTIC that gave its name to a group of similar antibiotics. It is used to treat many forms of infection caused by several types of micro-organism; conditions it is used particularly to treat include infections of the respiratory tract and acne. Administration is oral in the form of capsules, tablets and liquids, or by injection.
▲ side-effects: there may be nausea and vomiting, with diarrhoea. Occasionally there is sensitivity to light or other sensitivity reaction.
✚ warning: tetracycline should not be administered to patients who are aged under 12 years, or who have impaired kidney function.
Related articles: ACHROMYCIN; ACHROMYCIN V; AUREOCORT; DETECLO; ECONOMYCIN; TETRABID-ORGANON; TETRACHEL; TETREX.

tetracyclines are broad-spectrum ANTIBIOTICS used to treat infection by many organisms, but especially bacteria. They are particularly used in the treatment of infections of the respiratory tract and acne. However, perhaps through over-use of the drugs, bacterial resistance has grown considerably and the tetracyclines are no longer as efficacious as they once were. Moreover, most tetracyclines are more difficult to absorb in a stomach that contains milk, antacids, calcium salts or magnesium salts; they tend to make kidney disease worse; and they may be deposited on growing bone and teeth (causing staining and potential deformity), so they should not be administered to children aged under 12 years. Best known and most used

tetracyclines include tetracycline (which they were all named after),
doxycycline and oxytetracycline. Administration is oral in the form of
capsules, tablets or liquids.
see CHLORTETRACYCLINE; CLOMOCYCLINE SODIUM; DEMECLOCYCLINE
HYDROCHLORIDE; DOXYCYCLINE; LYMECYCLINE; MINOCYCLINE;
OXYTETRACYCLINE; TETRACYCLINE.

Tetralysal (*Farmitalia Carlo Erba*) is a proprietary broad-spectrum
ANTIBIOTIC, available only on prescription, used to treat many forms of
infection but particularly those of the skin and soft tissues, the ear,
nose or throat, or conditions such as pustular acne. Produced in the
form of capsules (in two strengths, the stronger under the name
Tetralysal 300), it is a preparation of the soluble TETRACYCLINE
complex lymecycline. It is not recommended for children aged under
12 years.
▲/✚ side-effects/warning: *see* LYMECYCLINE.

Tetrex (*Bristol-Myers*) is a proprietary broad-spectrum ANTIBIOTIC,
available only on prescription, used to treat many forms of infection
including acne. Produced in the form of capsules and tablets, it is a
preparation of the TETRACYCLINE tetracycline hydrochloride. It is not
recommended for children aged under 12 years.
▲/✚ side-effects/warning: *see* TETRACYCLINE.

T/Gel (*Neutrogena*) is a proprietary non-prescription medicated
shampoo designed to treat scaling skin on the scalp, as occurs with
dandruff or with psoriasis. Its principle constituent is COAL TAR.

Theo-Dur (*Astra*) is a proprietary non-prescription BRONCHODILATOR
used to treat conditions such as asthma. Produced in the form of
sustained-release tablets (in two strengths) for prolonged effect, Theo-
Dur has as its principal constituent the xanthine, theophylline.
▲/✚ side-effects/warning: *see* THEOPHYLLINE.

theophylline is a BRONCHODILATOR used mostly in sustained-release
forms of administration, generally to treat conditions such as asthma
over periods of around 12 hours at a time. It is also used to treat and
help prevent neonatal apnoea (a tendency to stop breathing).
Administration is oral in the form of tablets, capsules, or a liquid.
The liquid form is more suitable for small children, and since it does
not have sustained-release properties may need to be given more
frequently then every 12 hours. Blood level tests can be performed to
help optimize the dosage. Many proprietary preparations are not
recommended for children.
▲ side-effects: there may be nausea and gastrointestinal disturbances,
an increase or irregularity in the heartbeat, and/or insomnia. In
some cases theophylline can impair attention and therefore ability
at school.
✚ warning: treatment should initially be gradually progressive in the
quantity administered. Theophylline should be administered with
caution to patients who suffer from heart or liver disease, or peptic
ulcer.

Related articles: BIOPHYLLINE; NUELIN; SLO-PHYLLIN; THEO-DUR; UNIPHYLLIN CONTINUS.

Theraderm (*Westwood*) is a proprietary non-prescription preparation for the treatment of acne. Produced in the form of a gel for topical application (in two strengths), its active constituent is the KERATOLYTIC agent benzoyl peroxide.
▲/✚ side-effects/warning: *see* BENZOYL PEROXIDE.

thiabendazole is a drug used in the treatment of infestations by worm parasites, particularly those of the *Strongyloides* and *Ancylostoma* species that reside in the intestines but may migrate into the tissues. The usual course of treatment lasts for three days.
▲ side-effects: there may be nausea, vomiting, diarrhoea and weight loss; dizziness and drowsiness are not uncommon; there may also be headache and itching (pruritus). Possible hypersensitivity reactions include fever with chills, rashes and other skin disorders, and occasionally ringing in the ears (tinnitus) or liver damage.
✚ warning: thiabendazole should be administered with caution to patients with impaired kidney or liver function. Treatment should be withdrawn if hypersensitivity reactions occur.
Related article: MINTEZOL.

thiazides are effective DIURETICS used mainly to treat the symptoms of heart disease, such as fluid retention in the tissues and high blood pressure (hypertension) or to assist a failing kidney. They work by inhibiting the reabsorption of sodium and chloride ions within one specific part of the kidney. The result is a moderate diuresis that includes the excretion also of potassium. Potassium supplements are often administered simultaneously, or the thiazide may be combined with another type of diuretic that actively promotes the retention of potassium. Best known and most used thiazides include hydrochlorothiazide and bendrofluazide. Unlike some types of diuretics, the thiazides can be used for prolonged courses of treatment with no residual effects.
see BENDROFLUAZIDE; CYCLOPENTHIAZIDE; HYDROCHLOROTHIAZIDE.

thiopentone sodium is a widely used general ANAESTHETIC. It has no analgesic properties. Because the drug is exceptionally powerful, however, inadvertent overdosage does occur from time to time, causing respiratory depression and depression of the heart rate. Both initial induction of anaesthesia and awakening afterwards are smooth and rapid, although some sedative effects may endure for up to 24 hours. Administration is by injection.
▲ side-effects: there may be respiratory depression, and means for treating respiratory failure should be available. During induction with thiopentone sodium, sneezing, coughing and bronchial spasm may occur.
✚ warning: thiopentone sodium should not be given to patients whose respiratory tract is obstructed, those in severe shock, or those with porphyria (poor porphyrin metabolism). Caution should be taken

when administering the drug to patients with severe liver or kidney disease, or with metabolic disorders.
Related article: INTRAVAL SODIUM.

thyroxine sodium is a preparation of one of the natural thyroid HORMONES. It is used therapeutically to make up a hormonal deficiency on a regular maintenance basis, and to treat associated symptoms (myxoedema). It may also be used in the treatment of goitre. Administration is oral in the form of tablets.

Ticar (*Beecham*) is a proprietary ANTIBIOTIC, available only on prescription, used to treat serious infections such as septicaemia and peritonitis, in addition to infections of the respiratory tract or urinary tract. It may also be used to prevent infection in wounds. Produced in the form of a powder for reconstitution as a medium for injection, and in infusion bottles, Ticar is a preparation of the penicillin ticarcillin sodium.
▲/✚ side-effects/warning: *see* TICARCILLIN.

ticarcillin is an ANTIBIOTIC, one of the penicillins, used to treat serious infections such as septicaemia and peritonitis, in addition to infections of the respiratory tract or of the urinary tract. Administration is by injection or infusion.
▲side-effects: there may be sensitivity reactions ranging from a minor rash to urticaria and joint pains, and (occasionally) to high temperature of anaphylactic shock. High doses may in any case cause convulsions.
✚warning: ticarcillin should not be administered to patients known to be allergic to penicillins; it should be administered with caution to those with impaired kidney function.
Related articles: TICAR; TIMENTIN.

Tiempe (*DDSA Pharmaceuticals*) is a proprietary ANTIBACTERIAL, available only on prescription, used primarily to treat infections of the urinary or respiratory tracts. Produced in the form of tablets (in two strengths), it is a preparation of the antibacterial agent trimethoprim.
▲/✚ side-effects/warning: *see* TRIMETHOPRIM.

Timentin (*Beecham*) is a proprietary ANTIBIOTIC, available only on prescription, used to treat severe infections. (Patients with such conditions are generally in hospital.) Produced in the form of a powder for reconstitution as a medium for injection, Timentin is a compound preparation of the catalytic additive CLAVULANIC ACID with the penicillin ticarcillin.
▲/✚ side-effects/warning: *see* TICARCILLIN.

Timodine (*Lloyd-Hamol, Reckitt & Colman*) is a proprietary CORTICOSTEROID cream, available only on prescription, used for topical application on mild skin inflammation, especially where there is a yeast infection (such as candidiasis or thrush). It is a compound preparation that contains the steroid hydrocortisone, the ANTIFUNGAL

drug nystatin, the ANTISEPTIC benzalkonium chloride and the antifoaming agent dimethicone.
▲/✚ side-effects/warning: *see* HYDROCORTISONE; NYSTATIN.

Timoped (*Reckitt & Colman*) is a proprietary non-prescription cream for topical application to fungal skin infections (such as athlete's foot). Intended to be massaged into the affected area and allowed to dry to a white powder, the cream is a preparation of the ANTIFUNGAL drug tolnaftate with the ANTISEPTIC triclosan.

Tinaderm-M (*Kirby-Warrick*) is a proprietary non-prescription cream for topical application to fungal infections of the skin and nails. Intended to be applied two or three times a day, the cream is a preparation of the ANTIFUNGAL drugs tolnaftate and nystatin.
▲/✚ side-effects/warning: *see* NYSTATIN; TOLNAFTATE.

Tinset (*Janssen*) is a proprietary non-prescription ANTIHISTAMINE used in oral administration to treat allergic conditions such as hay fever and urticaria. Produced in the form of tablets, it is a preparation of the antihistamine oxatomide. It is not recommended for children aged under five years.
▲/✚ side-effects/warning: *see* OXATOMIDE.

tioconazole is a synthetic ANTIFUNGAL drug of the imidazole family, used principally in the topical treatment of infection by the *tinea* species known as ringworm (such as athlete's foot). Administration is in the form of a solution. To be effective treatment must be continued for more than six months. Rarely sensitivity reactions occur.

titanium dioxide paste is a non-proprietary formulation that combines the mild astringent titanium dioxide with a number of other mineral salts (including ZINC OXIDE) and water, forming a paste that is effective as a barrier preparation for topical application on the skin. There it protects, not only against infection and dirt, but also against ultraviolet radiation (providing what is known as a sunscreen).

Tixylix (*May & Baker*) is a proprietary non-prescription compound cough linctus that is not available from the National Health Service. Produced in the form of a syrup for dilution (the potency of the syrup once dilute is retained for 14 days), Tixylix is a preparation of the OPIATE ANTITUSSIVE pholcodine citrate and the ANTIHISTAMINE promethazine hydrochloride.
▲/✚ side-effects/warning: *see* PHOLCODINE; PROMETHAZINE HYDROCHLORIDE.

Tobralex (*Alcon*) is a proprietary preparation of the aminoglycoside ANTIBIOTIC drug tobramycin, available only on prescription, used in the form of eye-drops to treat bacterial infections of the eye.
▲/✚ side-effects/warning: *see* TOBRAMYCIN.

tobramycin is an ANTIBIOTIC, one of the aminoglycosides, effective against many forms of bacteria and against some other micro-

organisms. However, it is not absorbed from the intestine (except in
the case of local infection or liver failure) and so is administered by
injection when treating systemic disease. It is also produced in the
form of eye-drops to treat bacterial infections of the eye.

▲ side-effects: treatment must be discontinued if there are any signs
of deafness. There may be dysfunction of the kidneys.

✚ warning: tobramycin should not be administered to patients who
are already taking drugs that affect the neural system. It should be
administered with caution to those with impaired kidney function.
Prolonged or high dosage can cause deafness; blood levels should be
monitored.
Related articles: NEBCIN; TOBRALEX.

tocopherol is a general name for a group of substances known
collectively as VITAMIN E (and chemically classed as tocopherols and
tocotrienols). They have anti-oxidant properties, and are thought to
maintain the structure of cell membranes by preventing the oxidation
of their fatty acid constituents. Vitamin E deficiency may lead to a
form of anaemia through the rupture of red blood cells, particularly
in the very premature baby. Vitamin E deficiency can occur in
certain disorders of the liver and pancreas, such as cystic fibrosis. If
this is a long standing condition neurological problems can occur.
Good food sources include eggs, vegetable oils, wheat germ and green
vegetables. The form of tocopherol most used in therapy to make up
vitamin deficiency is alpha tocopheryl acetate. Administration is oral
in the form of tablets or capsules.
Related articles: EPHYNAL; VITA-E.

tocopheryl acetate (or alpha tocopheryl acetate) is one of the forms of
tocopherol (VITAMIN E) most used in vitamin replacement therapy.
see TOCOPHEROL.

Tofranil (*Geigy*) is a proprietary ANTIDEPRESSANT drug, available only on
prescription, with fewer sedative properties than many others, used to
treat depressive illness particularly in patients who are withdrawn
and apathetic. It may also be used to treat nocturnal bedwetting by
children (aged over seven years). Produced in the form of tablets (in
two strengths) and as a syrup for dilution (the potency of the syrup
once diluted is retained for 14 days), Tofranil is a preparation of
imipramine hydrochloride.
▲/✚ side-effects/warning: *see* IMIPRAMINE.

tolnaftate is a mild, synthetic, ANTIFUNGAL drug used principally in the
topical treatment of infections by the Tinea species known as
ringworm (such as athlete's foot). Administration is in the form of a
cream, a powder or a solution. Rarely, sensitivity reactions occur.
Related article: TIMOPED; TINADERM-N.

tolu linctus is a non-proprietary formulation that is a cough linctus
for children. Its various constituents (including citric acid and
GLYCEROL) are mixed in with a syrup derived from tolu balsam (itself
obtained from the bark of the South American tolu tree) which has
very mild ANTISEPTIC and EXPECTORANT action.

Tonivitan (*Medo*) is a proprietary multivitamin supplement, available on prescription only to private patients, used to treat overall VITAMIN deficiency. Produced in the form of capsules, it contains retinol (vitamin A), thiamine (vitamin B₁), nicotinic acid (of the B complex), ASCORBIC ACID (vitamin C), CALCIFEROL (vitamin D) and a dried preparation of yeast.

Tracrium (*Calmic*) is a proprietary SKELETAL MUSCLE RELAXANT, available only on prescription, used mainly under general anaesthesia during surgery. Produced in ampoules for injection, Tracrium is a preparation of atracurium besylate.
✚warning: see ATRACURIUM BESYLATE.

*tranquillizers are drugs that calm and soothe, and relieve anxiety. Many also cause some degree of sedation. They are often classified in two groups, major tranquillizers and minor. The major tranquillizers are used primarily to treat severe mental disorders – the psychoses (including schizophrenia and mania) – not only to relieve patients of their own private fears and terrors, but also to control violent behavioural disturbances that present a danger to the patients themselves and to those who look after them. The minor tranquillizers may also be used to treat mental disorders, such as neuroses, but are more commonly used in short-term therapies to treat anxiety and nervous tension. Best known and most used major tranquillizers include the PHENOTHIAZINES (such as CHLORPROMAZINE, thioridazine and PROCHLORPERAZINE) and such drugs as haloperidol, fluspirilene and flupenthixol. Best known and most used minor tranquillizers include the BENZODIAZEPINES (such as DIAZEPAM and chlordiazepoxide) and such drugs as meprobamate. Prolonged treatment with some minor tranquillizers can lead to dependence (addiction).

Travasept (*Travenol*) is a proprietary non-prescription DISINFECTANT for use in cleaning wounds and burns. Produced in sachets of solution (not for further dilution), Travasept is a compound preparation of the ANTISEPTICS cetrimide and chlorhexidine acetate (in two strengths, under the trade names Travasept 30 and Travasept 100).

Tri-Adcortyl (*Squibb*) is a proprietary preparation for topical application in the treatment of severe non-infective skin inflammation (such as eczema), especially in cases that have not responded to less powerful therapies. Available only on prescription, and produced in the form of a cream and an ointment, it is a compound of the CORTICOSTEROID triamcinolone acetonide together with the ANTIFUNGAL drug nystatin, and the ANTIBIOTICS gramicidin and neomycin. A form of the ointment prepared especially for the topical treatment of infection of the outer ear is also available (under the name Tri-Adcortyl Otic).
▲/✚ side-effects/warning: *see* NYSTATIN; TRIAMCINOLONE ACETONIDE.

triamcinolone is a synthetic CORTICOSTEROID used to suppress the symptoms of inflammation, especially when caused by allergic disorders. It is administered in the form of tablets, or by injection.

▲ side-effects: treatment of susceptible patients may engender a euphoria – or a state of confusion or depression. Rarely, there is peptic ulcer.

✚ warning: triamcinolone should not be administered to patients who suffer from psoriasis. In children, administration may lead to stunting of growth. Prolonged use may cause muscular weakness. As with all corticosteroids, triamcinolone treats only inflammatory symptoms; an undetected and potentially serious infection may have its effects masked by the drug until it is well established. *Related article:* LEDERCORT.

triamcinolone acetonide is a synthetic CORTICOSTEROID used to suppress the symptoms of inflammation, especially when caused by allergic disorders. It is administered sometimes as a systemic medication (in the form of an injection) to relieve such conditions as hay fever or asthma but, more commonly, is applied by local injection to treat skin inflammations or such conditions as rheumatoid arthritis and bursitis. Several proprietary preparations are in the form of a cream for topical application, mostly in the treatment of severe non-infective eczema, but one or two are for treating inflammations in the mouth.

▲ side-effects: systemic treatment of susceptible patients may engender a euphoria – or a state of confusion or depression. Rarely, there is peptic ulcer.

✚ warning: triamcinolone acetonide should not be administered to patients with psoriasis. In children, systemic administration may lead to stunting of growth. Prolonged use may cause muscular weakness, and in any case should be avoided. As with all corticosteroids, triamcinolone acetonide treats only inflammatory symptoms; an undetected and potentially serious infection may have its effects masked by the drug until it is well established. *Related articles:* ADCORTYL; AUDICORT; AUREOCORT; KENALOG; LEDERCORT; NYSTADERMAL; TRI-ADCORTYL.

triamcinolone hexacetonide is a synthetic CORTICOSTEROID used to suppress the symptoms of inflammation. It is administered by local injection to treat skin inflammation or such conditions as rheumatoid arthritis and bursitis.

▲ side-effects: systemic treatment of susceptible patients may engender a euphoria – or a state of confusion or depression. Rarely, there is peptic ulcer.

✚ warning: triamcinolone hexacetonide should not be administered to patients with psoriasis. In children, administration may lead to stunting of growth. Prolonged use may cause muscular weakness, and in any case should be avoided. As with all corticosteroids, triamcinolone hexacetonide treats only inflammatory symptoms; an undetected and potentially serious infection may have its effects masked by the drug until it is well established. *Related article:* LEDERSPAN.

Tribiotic (*Riker*) is a proprietary ANTIBIOTIC, available only on prescription, used as a spray in topical application to infections of the skin. Produced in aerosol units, it is a compound preparation of three antibiotics: neomycin sulphate, polymyxin B sulphate and bacitracin zinc.

Tri-Cicatrin (*Calmic*) is a proprietary ANTIBIOTIC drug also containing the CORTICOSTEROID hydrocortisone, used in topical applications to treat mild skin inflammmation where there is also infection. Produced in the form of an ointment, its major active constituents include the ANTISEPTICS neomycin sulphate, bactracin zinc and the ANTIFUNGAL agent nystatin.

▲/✚ side-effects/warning: *see* HYDROCORTISONE; NEOMYCIN.

trichloroethylene is an inhalant general ANAESTHETIC with powerful ANALGESIC properties used primarily in combination with nitrous oxide-oxygen mixtures, but it has rather poor MUSCLE RELAXANT properties. It is normally administered only after anaesthesia has been initially induced with some other agent.

▲ side-effects: side-effects are rare (in fact the drug helps stabilize several body functions, such as blood pressure). But the respiratory rate may increase, and post-operative vomiting is not uncommon. It may decrease the function of the liver and kidneys.

✚ warning: trichloroethylene is not suitable for induction of anaesthesia; moreover, administration of the drug should be discontinued some time before the end of surgery because the recovery rate from the drug afterwards is comparatively slow.

triclofos sodium is a derivative of the soluble SEDATIVE chloral hydrate, used as a HYPNOTIC to treat insomnia. Administration is oral in the form of an elixir; the liquid is less irritant to the stomach lining than chloral hydrate.

▲ side-effects: concentration and speed of thought and movement are affected. There is commonly drowsiness, dry mouth and gastric irritation; there may also be sensitivity reactions (such as a rash) and, in the elderly, a mild state of confusion.

✚ warning: triclofos sodium should be administered with caution to those with lung disease, particularly if there is depressed breathing. Withdrawal of treatment should be gradual. Prolonged use may lead to tolerance and dependence (addiction).

*tricyclic drugs are one of the two main classes of ANTIDEPRESSANT, and often have SEDATIVE and TRANQUILLIZER effects. In children they may be used to treat bedwetting (eneuresis). Chemically, they are dibenzazipine or debenzocycloheptone derivatives. Examples include AMITRIPTYLINE and lofepramine.

Tridesilon (*Lagap*) is a proprietary CORTICOSTEROID preparation, available only on prescription, used in topical application to treat severe non-infective skin inflammation (such as eczema), especially when therapy with less powerful corticosteroids has failed. Produced in the form of a water-miscible cream and a paraffin-based ointment, Tridesilon's major active constituent is the steroid desonide.

▲/✚ side-effects/warning: *see* DESONIDE.

triiodothyronine is a natural thyroid HORMONE, administered therapeutically in the form of liothyronine sodium to make up a hormonal deficiency (hypothyroidism) and to treat associated symptoms (myxoedema). It may also be used in the treatment of goitre.
see LIOTHYRONINE SODIUM.

Triludan (*Merrell*) is a proprietary non-prescription ANTIHISTAMINE used to treat the symptoms of allergic disorders such as hay fever and urticaria. Produced in the form of tablets and as a suspension for dilution (the potency of the suspension once dilute is retained for 14 days), it is a preparation of terfenadine.
▲/✚ side-effects/warning: *see* TERFENADINE.

Triludan Forte (*Merrell*) is a proprietary non-prescription ANTIHISTAMINE used to treat the symptoms of allergic disorders, such as hay fever and urticaria. Produced in the form of tablets it is the the stronger form of Triludan and is a preparation of terfenadine. It is not recommended to children under two years.
▲/✚ side-effects/warning: *see* TERFENADINE.

trimeprazine tartrate is an ANTIHISTAMINE that has additional SEDATIVE properties. It is used to treat the symptoms of allergic disorders (particularly rashes and itching), as a premedication prior to surgery, and sometimes even as an ANTI-EMETIC. It is often used as a sedative and is also used in atopic eczema to relieve itching. Administration is oral in the form of tablets or as a dilute syrup.
▲ side-effects: there may be headache, drowsiness and dry mouth. Some patients experience sensitivity reactions on the skin.
Related article: VALLERGAN.

trimethoprim is an ANTIMICROBIAL, used to treat and to prevent the spread of many forms of bacterial infection but particularly those of the urinary and respiratory tracts. It is often used in a small dose at night-time to help prevent urinary infection in children with urinary abnormalities which predispose them to kidney infection. It is peculiarly effective in combination with a sulphonamide drug, for the combined effect is greater than twice the individual effect of either partner. This is the basis of the medicinal compound CO-TRIMOXAZOLE (which forms the active constituent of many proprietary preparations). Administration of trimethoprim is oral in the form of tablets or a dilute suspension, or by injection.
▲ side-effects: there may be nausea, vomiting and gastrointestinal disturbances; rashes may break out, with itching (pruritus).
✚ warning: trimethoprim should not be administered to newborn babies, or to patients who have severely impaired kidney function. Dosage should be reduced for patients with poor kidney function.
Related articles: IPRAL; MONOTRIM; SYRAPRIM; TIEMPE; TRIMOGAL; TRIMOPAN.

Trimogal (*Lagap*) is a proprietary ANTIMICROBIAL, available only on prescription, used to treat and to prevent the spread of many forms of bacterial infection but particularly those of the urinary and respiratory tracts. Produced in the form of tablets (in two strengths), it is a preparation of trimethoprim.

▲/✚ side-effects/warning: *see* TRIMETHOPRIM.

Trimopan (*Berk*) is a proprietary ANTIMICROBIAL agent, available only on prescription, used to treat and to prevent the spread of many forms of bacterial infection, but particularly those of the urinary and respiratory tracts. Produced in the form of tablets (in two strengths), and as a sugar-free suspension for dilution (the potency of the suspension once dilute is retained for 14 days), it is a preparation of trimethoprim.

▲/✚ side-effects/warning: *see* TRIMETHOPRIM.

Trimovate (*Glaxo*) is a proprietary CORTICOSTEROID and ANTIBIOTIC preparation, available only on prescription, used in topical application to treat severe skin inflammation, especially when therapy with less powerful corticosteroids has failed. Produced in the form of a water-miscible cream and a paraffin-based ointment, Trimovate's major active constituents are the steroid clobetasone butyrate, the ANTIFUNGAL drug nystatin, and the TETRACYCLINE antibiotic chlortetracycline hydrochloride.

▲/✚ side-effects/warning: *see* CHLORTETRACYCLINE; CLOBETASONE BUTYRATE; NYSTATIN.

Triominic (*Beecham*) is a proprietary non-prescription nasal DECONGESTANT that is not available from the National Health Service. Unlike many decongestants, however, it is produced in the form of tablets and as a sugar-free syrup for dilution (the potency of the syrup once dilute is retained for 14 days). Both forms are preparations of the ANTIHISTAMINE pheniramine maleate in combination with the sympathomimetic phenylpropanolamine hydrochloride.

▲/✚ side-effects/warning: *see* PHENIRAMINE MALEATE; PHENYLPROPANOLAMINE HYDROCHLORIDE.

Triosorbon (*Merck*) is a proprietary non-prescription dietary supplement for patients who are severely undernourished (as with anorexia nervosa) or who have serious problems with the absorption of food. It consists of a gluten-, sucrose- and galactose-free, lactose-low powder that contains protein, carbohydrates, fats, vitamins and minerals. It is not suitable for children aged under five years.

Triplopen (*Glaxo*) is a proprietary ANTIBIOTIC, used in the treatment or prevention of many forms of bacterial infection. Produced in the form of powder for reconstitution as a medium for injection, it is a compound preparation of three penicillin-type antibiotics: benzylpenicillin sodium, procaine penicillin and benethamine penicillin. The injection can be painful.

▲/✚ side-effects/warning: *see* BENETHAMINE PENICILLIN; BENZYLPENICILLIN; PROCAINE PENICILLIN.

triprolidine is an ANTIHISTAMINE used to treat the symptoms of allergic disorders such as hay fever and urticaria. A long-acting drug, its effect may last for more than 12 hours. Administration (in the form of triprolidine hydrochloride) is oral as tablets, sustained-release tablets, and a dilute elixir.

▲ side-effects: there may be headache, drowsiness and dry mouth. Some patients experience sensitivity reactions on the skin.
Related article: ACTIDIL.

Tritamyl (*Procea*) is the name of a brand of gluten-free starch-based self-raising flour with which foods such as bread can be made for patients who cannot tolerate dietary gluten (as with coeliac disease and other amino acid deficiencies). A low-protein version is also available under the name Tritamyl PK.

Trivax (*Wellcome*) is a proprietary preparation of the triple vaccine diphtheria-pertussis-tetanus (DPT) vaccine, consisting of a combination of the toxoids (antibodies produced in response to the toxins) of the diphtheria and tetanus bacteria with pertussis vaccine. It is produced in ampoules for injection.
see DIPHTHERIA-PERTUSSIS-TETANUS (DPT) VACCINE.

Trivax-AD (*Wellcome*) is a proprietary preparation of the triple vaccine diphtheria-pertussis-tetanus (DPT) vaccine, consisting of a combination of the toxoids (antibodies produced in response to the toxins) of the diphtheria and tetanus bacteria with pertussis vaccine, all adsorbed on to a mineral carrier (in the form of aluminium hydroxide). It is produced in ampoules for injection.
see DIPHTHERIA-PERTUSSIS-TETANUS (DPT) VACCINE.

tropicamide is a short-acting ANTICHOLINERGIC drug used (in mild solution) to dilate the pupil of the eye for ophthalmic examination. Administration is in the form of eye-drops.

▲ side-effects: vision is blurred or otherwise disturbed. Overdosage may lead to increased heart rate and to behavioural changes in susceptible patients.

✚ warning: tropicamide should not be administered to patients with certain forms of glaucoma, or who are known to have soft lenses.
Related articles: MINIMS; MYDRIACYL.

Trosyl (*Pfizer*) is a proprietary ANTIFUNGAL preparation available only on prescription for topical application to fungal infections of the nails. Produced in the form of a solution with an applicator brush. Trosyl is a preparation of the antifungal drug tioconazole.

▲/✚ side-effects/warning: *see* TIOCONAZOLE.

Trufree (*Cantassium*) is a proprietary brand of gluten-free flours which are used in baking for patients who cannot tolerate gluten (as in the case of coeliac disease).

Tryptizol (*Morson*) is a proprietary ANTIDEPRESSANT drug, available only on prescription, used in the treatment of depressive illness and especially in cases where its additional SEDATIVE properties may be advantageous to the patients or to those that care for them. However,

the drug is additionally used to prevent bedwetting at night in children. Produced in the form of tablets (in three strengths), as sustained-release capsules, as a sugar-free liquid for dilution (the potency of the liquid once dilute is retained for 14 days), and in vials for injection, Tryptizol is a preparation of amitryptiline hydrochloride.
▲/✚ side-effects/warning: *see* AMITRYPTILINE.

Tubarine Miscible (*Calmic*) is a proprietary preparation of the SKELETAL MUSCLE RELAXANT tubocurarine chloride, used under general anaesthesia for medium- or long-duration paralysis. Available only on prescription, it is produced in ampoules for injection.
▲/✚ side-effects/warning: *see* TUBOCURARINE.

tubocurarine is a SKELETAL MUSCLE RELAXANT used primarily (in the form of tubocurarine chloride) under general anaesthesia for medium- or long-duration paralysis. It is the paralytic factor in the well-known South American poison curare. Apart from its use in surgical operations, the drug may also be used occasionally to treat the spasm associated with tetanus or with some mental disorders. Administration is ordinarily by injection.
▲ side-effects: following injection, a rash may appear on the chest and neck, due to the release of histamine. Onset of the paralysis may be accompanied by hypotension.
Related articles: JEXIN; TUBARINE MISCIBLE.

Turbohaler (*Astra*) is a form of dry powder inhaler. It comes as a self-contained unit and each inhaler has 200 doses. The unit is disposable after use and dispenses pure drug, in this case the BRONCHODILATOR BRICANYL (terbutaline). Many other dry powder inhalers use a vehicle such as lactose to carry the active ingredient, which can make some children cough. To use a new dose the inhaler is twisted until a click is heard.

typhoid vaccine is a suspension of dead typhoid bacteria, administered by deep subcutaneous or intramuscular injection. Full protection is, however, not guaranteed, and travellers at risk are advised not to eat prepared but uncooked food or to drink untreated water. Dosage is normally repeated after 4 to 6 weeks – unless reactions have been severe. Some reaction is to be expected: swelling, pain and tenderness occur after a couple of hours, followed by high temperature and malaise, possibly with a headache.

Tyrozets (*Merck, Sharp & Dohme*) is a proprietary non-prescription brand of ANTISEPTIC lozenges used to sanitize and relieve pain in the mouth and throat. They contain the local ANAESTHETIC benzocaine together with the ANTIBACTERIAL compound tyrothricin.
▲/✚ side-effects/warning: *see* BENZOCAINE.

Ultrabase (*Schering*) is a proprietary water-miscible cream used as a skin emollient (softener and soother) and as a medium for various other skin preparations. Available without prescription, it contains liquid paraffin, stearyl alcohol and white soft paraffin.

Ultradil Plain (*Schering*) is a proprietary CORTICOSTEROID preparation, available only on prescription, in the form of either a water-miscible cream or a more oily ointment. Its active constituents are fluocortolone hexanoate and fluocortolone pivalate, which are effective in treating inflammatory skin conditions such as eczema and psoriasis. In made-up dilute form, either version retains its potency for 14 days.
▲/✚ side-effects/warning: *see* FLUOCORTOLONE.

Ultralanum Plain (*Schering*) is a proprietary CORTICOSTEROID preparation, available only on prescription, in the form of either a water-miscible cream of a more oily ointment. Its active constituents are fluocortolone hexanoate and fluocortolone pivalate at higher concentrations than present in ULTRADIL PLAIN. Ultralanum is also used to treat inflammatory skin conditions, and in made-up dilute form also retains its potency for 14 days.
▲/✚ side-effects/warning: *see* FLUOCORTOLONE.

Ultratard, MC (*Novo*) is a proprietary preparation of INSULIN zinc suspension, available in ampoules for injection by diabetics according to individual requirements.

Unguentum Merck (*Merck*) is a proprietary, non-prescription skin emollient (softener and soother) and barrier ointment, also used as a medium for other skin preparations. Because it contains similar proportions of fats and water it is particularly stable; its principal constituent is white soft paraffin. One of the safest of all ointments, its complex formula includes no known allergen.

Unigesic (*Unimed*) is a proprietary compound ANALGESIC, not available on a National Health Service prescription, that principally consists of a mixture of paracetamol and caffeine.
▲/✚ side-effects/warning: *see* CAFFEINE; PARACETAMOL.

Unimycin (*Unigreg*) is a proprietary ANTIBIOTIC, available only on prescription, containing oxytetracycline hydrochloride; it is administered in the form of capsules, and is effective against a wide range of infections. It is not recommended for the treatment of children aged under 12 years.
▲/✚ side-effects/warning: *see* OXYTETRACYCLINE.

Uniphyllin Continus (*Napp*) is a proprietary, slow release BRONCHODILATOR consisting of tablets containing theophylline. It is used to treat respiratory symptoms caused by bronchial asthma. There is a half-strength children's version − Uniphyllin Paediatric Continus − although even this is not advised for children aged under 12 months.
▲/✚ side-effects/warning: *see* THEOPHYLLINE.

Unisept (*Schering*) is a proprietary non-prescription DISINFECTANT and wound cleanser that is available in sachets; each sachet contains chlorhexidine gluconate in very dilute solution.
▲/✚ side-effects/warning: *see* CHLORHEXIDINE.

Urantoin (*DDSA Pharmaceuticals*) is a proprietary form of the antimicrobial drug nitrofurantoin, used specifically to treat infections of the urinary tract. Produced as tablets, Urantoin is available only on prescription.
▲/✚ side-effects/warning: *see* NITROFURANTOIN.

Uriben (*RP Drugs*) is a proprietary ANTIBACTERIAL agent, available only on prescription, in the form of a syrupy suspension of nalidixic acid. Used in solution to treat gastrointestinal infections and infections of the urinary tract, once made up its potency is retained for 14 days.
▲/✚ side-effects/warning: *see* NALIDIXIC ACID.

Uticillin (*Beecham*) is a proprietary ANTIBACTERIAL drug, available only on prescription, in the form of tablets containing carfecillin sodium. The tablets are prescribed to treat infections of the urinary tract.
▲/✚ side-effects/warning: *see* CARFECILLIN SODIUM.

*vaccines confer active immunity against specific diseases: that is, they cause a patient's own body to create a defence (in the form of antibodies against the disease). Most are administered in the form of a suspension of dead viruses (as in flu vaccine) or bacteria (as in typhoid vaccine), or of live but attenuated viruses (as in rubella vaccine) or bacteria (As in BCG vaccine against tuberculosis). A third type is a suspension containing extracts of the toxins emitted by the invading organism that also cause the formation of antibodies (as in tetanus vaccine). Vaccines that incorporate dead micro-organisms generally require a series of administrations (most often three) to build up a sufficient supply in the body of antibodies; booster shots may thereafter be necessary at regular intervals to reinforce immunity. Vaccines that incorporate live micro-organisms may confer immunity with a single dose, because the organisms multiply within the body, although some vaccines still require three administrations (as in oral poliomyelitis vaccine).

▲ side-effects: side-effects range from little or no reactions to severe discomfort, high temperature and pain.

✚ warning: vaccination should not be administered to patients who have a febrile illness or any form of infection. Vaccines containing live material should not be administered routinely to patients who are pregnant, or who are known to have an immunodeficiency disorder.

Valium (*Roche*) is a proprietary form of the powerful BENZODIAZEPINE diazepam, it is mainly used by injection into a vein to stop a convulsion. By mouth it is sometimes used to treat anxiety or as a skeletal muscle relaxant.

▲/✚ side-effects/warning: *see* DIAZEPAM.

Vallergan (*May & Baker*) is a proprietary ANTIHISTAMINE, available only on prescription, consisting of timeprazine tartrate in the form of either of tablets or of syrup for dilution (the syrup once diluted retains potency for 14 days). Vallergan is prescribed to treat various types of allergic reaction, particularly those which include itching skin. It has SEDATIVE effects as with most antihistamines.

▲/✚ side-effects/warning: *see* TRIMEPRAZINE TARTRATE.

Valoid (*Calmic*) is a proprietary form of ANTIHISTAMINE prescribed to treat vomiting, motion sickness and loss of the sense of balance (labyrinthitis). It comes in two forms: tablets, containing cyclizine hydrochloride and available without prescription; and ampoules for injection, containing cyclizine lactate and available only on prescription.

▲/✚ side-effects/warning: *see* CYCLIZINE.

Vamin (*Kabi Vitrum*) is the name of a selection of proprietary infusion fluids for the intravenous nutrition of a patient in whom feeding via the alimentary tract is not possible. All contain amino acids and provide energy, some in the form of glucose, others in the form of various electrolytes.

Vancocin (*Lilly*) is the name of a selection of proprietary forms of the ANTIBIOTIC vancomycin hydrochloride. Available only on prescription, there are capsules (produced under the name Matrigel) and powdered forms for use in solution orally and as injections.
▲/✚ side-effects/warning: *see* VANCOMYCIN.

vancomycin is an ANTIBIOTIC most commonly administered orally to treat certain forms of colitis, but also used in intravenous infusion to treat endocarditis and other serious infections. Because incautious use may have deleterious effects on the organs of the ear, on the kidney, and on the tissues at the site of injection, blood counts and tests on liver and kidney functions are necessary during treatment.
▲ side-effects: infusion may cause high body temperature and a rash; incautious use may lead to ringing in the ears (tinnitus) and even to kidney disease.
✚ warning: vancomycin should be administered with caution to patients with impaired kidney function or who are deaf.
Related article: VANCOCIN.

*vasoconstrictors cause a narrowing of the blood vessels, and thus a reduction in the rate of blood flow and an increase in blood pressure. They are used to increase blood pressure in circulatory disorders, in cases of shock, or in cases where pressure has fallen during lengthy or complex surgery. Different vasoconstrictors work in different ways; vasoconstrictors that have a marked or local effect on mucous membranes, for example, may be used to relieve nasal congestion. Some are used to prolong the effects of local anaesthetics. Best known and most used vasoconstrictors include PHENYLEPHRINE, xylometazoline and methoxamine.

Vasogen (*Pharmax*) is a proprietary non-prescription barrier cream, used to soothe and dress nappy rash, bedsores, and rashes in excretory areas. Active constituents are CALAMINE, DIMETHICONE and ZINC OXIDE.

vasopressin is a natural body HORMONE secreted by the posterior lobe of the pituitary gland; it is known also as antidiuretic hormone, or ADH. In therapy, vasopressin — a VASOCONSTRICTOR — is used mostly to treat pituitary-originated diabetes insipidus. There are two main forms: DESMOPRESSIN and LYPRESSIN; TERLIPRESSIN is another derivative. Preparations include nose-drops, nasal spray, injections and solutions for infusion.
✚ warning: doses should be adjusted to individual response, to balance water levels in the body.
Related article: PITRESSIN.

V-Cil-K (*Lilly*) is a proprietary preparation of the penicillin-type ANTIBIOTIC phenoxymethylpenicillin, used mainly to treat infections of the head and throat, and some skin conditions. Available only on prescription, it is produced in the form of capsules, tablets (in two strengths), a syrup for dilution, and a children's syrup (in two strengths) for dilution (the potency of the diluted syrup is retained for seven days).

▲/✚ side-effects/warning: *see* PHENOXYMETHYLPENICILLIN.

vecuronium bromide is a relatively recently derived SKELETAL MUSCLE RELAXANT, of the type known as non-depolarizing or competitive. Administration is by injection, commonly under general anaesthetic during surgery.

✚warning: patients treated with vecuronium bromide must have their respiration controlled and monitored until the drug has been inactivated or antagonized. The effect of repeated large doses is cumulative.
Related article: NORCURON.

Velbe (*Squibb*) is a proprietary form of the CYTOTOXIC drug vinblastine sulphate, produced in the form of the powdered sulphate together with an ampoule of diluent. Available only on prescription, Velbe is used to treat cancer particularly lymphomas, Hodgkin's disease and some neoplasms.

▲/✚ side-effects/warning: *see* VINBLASTINE SULPHATE.

Velosef (*Squibb*) is a proprietary form of the CEPHALOSPORIN ANTIBIOTIC cephradine, available only on prescription, as capsules (in two strengths), a syrup (for dilution) or a powdered form for use in solution as injections. The potency of the syrup once diluted is retained for seven days.

▲/✚ side-effects/warning: *see* CEPHRADINE.

Velosulin (*Nordisk Wellcome*) is a proprietary form of INSULIN, derived from pigs and highly purified, for use in treating and maintaining diabetic patients. It is produced in the form of ampoules for injection.
Related article: HUMAN VELOSULIN.

Venos (*Beecham Health Care*) is a proprietary non-prescription cough mixture produced in the form of an antitussive formula and as an EXPECTORANT. The active constituents of the antitussive is the cough suppressant noscapine, and the expectorant contains guaiphensin, aniseed oil, capsicum and camphor.

Ventide (*Allen & Hanburys*) is a proprietary CORTICOSTEROID compound, available only on prescription, used to treat the symptoms of asthma. It is produced in the form of an aerosol inhalant containing the steroid beclomethasone dipropionate with the BRONCHODILATOR salbutamol. It is not commonly used in paediatrics; it is preferable to use separate inhalers for both medications.

▲/✚ side-effects/warning: *see* BECLOMETHASONE DIPROPIONATE; SALBUTAMOL.

Ventodisks (*A&A*) is a proprietary form of the selective BETA-RECEPTOR STIMULANT salbutamol, used as a BRONCHODILATOR in patients with asthma. Available only on presription Ventodisks are produced in the form of powder contained in discs, supplied with an inhaler called a diskhaler.

▲/✚ side-effects/warning: *see* SALBUTAMOL.

Ventolin (*Allen & Hanburys*) is a proprietary form of the selective
BETA-RECEPTOR STIMULANT salbutamol, used as a BRONCHODILATOR in
patients with asthma. Available only on prescription, Ventolin
appears in many forms: as tablets (in three strengths, one form under
the name Spandets), as sugar-free syrup (for dilution, potency once
diluted is retained for 28 days), as ampoules for injection (in two
strengths), as infusion fluid (after dilution), as aerosol inhalant, as
ampoules for nebulization spray, and as a solution (for further
dilution). In young children the aerosol inhaler can be given via a
spacer device called a Volumatic. Ventolin can also be given by two
different dry powder inhalers (Rotahaler and Diskhaler).
▲/✚ side-effects/warning: *see* SALBUTAMOL.

Ventolin CR (*Allen & Hanburys*) is a proprietary form of the selective
BETA-RECEPTOR STIMULANT salbutamol, used as a BRONCHODILATOR in
patients with asthma. Available only on prescription Ventolin CR it
is produced in the form of continuous release tablets of two strengths.
This continuous release property may be helpful to prevent or relieve
night-time symptoms when the patient is asleep.
▲/✚ side-effects/warning: *see* SALBUTAMOL.

verapamil hydrochloride is a calcium antagonist ANTIARRHYTHMIC
drug used to treat heartbeat irregularities, it can be given by
injection or orally.
▲ side-effects: potential side-effects include nausea, vomiting and
constipation; infusion may result in low blood pressure. Very rarely
there is liver damage.
✚ warning: verapamil hydrochloride should not be administered to
patients already taking beta-blockers, or who have heart block of
heart failure, or to those with bradycardia (slow heartbeat).

Verkade (*G F Dietary Supplies*) is the name of a proprietary non-
prescription brand of gluten-free biscuits, produced for patients who
suffer from coeliac disease and other forms of gluten sensitivity.

Vermox (*Janssen*) is a proprietary ANTHELMINTIC drug, available only
on prescription, used to treat infestation by pinworms (threadworms)
and similar intestinal parasites. Comprising mebendazole, Vermox is
produced in two forms: as tablets and in suspension.
▲/✚ side-effects/warning: *see* MEBENDAZOLE.

Verrugon (*Pickles*) is a proprietary non-prescription ointment
consisting of salicylic acid in a paraffin base, used to treat warts and
remove hard, dead skin.
✚ warning: see SALICYLIC ACID.

Vertigon (*Smith, Kline & French*) is a proprietary ANTI-EMETIC,
available only on prescription, used to relieve the symptoms of nausea
caused by the vertigo and loss of balance experienced in infections of
the inner and middle ears, or as a result of the administration of
CYTOTOXIC drugs in the treatment of cancer. It is produced as

spansules (soluble capsules) containing the major TRANQUILLIZER prochlorperazine (in two strengths).

▲/✚ side-effects/warning: *see* PROCHLORPERAZINE.

Verucasep (*Galen*) is a proprietary non-prescription gel containing the KERATOLYTIC glutaraldehyde, used to treat warts and remove hard, dead skin.

✚ warning: see GLUTARALDEHYDE.

Vibramycin (*Pfizer*) is a proprietary form of the TETRACYCLINE ANTIBIOTIC doxycycline, available only on prescription, as capsules (in two strengths), a sugar-free syrup (for dilution) or − under the separate name Vibramycin-D − soluble (dispersible) tablets. Vibramycin is prescribed to treat many bacterial and microbial infections. It is not recommended for children under 12 years.

▲/✚ side-effects/warning: *see* DOXYCYCLINE.

Vicks Coldcare (*Richardson-Vicks*) is a proprietary non-prescription cold relief preparation in the form of capsules, which contain paracetamol, the ANTITUSSIVE dextromethorphan and the DECONGESTANT phenylpropanolamine.

▲/✚ side-effects/warning: *see* DEXTROMETHORPHAN; PARACETAMOL.

vidarabine is an ANTIVIRAL drug used to treat serious infections by herpes viruses (such as chickenpox and shingles) in patients whose immune systems are already suppressed by other drugs (acyclovir is more commonly used for this purpose). Administration is by intravenous infusion.

▲ side-effects: there may be nausea and vomiting, diarrhoea and/or anorexia; a tremor may become apparent, with dizziness or a state of confusion; in the blood, white cells and platelets may decrease.

✚ warning: careful monitoring of blood count and kidney function is required: dosage should be balanced at an optimum.

Related article: VIRA-A.

Videne (*Riker*) is a proprietary non-prescription skin disinfectant and cleanser containing povidone-iodine. Much used in hospitals, several forms are available: a water-based solution, a detergent-based surgical scrub, a tincture in methylated spirit (for washing skin preparatory to surgery), and dusting powder (for direct application to minor wounds).

▲/✚ side-effects/warning: *see* POVIDONE-IODINE.

Vidopen (*Berk*) is a proprietary form of the broad-spectrum PENICILLIN called ampicillin, available only on prescription. It is an ANTIBIOTIC used mainly to treat infections of the respiratory passages and the middle ear. Vidopen is produced as capsules (in two strengths) and as a syrup (in two strengths, for dilution); the potency of the syrup once diluted is retained for seven days.

▲/✚ side-effects/warning: *see* AMPICILLIN.

Vigranon B (*Wallace*) is a proprietary non-prescription compound of B complex VITAMINS that is not available from the National Health

Service. Produced in the form of a syrup, it contains thiamine (vitamin B₁), riboflavine (vitamin B₂), PYRIDOXINE (vitamin B₆), nicotinamide and pantothenic acid (panthenol).

vinblastine sulphate is a CYTOTOXIC drug, one of the VINCA ALKALOIDS. Available in its proprietary forms only on prescription, its ability to halt the process of cell reproduction means that it is used to treat cancer, particularly Hodgkin's disease, lymphomas and some neoplasms. But treatment with vinblastine sulphate may cause unpleasant side-effects, and even handling the material may cause problems: it is an irritant to tissue.
▲ side-effects: as part of chemotherapy for cancer, its inevitable toxicity may produce unpleasant side-effects. These range from nausea and vomiting, depression of the bone-marrow's ability to produce red blood cells, and hair loss, to loss of sensation at the extremities, abdominal bloating and serious constipation.
✚ warning: the use of vinblastine sulphate must be closely monitored in relation to each individual patient's tolerance of the toxicity of the drug.
Related article: VELBE.

vinca alkaloids are a type of CYTOTOXIC drug; they work by halting the process of cell reproduction and are thus used to treat cancer, especially leukaemia, lymphomas and some sarcomas. But their toxicity inevitably causes some serious side-effects, in particular some loss of neural function at the extremities, and such symptoms may become so severe as to oblige a reduction in dosage.
Related articles: ONCOVIN; VELBE; VINBLASTINE SULPHATE; VINCRISTINE SULPHATE.

vincristine sulphate is a CYTOTOXIC drug, one of the VINCA ALKALOIDS. Available in its proprietary forms only on prescription, its ability to halt the process of cell reproduction means that it is used to treat cancer, particularly acute leukaemia, Hodgkin's disease and other lymphomas. But treatment with vincristine sulphate may cause unpleasant side-effects, and even handling the material may cause problems: it is an irritant to tissue.
▲ side-effects: as part of chemotherapy for cancer, its inevitable toxicity may produce unpleasant side-effects. These range from nausea and vomiting, constipation and hair loss, to loss of sensation at the extremities, neural failure and abdominal bloating.
✚ warning: the use of vincristine sulphate must be closely monitored in relation to each individual patient's tolerance of the toxicity of the drug.
Related article: ONCOVIN.

Vioform-Hydrocortisone (*Ciba*) is a proprietary ANTIBACTERIAL ANTIFUNGAL steroid compound preparation of hydrocortisone and clioquinol used to treat inflammatory skin disorders when infection is not the cause of the inflammation. It is produced as a water-based cream (for further dilution) and a more oily white soft paraffin-based ointment (also for dilution); the potency of either form in dilution is retained for 14 days.

▲/✚ side-effects/warning: *see* HYDROCORTISONE.

Vira-A (*Parke-Davis*) is a proprietary ANTIVIRAL drug, available only on prescription, used to treat herpes infections. It is produced in two forms: as a concentrated fluid for dilution before intravenous infusion or injection, and as an eye ointment. In both cases the active constituent is vidarabine.

▲/✚ side-effects/warning: *see* VIDARABINE.

Virudox (*Ferring*) is a proprietary ANTIVIRAL drug, available only on prescription. It is used to treat infections of the skin by herpes simplex (cold sores, fever sores) or by herpes zoster (shingles). Produced in the form of a lotion or paint for topical application with a brush. Virudox is a solution of idoxuridine in the organic solvent dimethyl sulpoxide (DMSO).

▲/✚ side-effects/warning: *see* IDOXURIDINE.

Vista-Methasone (*Daniel*) is a proprietary ANTI-INFLAMMATORY steroid drug, available only on prescription, in the form of drops to treat inflammation in the ear, eye or nose. Used solely where infection is not the cause of the inflammation, its active constituent is betamethasone sodium phosphate. A second version – called Vista-Methasone N – additionally contains the ANTIBIOTIC neomycin sulphate.

▲/✚ side-effects/warning: *see* BETAMETHASONE SODIUM PHOSPHATE.

Vita-E (*Bioglan*) is a proprietary non-prescription form of vitamin E (TOCOPHEROL) supplements. Vita-E Gels are capsules containing alpha tocopheryl acetate, and are produced in three strengths; Vita-E Gelucaps also contain alpha tocopheryl acetate but are chewy tablets; Vita-E Succinate is in the form of tablets containing alpha tocopheryl succinate. There is also Vita-E Ointment, a paraffin-based ointment containing alpha tocopheryl acetate, for treating bedsores and similar conditions.

vitamin B is the collective term for a number of water-soluble vitamins found particularly in dairy products, cereals and liver.
see FOLIC ACID; PYRIDOXINE.

vitamin C is another term for ascorbic acid.
see ASCORBIC ACID.

vitamin D is another term for calciferol; it occurs naturally in plants (ergocalciferol) and through the action of sunlight on the skin (cholecalciferol).
see CHOLECALCIFEROL; ERGOCALCIFEROL.

vitamin E is a group of chemically-related oxidant compounds consisting of tocopherols and tocotrienols. Their main effect is thought to be to increase the stability of cell membranes. Good food sources

are dairy products, vegetable oils and cereals; deficiency is rare.
Related article: VITA-E.

vitamin K is a fat-soluble vitamin that occurs naturally in plants
(phytomenadione) and in animals (menaquinone) and derived in the
diet from fresh green vegetables, fruit and egg-yolk. It is essential to
the process of blood clotting. Deficiency of the vitamin is very rare
except in some newborn babies (most hospitals give it routinely to all
newborn infants). Deficiency can also occur in association with certain
forms of liver disease (due to malabsorption).
see PHYTOMENADIONE.

vitamins are substances required in small quantities for healthy
growth, development and metabolism; lack of any one vitamin causes
a specific deficiency disorder. Because they cannot usually be
synthesized by the body, vitamins have to be absorbed or ingested
from external sources – generally these are food substances.

Vitlipid (*KabiVitrum*) is a proprietary form of liquid VITAMIN
supplement for intravenous infusion into patients who cannot be
adequately fed via the alimentary canal. An emulsion intended to be
combined with a lipid-based intravenous infusion, Vitlipid is a
compound of retinol (vitamin A), ERGOCALCIFEROL (vitamin D) and
PHYTOMENADIONE (vitamin K). It is produced in two strengths: one for
adults, the other for children.

Vitrimix KV (*KabiVitrum*) is an infusion fluid for the intravenous
nutrition of a patient in whom feeding via the alimentary tract is not
possible. It is produced in the form of a combined pack of INTRALIPID
and VAMIN, and contains amino acids, glucose and electrolytes.

Voltarol (*Geigy*) is a proprietary non-steroidal ANTI-INFLAMMATORY non-
narcotic ANALGESIC, available only on prescription, used to treat
arthritic and rheumatic pain and other musculo-skeletal disorders. Its
active constituent is diclofenac sodium, and it is produced in the form
of tablets (in either of two strengths, plus a sustained-release version
called Voltarol Retard), ampoules for injection, and anal suppositories
(in either of two strengths).
▲/✚ side-effects/warning: *see* DICLOFENAC SODIUM.

Volumatic (*Allen & Hanburys*) is a large-volume inhaler device for
use with the antiasthma medications BECLOFORTE, BECOTIDE, VENTIDE
and VENTOLIN, all of which rely on the corticosteroid BECLOMETHASONE
DIPROPIONATE and/or the sympathomimetic SALBUTAMOL.

Wallachol (*Wallace*) is a proprietary non-prescription compound primarily of B complex VITAMINS that is not available from the National Health Service. Produced in the form of tablets and a syrup, Wallachol contains thiamine (vitamin B₁), riboflavine (vitamin B₂), PYRIDOXINE (vitamin B₆), cyanocobalamin (vitamin B₁₂), nicotinamide and other metabolic constituents.

Waxsol (*Norgine*) is a proprietary non-prescription form of ear-drops designed to soften and dissolve ear-wax (cerumen), and commonly prescribed for use at home two nights consecutively before syringing of the ears in a doctor's surgery. Its solvent constituent is dioctyl sodium sulphosuccinate (also called docusate sodium).
✚warning: *see* DIOCTYL SODIUM SULPHOSUCCINATE.

Welldorm (*S & N Pharm*) is a proprietary HYPNOTIC and SEDATIVE available only on prescription, used to treat insomnia. It is produced in the form of tablets, the active ingredient of which is chloral betaine, and as an elixir, active ingredient chloral hydrate. Previous formulations of Welldorm tablets and elixir contained dichlorophenazane, a derivative of chloral hydrate.
▲/✚ side-effects/warning: *see* CHLORAL HYDRATE.

Whitfield's ointment is a common name for the non-proprietary compound benzoic acid ointment, used most commonly to treat patches of the fungal infection ringworm.
see BENZOIC ACID OINTMENT.

Wysoy (*Wyeth*) is a soya-based milk substitute which does not contain the milk-sugar lactose. It is therefore suitable for babies who are allergic to cows' milk or who cannot tolerate lactose (this can sometimes temporarily occur after gastroenteritis). Produced in the form of powder, for reconstitution, Wysoy provides a virtually complete diet, containing protein, carbohydrate, fat, vitamins, minerals and trace elements; it is – naturally – free of cow's milk protein and lactose, but it is also gluten-free.

Xylocaine (*Astra*) is a series of proprietary preparations of the local ANAESTHETIC lignocaine, mostly available only on prescription. In the form of anhydrous lignocaine hydrochloride, Xylocaine is produced in ampoules for injection, in various strengths, with and without ADRENALINE (which increases duration of effect). Cartridges of this form of Xylocaine are also available for use in dental surgery, as are (non-prescription) tubes or syringes of Xylocaine Gel (with and without CHLORHEXIDINE gluconate). In addition, there is (non-prescription) Xylocaine Viscous solution and Xylocaine 4% Topical solution for local use on skin or mucous membranes. Containing lignocaine – as opposed to the hydrochloride – there is (non-prescription) Xylocaine Ointment and Xylocaine Spray (with cetylpyridinium chloride).
▲/✚ side-effects/warning: *see* LIGNOCAINE.

Xylotox (*Astra*) is a proprietary dental local ANAESTHETIC, available only on prescription, containing lignocaine hydrochloride and ADRENALINE (the latter to add duration to the effect). It is produced in cartridges for easy attachment to a dentist's hypodermic.
▲/✚ side-effects/warning: *see* LIGNOCAINE.

Yomesan (*Bayer*) is a proprietary, non-prescription form of the ANTHELMINTIC drug niclosamide, used to treat infestation by tapeworms; it is produced as chewy yellow tablets. Careful monitoring of the infestation is required, together with reassuring counselling of the patient.

▲/✚ side-effects/warning: *see* NICLOSAMIDE.

Zaditen (*Sandoz*) is a proprietary drug, available only on prescription, intended to reduce the incidence of asthmatic attacks, or to treat allergic rhinitis or conjunctivitis. However, trials have shown its effect in preventing asthma to be disappointing. It is produced in the form of capsules, tablets, and an elixir for dilution. (The potency of the dilute elixir is retained for 14 days.) Zaditen's active constituent is ketotifen (in the form of the fumarate), which may take several weeks of treatment to achieve its full effect in the body.
▲/✚ side-effects/warning: *see* KETOTIFEN.

Zadstat (*Lederle*) is a proprietary ANTIBIOTIC and ANTIPROTOZOAL drug, available only on prescription, used to treat infections by anaerobic bacteria, amoebae and protozoa, particularly infections of the rectum, colon and vagina. It may also be used to treat ulcerative infections of the gums. Produced in the form of tablets, suppositories (in either of two strengths), and in a Minipack for intravenous infusion, Zadstat is a preparation of the drug metronidazole.
▲/✚ side-effects/warning: *see* METRONIDAZOLE.

Zagreb Antivenom (*Regent*) is a proprietary antidote to the poison injected by an adder. The systemic effects of an adder's bite are rarely serious enough to warrant the use of the antivenom (which has to be diluted with saline solution), but severely low blood pressure, heart arrhythmia or extensive swelling of the bitten limb are indications that more than cleaning, dressing and immobilization is required. Antivenoms for other snakes' poisons are available from the National Poisons Information Centre in London, and the Walton Hospital in Liverpool.

Zantac (*Glaxo*) is a proprietary form of the anti-ulcer drug ranitidine hydrochloride, available only on prescription, used to reduce the acidity of stomach juices. It is used in the treatment of peptic ulcers and of heartburn caused by peptic disturbance. It is produced in the form of tablets (in either of two strengths), soluble (dispersible) tablets, or ampoules for injection. Treatment is not recommended for children aged under eight years.

Zarontin (*Parke-Davis*) is a proprietary form of the anti-epileptic drug ethosuximide, available only on prescription, used to treat and suppress petit mal ("absence") seizures. Available in the form of capsules and an elixir for dilution (the potency of the dilute elixir is retained for 14 days), monitoring of blood levels following the initiation of treatment with Zarontin can help establish an optimum treatment level.
▲/✚ side-effects/warning: *see* ETHOSUXIMIDE.

ZeaSORB (*Stiefel*) is a proprietary non-prescription dusting powder, used to dry and soothe skin in folds or on surfaces where friction may occur. Active constituents include CHLOROXYLENOL (a DISINFECTANT cleanser).

Zinacef (*Glaxo*) is a proprietary broad-spectrum ANTIBIOTIC, available only on prescription, used to treat bacterial infections and to retain

Z

asepsis during surgery. Produced in the form of powder for reconstitution as a medium for injections, Zinacef is a preparation of the CEPHALOSPORIN cefuroxime.
▲/✚ side-effects/warning: *see* CEFUROXIME.

Zinamide (*Merck, Sharp & Dohme*) is a proprietary ANTITUBERCULAR drug, available only on prescription, consisting of tablets containing pyrazinamide. It is usually prescribed in combination with other antitubercular drugs.
▲/✚ side-effects/warning: *see* PYRAZINAMIDE.

zinc is a trace element, necessary in tiny quantities in a daily diet. Deficiency demanding the administration of zinc supplements is rare, however, but occurs with inadequate diet, in cases of malabsorption of ingested food, and where trauma causes loss of zinc from the blood. Conversely, zinc supplements cause some uncomfortable side-effects such as dyspepsia.
Related articles: ZINC OXIDE; ZINC SULPHATE.

zinc oxide is a mild astringent used primarily to treat skin disorders such as nappy rash, urinary rash and eczema. It is available (without prescription) in any of a number of compound forms − as a water-based cream (with arachis oil, oleic acid and wool fat); as an ointment, and as an ointment with castor oil; as dusting powder (with starch and talc); as a paste (with starch and white soft paraffin; or with starch and salicylic acid − Lassar's paste), sometimes in impregnated bandages.
Related article: ZINC PASTE.

zinc paste is a non-proprietary compound made up of ZINC OXIDE, starch and white soft paraffin, which is slightly astringent and is used as a base to which other active constituents can be added, especially within impregnated bandages. Of all such pastes (compounded to treat and protect the lesions of skin diseases such as eczema and psoriasis), zinc paste is the standard type.

zinc sulphate is one form in which zinc supplements can be administered in order to make up a ZINC deficiency in the body. There are several proprietary preparations, all different in form although all oral in administration.
▲ side-effects: there may be abdominal pain or mild gastrointestinal upsets.
Related articles: SOLVAZINC; ZINCOMED; Z SPAN.

Zincaband (*Seton*) is a proprietary non-prescription form of impregnated bandaging, impregnated with gelatinous ZINC PASTE and used to treat eczema, varicose veins and skin ulcers. (Further bandaging is required to hold it in place.)

Zincomed (*Medo*) is a proprietary non-prescription form of ZINC supplement, used to treat zinc deficiency in the body. It is produced in the form of capsules containing zinc sulphate.
▲/✚ side-effects/warning: *see* ZINC SULPHATE.

Zovirax (*Wellcome*) is a proprietary form of the ANTIVIRAL drug acyclovir, available only on prescription, used to treat infection by herpes simplex and herpes zoster organisms. It is available in the form of tablets (in either of two strengths), a suspension (for dilution with syrup or sorbitol; the potency of the dilute suspension is retained for 28 days), and a powder for reconstitution as an intravenous infusion. To treat one form of herpes simplex, there is also an eye ointment; urogenital forms of herpes are treated by a water-based cream. Treatment by any of these preparations is required at least four times a day.
▲/✚ side-effects/warning: *see* ACYCLOVIR.

Z Span (*Smith, Kline & French*) is a proprietary non-prescription form of ZINC supplement, used to treat zinc deficiency in the body. Produced in the form of spansules (slow-release capsules) containing zinc sulphate monohydrate, Z Span is not recommended for children aged under 12 months.
▲/✚ side-effects/warning: *see* ZINC SULPHATE.

Zyloric (*Calmic*) is a proprietary form of the xanthine-oxidase inhibitor allopurinol, used to treat high levels of uric acid in the bloodstream. Available only on prescription, Zyloric is produced for oral administration in the form of tablets.
▲/✚ side-effects/warning: *see* ALLOPURINOL.

Zymafluor (*Zyma*) is a proprietary non-prescription form of fluoride supplement for administration in areas where the water supply is not fluoridated, especially to growing children. Produced in the form of tablets (in either of two strengths, to correspond with local water fluoridation levels), Zymafluor's active constituent is sodium fluoride.